Handbook of
Osteology

THIRD EDITION

Handbook of
Osteology

THIRD EDITION

Nafis Ahmad Faruqi

MBBS, MS, MNYAS (USA), Man of YK2 (USA)

Professor
Department of Anatomy
JN Medical College, AMU
Aligarh-202002, India

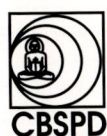

CBSPD

CBS Publishers & Distributors Pvt Ltd

New Delhi • Bengaluru • Chennai • Kochi • Kolkata • Lucknow • Mumbai
Hyderabad • Jharkhand • Nagpur • Patna • Pune • Uttarakhand

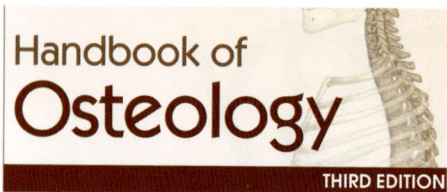

ISBN: 978-93-86478-18-4

Third Edition: 2018

Reprint: 2023

First Edition: 2007

Second Edition: 2012

Published by Satish Kumar Jain and Produced by Varun Jain for

CBS Publishers & Distributors Pvt Ltd

4819/XI Prahlad Street, 24 Ansari Road, Daryaganj, New Delhi 110 002, India

Ph: 011-23289259, 23266861

Website: www.cbspd.com

e-mail: delhi@cbspd.com

Corporate Office: 204 FIE, Industrial Area, Patparganj, Delhi 110 092, India

Ph: 011-4934 4934   Fax: 011-4934 4935   e-mail: publishing@cbspd.com; publicity@cbspd.com

Branches

- **Bengaluru:** Seema House 2975, 17th Cross, K.R. Road, Banasankari 2nd Stage, Bengaluru 560 070, Karnataka, India
  Ph: +91-80-26771678/79   Fax: +91-80-26771680   e-mail: bangalore@cbspd.com
- **Chennai:** 7, Subbaraya Street, Shenoy Nagar, Chennai 600 030, Tamil Nadu, India
  Ph: +91-44-26680620, 26681266   Fax: +91-44-42032115   e-mail: chennai@cbspd.com
- **Kochi:** 42/1325, 1326, Power House Road, Opp KSEB, Power House, Ernakulam 682 018, Kerala, India
  Ph: +91-484-4059061-65,67   Fax: +91-484-4059065   e-mail: kochi@cbspd.com
- **Kolkata:** 147, Hind Ceramics Compound, 1st Floor, Nilgunj Road, Belghoria, Kolkata 700 056, West Bengal, India
  Ph: +91-33-25633055/56   e-mail: kolkata@cbspd.com
- **Lucknow:** Basement, Khushnuma Complex, 7-Meerabai Marg (Behind Jawahar Bhawan), Lucknow 226 001, UP, India
  Ph: 0522-4000032   e-mail: tiwari.lucknow@cbspd.com
- **Mumbai:** PWD Shed. Gala no. 25/26, Ramchandra Bhatt Marg, Next to JJ Hospital Gate no. 2,
  Opp. Union Bank of India, Noorbaug Mumbai 400 009, Maharashtra, India
  Ph: 022-66661880/89   e-mail: mumbai@cbspd.com

Representatives

• **Hyderabad**	0-9885175004	• **Jharkhand**	0-9811541605	• **Nagpur**	0-9421945513
• **Patna**	0-9334159340	• **Pune**	0-9923910676	• **Uttarakhand**	0-9716462459

Printed at: HT Media Ltd. Greater Noida, UP, India

To

My wife Roshan Ara whose encouraging attitude was great force in compiling this book although she was one who suffered most during its preparation.

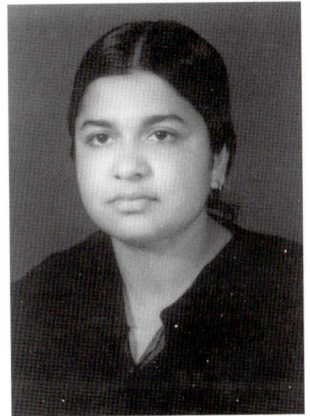

Roshan Ara
Professor
Department of Philosophy
Faculty of Arts, Aligarh Muslim University
Aligarh, UP

Preface to the Third Edition

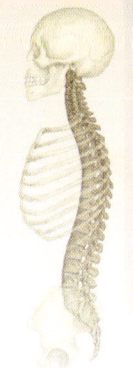

The third edition of **Handbook of Osteology** is thoroughly revised in the light of recent advances on the subject. All the diagrams have been redrawn and made coloured to make them more accurate and attractive. A large number of new diagrams in all the chapters has made the book more useful and graspable. Mnemonics have been added at several places to simplify the memorising of hard facts.

I request all the readers to provide me their suggestions so that the book may be further improved in subsequent editions.

Nafis Ahmad Faruqi

Reader's Comments

Dear Reader,

I will feel honoured if you spare a few minutes from your precious time and comment on this book. Your suggestions will go long way in improving this book in subsequent editions.

Address

Dr. Nafis Ahmad Faruqi
Gulfishan
Allahwali Kothi
Dodhpur, Civil Lines
Aligarh-202001
Mob. 09358256504
WhatsApp no. 07060888167
Email: drnafisahmad@rediffmail.com

Acknowledgements

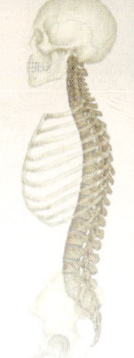

It is my moral duty to acknowledge all those people who helped me in bringing out the third edition of my book *Handbook of Osteology*. Although only few of them are directly involved, I feel pleasure in mentioning the names of many others whose loving and encouraging attitude infused great force in me to work hard for fulfilling the dream of Sir Syed Ahmad Khan, the founder of Aligarh Muslim University, Aligarh, UP, India.

1. First and foremost I sincerely thank to Lt. Gen. (Retd.) Zameer Uddin Shah (Vice-Chancellor, AMU, Aligarh) who made history by not declaring sine die during his five years tenure and created congenial academic atmosphere.

2. I am zero without the help of following members of CBS team, **Mr SK Jain** (*CMD*), **Mr YN Arjuna** (*Senior Vice President—Publishing, Editorial and Publicity*), **Mrs Ritu Chawla** (*AGM—Publishing*), **Ms Ritu Tiwai** (*DTP Operator*), **Mr Sanjay Kishan Chauhan** (*Graphic Designer*), **Mr Neeraj Prasad** (*Cover and Graphic Designer*) and **Mr Kshirod Kumar Sahoo and Mr Ananda Mohanty** (*Readers*).

3. Dr Krishna Garg, ex-Professor and Head, Department of Anatomy, Lady Hardinge Medical College, New Delhi, and Chief Editor of BD Chaurasia's Human Anatomy and author of many other books. She was one who inspired me most.

4. Dr Khursheed Alam, Professor and Head, Department of Anatomy, Patna Medical College, Patna, who introduced my books to his undergraduate and postgraduate medical students. I realy feel obliged.

5. Dr Shoukat Nijamsaheb Kazi, Principal, Prasad Institute of Medical Sciences, Sarai Shahajadi, Banthara, Kanpur Road, Lucknow, UP.

6. Colleagues Prof. Tariq Zaidi (Head of the Department), Prof. Aijaz Ahmed Khan, Prof. SM Yunus, Dr SM Dawar Husain, Dr Farhan Kirmani, Dr Fazal Ur Rehman, Dr Farah Ghaus, Dr Nema Usman, Dr Mohd Imran, Dr Mohd Ajmal (SR), Dr Israr Ahmad Khan (SR), Dr Ragya Bharadwaj (SR).

7. Postgraduate students, Dr Pallavi Ranjan Anand, Dr Fayezah Ahsan Khan, Dr Mahammad Asif Khan, Dr Waqar Akram.

8. Prof. PK Sharma, Department of Anatomy, Era's Lucknow Medical College and Hospital, Lucknow, UP.

9. Dr Makandar UK, C/O AM Pathan, Behind SP Office, Kumbar Galli, Jorapur Peth, Vijaypur, Karnataka.

10. Prof. Namita Malhotra, Department of Anatomy, SHKM Medical College, Mewat, Haryana.

11. Dr Saim Hasan, Department of Anatomy, SHKM Medical College, Mewat, Haryana.

12. Dr Tarun Maheshwari, Department of Anatomy, Govt. Doon Medical College, Dehradun, Uttarakhand.

13. Prof. Harsh Chaturvedi, Department of Anatomy, Shridev Suman Subharti Medical College, Subhartipuram, Nanda Ki Chawki, Premnagar, Dehradun, Uttarakhand.

14. Dr Faisal Taufiq, Department of Anatomy, Shridev Suman Subharti Medical College, Subhartipuram, Nanda Ki Chwki, Premnagar, Dehradun, Uttarakhand.

15. Dr Rati Tandon, Department of Anatomy, All India Institue of Medical Sciences, New Delhi.

16. Dr Mohd Arshad, Department of Anatomy, Glocal Medical College, Superspeciality Hospital and Research Centre, Saharanpur, UP.

17. Prof. (Colonel) Arvind Kishor Shukla, Sena Medal, Principal and Dean, Jauhar Institute of Medical Sciences, Mohammad Ali Jauhar University, Jauhar Nagar, Rampur, UP.

18. Prof. Anand Mishra, Department of Anatomy, IMS, BHU, Varansi, UP.

19. Prof. Naresh Chandra, Head, Department of Anatomy, Hind Institute of Medical Sciences, Safedabad, Barabanki, UP.

20. Prof. Shah Alam Khan, Department of Orthopaedics, AIIMS, Ansari Nagar, New Delhi.

21. Dr Nidhi Sharma, Department of Anatomy, TMMC, NH-24, Muradabad.

22. Dr Devendra Nath Sinha, B9/84B, Udai Giri Apartment 2, Sector 34, Noida, GB Nagar, UP.

23. Dr Manisha Upadhyay, Department of Anatomy, Govt. Medical College, Chakranpur, Azamgarh.

24. Prof. Riazul Qamar, Department of Anatomy, MAMC, New Delhi.

25. Prof. Brijendra Singh, Department of Anatomy, AIIMS, Rishikesh, UK.

26. Dr Royana Singh, Department of Anatomy, IMS, BHU, Varanasi.

27. Prof Awadhesh Kumar Singh, Department of Anatomy, MLN Medical College, Allahabad.

28. Dr Nishtha Singh, Department of Anatomy, MLN Medical College, Allahabad.

29. Prof. NN Srivastava, Department of Anatomy, UPRIMS and R, Safai, Etawah.

30. Prof. TC Singel, Department of Anatomy, MES Medical College, Jamnagar, Gujarat.

31. Prof. S.K. Pandey, Department of Anatomy, IMS, BHU, Varanasi, UP.

32. Dr Zeba Alam, Department of Anatomy, AIIMS, Patna, Bihar.

33. Prof. DK Sharma, Department of Anatomy, AIIMS, Raipur, Chhattisgarh.

34. Dr VK Konuri, Department of Anatomy, AIIMS, Raipur, Chhattisgarh.

35. Dr Azmi Mohsin, MSDS Medical College and Hospital, Farukhabad, UP.

36. Prof. Daxa Dixit, Department of Anatomy, JNMC, Nehru Nagar, Belagavi, Karnataka.

37. Dr Alka Udainia, Department of Anatomy, Govt. Medical College, Surat, Gujarat.

38. Dr K Sandhya, Department of Anatomy, RIMS, Ranchi, Jharkhand.

39. Prof. Renu Prasad, Department of Anatomy, RIMS, Ranchi, Jharkhand.

40. Prof. Narendra Thakur, Department of Anatomy, RIMS, Ranchi, Jharkhand.

41. Prof. SHH Zaidi, Department of Anatomy, Rohilkhand Medical College, Bareilly, UP.

42. Prof. RK Srivastava, Principal, Rama Medical College, Kanpur, UP.

43. Dr Upendra Kumar Gupta, Professor and Head, Department of Anatomy, National Institute of Medical Sciences and Research, NIMS University, Jaipur, Rajasthan.

44. Dr Shikky Garg, Department of Anatomy, Sarojini Naidu Medical College, Agra, UP.

45. Prof. SL Jethani, Department of Anatomy, Himalayan Institute of Medical Sciences, SRHU, Jolly Grant, Dehradun, Uttarakhand.

46. Prof. RK Rohatgi, Department of Anatomy, Himalayan Institute of Medical Sciences, SRHU, Jolly Grant, Dehradun, Uttarakhand.

47. Dr Aksh Dubey, Department of Anatomy, Himalayan Institute of Medical Sciences, SRHU, Jolly Grant, Dehradun, Uttarakhand.

48. Prof. Suniti Raj Mishra, Department of Anatomy, GSVM Medical College, Kanpur, UP.

49. Dr Zeba Khan, Department of Anatomy, Grant Government Medical College and Sir JJ Group of Hospitals, Byculla, Mumbai, Maharashtra.

50. Dr Prerna Gupta, Department of Anatomy, Integral Institute of Medical Sciences and Research, Integral University, Lucknow, UP.

51. Prof. Mehboobul Haque, Department of Anatomy, Integral Institute of Medical Sciences and Research, Integral University, Lucknow, UP.

52. Prof. Neel Kamal Arora, Head, Department of Anatomy, Shri Ram Murti Smarak Institute of Medical Sciences, Bareilly Nainital Road, Bhojipura, Bareilly, UP.

53. Dr AK Srivastava, Professor and Head, Department of Anatomy, HIMS, Mau, Ataria, Sitapur, UP.

54. Dr Bindu Singh, Department of Anatomy, BRD Medical College, Gorakhpur, UP.

55. Muktyaz Hussein, Department of Anatomy, Govt. Medical College, Nausera Ujjani Road, Badaun, UP.

56. Dr Ashwani Bilandu, Department of Orthopaedics, City Hospital, Karolbagh, New Delhi.

57. Prof. Satyam Khare, Head, Department of Anatomy, Subhart Medical College, Meerut, UP.

58. Dr Shailesh M Patel, Professor and Head, Department of Anatomy, Govt. Medical College, Bhavnagar, Gujarat

59. Dr Rekha Parashar, Department of Anatomy, National Institute of Medical Sciences and Research, NIMS University, Jaipur, Rajasthan.

60. Dr Bashir Karim Khan, Department of Anatomy, Govt. Medical College, Dhule, Maharashtra.

61. Prof. A Shariff, Department of Anatomy, AIIMS, New Delhi.

62. Prof. Navneet Kumar, Department of Anatomy, KGMU, Lucknow, UP.

63. Dr RK Diwan, Department of Anatomy, KGMU, Lucknow, UP.

64. Dr Manjula Singh, Department of Anatomy, Govt. Medical College, Kannauj, UP.

65. Prof. Anita Rani, Deaprtment of Anatomy, KGMU, Lucknow, UP.

66. Dr Rekha Lalwani, Department of Anatomy, AIIMS, Bhopal, MP.

67. Prof. Punita Manik, Department of Anatomy, KGMU, Lucknow, UP.

68. Dr Badal Singh, Department of Anatomy, MLN Medical College, Allahabad, UP.

69. Prof. Jyoti Chopra, Department of Anatomy, KGMU, Lucknow, UP.

70. Prof. Mukesh Singla, Department of Anatomy, AIIMS, Rishikesh, UK.

71. Dr Tabinda Hasan, Al Matefa College of Medicine, Riyadh, KSA.

72. Porf. Mujahid Beg, Department of Medicine, JNMC, AMU, Aligarh, UP.

73. Prof. Tabassum Shahab, Department of Paediatrics, JNMC, AMU, Aligarh, UP.

74. Prof. Javed Akhtar, Registrar, AMU, Aligarh, UP.

Contents

General Considerations of Bone

DEFINITION

Bone is the hard part of the body providing dynamic framework to it.

PROPERTIES

1. Bone is a living tissue.
2. Bone is supplied by arteries and nerves.
3. Bone is drained by veins.
4. Bone grows with age.
5. Bone is subject to disease.
6. Bone regenerates when damaged. It has greater regenerative power than any other tissue of the body, except blood.
7. Fractured bone heals leading to union.
8. Bone can undergo remodelling.
9. Bone can withstand strains and stresses.
10. Bone can atrophy or hypertrophy.

FUNCTIONS

1. Bones provide framework to the body.
2. Bones accord shape to the body.
3. Bones act as levers for muscles and, therefore, help in the movements of the body.
4. Bones provide protection to number of viscera, e.g. brain, lungs and heart.
5. Bone is site of blood formation.

6. Bone plays important role in the immune responses of body by producing cells of reticuloendothelial system.
7. Bones are store houses of calcium and phosphorus.

CHEMICAL COMPOSITION

Bone is one-third organic and two-thirds inorganic. Inorganic calcium salts [calcium phosphate, calcium carbonate and crystals of hydroxyapatite, i.e. Ca_{10} {PO_4}$_4$ $(OH)_2$] make it hard and rigid. The organic connective tissue (collagen fibres) makes it tough and resilient. The collagen protein of collagen fibres is characterised by hydroxyproline amino acid.

STRUCTURE OF BONE

I. Macroscopically

There are two types of bones, spongy or cancellous bone and compact or dense bone. Outer covering of all bones is made up of compact bone (Fig. 1.1). Cancellous bone fills up the interior of the bone except the following.

i. In the shaft of long bone it is replaced by medullary cavity. This is filled with red marrow in newborn but replaced by yellow or fatty marrow in adults.

IV. Regional classification

Bones may be classified regionally as:

a. Axial bones

It includes 80 bones as shown below:

i. Skull bones	–	22
ii. Vertebrae	–	26
iii. Ribs	–	24
iv. Sternum	–	1
v. Auditory ossicles	–	6
vi. Hyoid	–	1

b. Appendicular bones

It includes 126 bones which are further subgrouped as:

    i. Upper limb bones – 64
    ii. Lower limb bones – 62
       Total number of bones is 206

V. Miscellaneous classification

a. Accessory bones

An accessory bone is a small piece of bone which develops from a separate centre of ossification but fails to unite with the main mass of bone, e.g. sutural (Wormian) bones and interparietal bones (Fig. 1.4).

b. Sesamoid bones (Table 1.1)

A sesamoid bone is a bone usually small, developing in the tendon of a muscle, ligament or joint capsule. They ossify after birth and are devoid of periosteum. Sesamoid bones possibly resist pressure, they alter the direction of pull of muscle and minimize the friction.

Table 1.1: Some examples of sesamoid bones

Sesamoid bone	Tendon of muscle
i. Patella	Quadriceps
ii. Pisiform	Flexor carpi ulnaris
iii. Fabella	Lateral head of gastrocnemius
iv. Rider's bone	Adductor longus

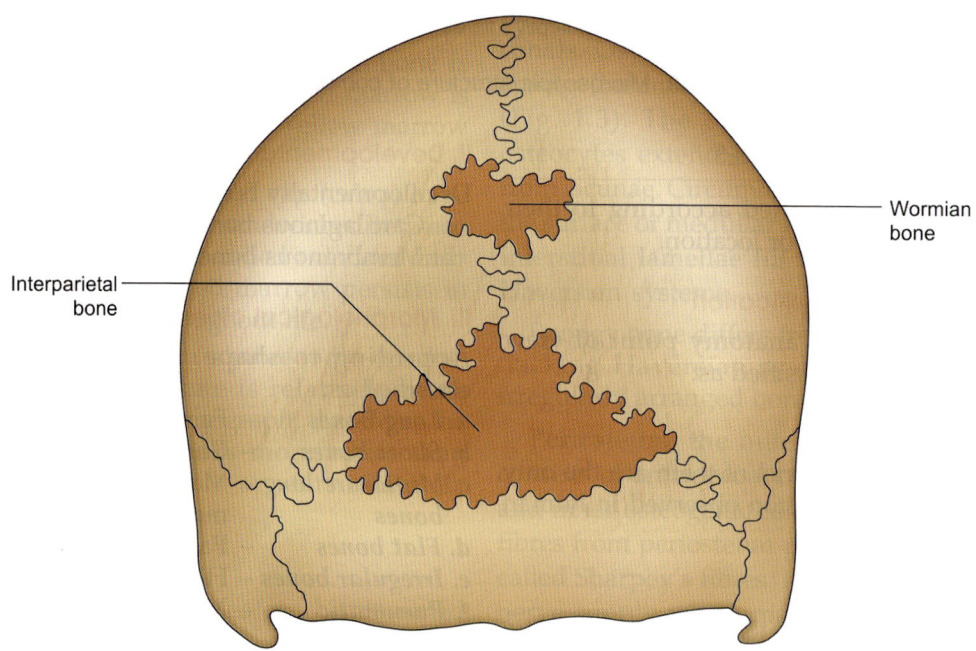

Fig. 1.4: Accessory bones

Wormian bone

Interparietal bone

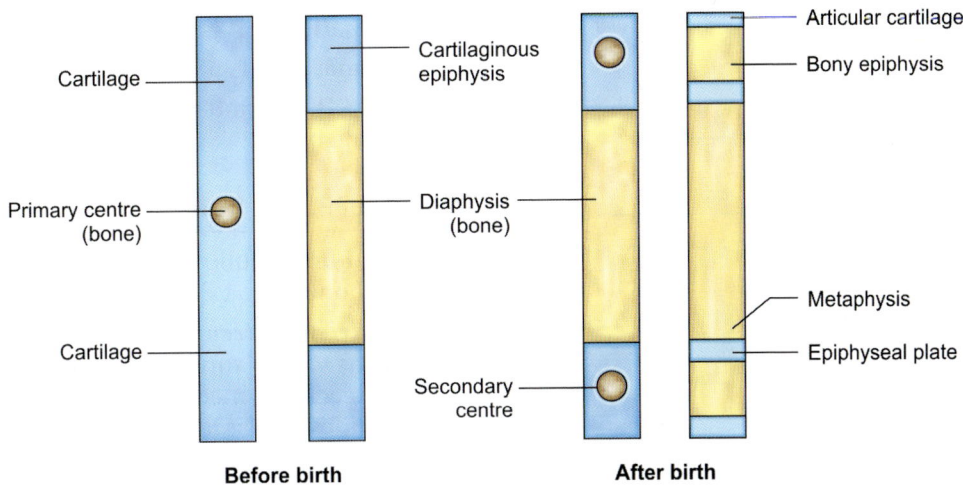

Fig. 1.5: Developing long bone

PARTS OF A YOUNG LONG BONE

1. Epiphysis (Greek epi: upon + physis: growth)

At birth both the ends of a long bone are cartilaginous, known as *cartilaginous epiphyses*. After birth these ends undergo ossification resulting into formation of *bony epiphyses*. Epiphysis can be classified as:

   i. *Pressure epiphysis:* Located adjacent to articulation and helps in transmission of weight, e.g. head of femur, lower end of radius, talus.

   ii. *Traction epiphysis (apophysis):* Located at the site of attachment of tendon, e.g. lesser trochanter, tibial tuberosity, tubercles of humerus.

   iii. *Atavistic epiphysis:* Located in that part of a developing bone which was phylogenetically an independent bone, e.g. coracoid process of scapula and os trigonum (lateral tubercle) of talus.

   iv. *Aberrant epiphysis:* It is not always present, e.g. epiphysis at the head of 1st metacarpal and bases of other metacarpals.

2. Diaphysis (Greek dia: in between + physis: growth)

It is the region between the two epiphyses of a developing long bone. It corresponds to the shaft of a long bone (Fig. 1.5).

3. Epiphyseal plate (Growth cartilage, Growth plate, Physis)

The cartilaginous plate between epiphysis and diaphysis is called the epiphyseal plate. This is responsible for longitudinal growth of long bones. Epiphyseal plate is nourished by both epiphyseal and metaphyseal arteries.

4. Metaphysis

The epiphyseal end of diaphysis is called metaphysis.

FEATURES OF BONES (Fig. 1.6)

1. **Articular surface:** This is smooth surface participating in the formation of a joint.

2. **Condyle:** This is a large portion at the end of a long bone which is partly articular.

3. **Epicondyle:** It is a small projection from the condyle.

4. **Facet:** It is a small articular surface.

5. **Fossa:** This is a localized depression on the surface.

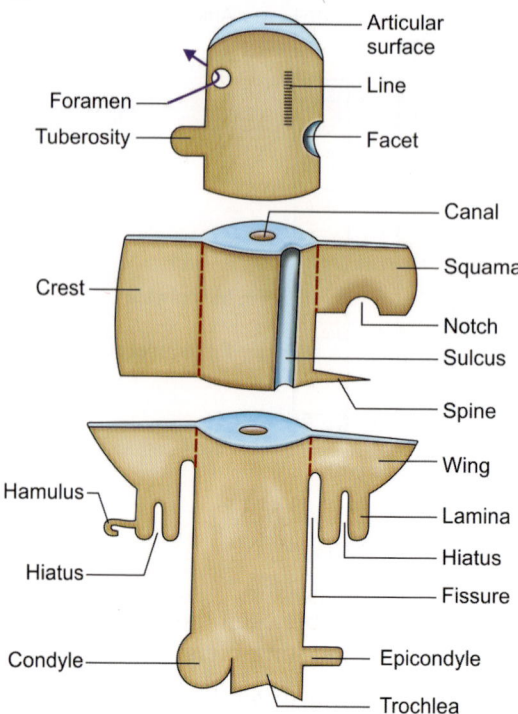

Articular surface
Line
Foramen
Tuberosity
Facet
Canal
Crest
Squama
Notch
Sulcus
Spine
Wing
Hamulus
Lamina
Hiatus
Hiatus
Fissure
Condyle
Epicondyle
Trochlea

Fig. 1.6: Features of bones

6. **Sulcus/Groove:** This is a linear depression.

7. **Tuberosity/Tubercle/Trochanter/Process:** This is a localized projection.

8. **Trochlea:** A structure which is pulley like.

9. **Foramen:** This is an entry point in the bone.

10. **Canal:** It is a tunnel in the bone.

11. **Notch/Incisure:** This is a marked depression along margin.

12. **Hiatus:** This is a gap in the bone.

13. **Fissure:** A cleft between two adjacent bones is called fissure.

14. **Spine:** It is a pointed process.

15. **Hamulus/Cornu:** This is a hook like projection.

16. **Line:** It is a linear roughness on the surface of bone.

17. **Crest:** This is an elongated flat projection.

18. **Lamina/Plate:** It is a flat piece of bone.

19. **Squama:** This is a large lamina.

20. **Wing:** It is a lateral projection from a midline bone.

BLOOD SUPPLY OF BONES

I. **Long bones:** Following arteries supply a long bone (Fig. 1.7):

  a. **Nutrient artery:** It enters the *nutrient foramen* and runs in the nutrient canal to reach the medullary cavity where it divides into ascending and descending branches (nutritiae). It supplies medullary cavity, inner 2/3rd of the compact bone and metaphysis. It is tortuous to allow the movement of bone.

  b. **Periosteal arteries:** Several periosteal arteries supply the periosteum and outer 1/3rd of compact bone of diaphysis. Periosteal arteries are especially numerours beneath the ligamentous and muscular attachments.

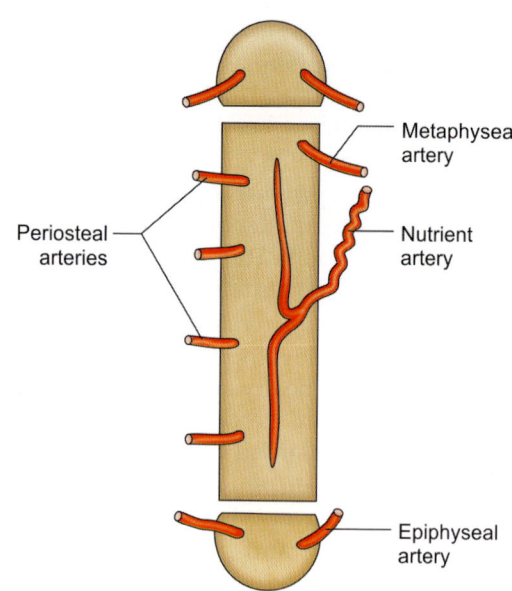

Metaphyseal artery
Periosteal arteries
Nutrient artery
Epiphyseal artery

Fig. 1.7: Arteries supplying a long bone

c. *Epiphyseal arteries:* These are derived from periarticular vascular arcades (circulus vasculosus articuli). These supply the epiphysis.

d. *Metaphyseal arteries:* These are derived from neighbouring systemic vessels to supply the metaphysis.

II. Short bones

These are supplied by numerous periosteal vessels.

III. Vertebrae

The body of vertebra is supplied by the anterior and posterior vessels (Fig. 1.8). The vertebral arch is supplied by large vessels entering through the bases of transverse processes.

IV. Ribs: These are supplied by nutrient and periosteal vessels.

V. Flat bones: These are supplied by nutrient and periosteal vessels.

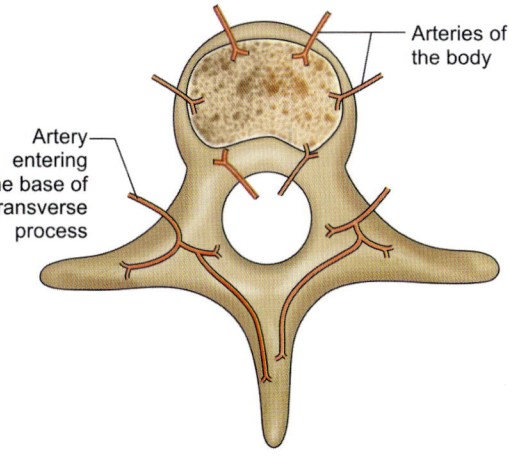

Arteries of the body

Artery entering the base of transverse process

Fig. 1.8: Arterial supply of vertebra

NERVE SUPPLY OF BONES

Nerves accompany the blood vessels of bone. Periosteal nerves are sensory (carry pain) while others are vasomotor in nature.

LYMPHATIC DRAINAGE OF BONES

Lymphatics have not been demonstrated within bone but these are very much present in periosteum which drain into regional lymph nodes.

OSSIFICATION OF BONES

1. Bones ossify from centres of ossification from where laying down of long lamellae starts by osteoblasts.

2. Centres of ossification may be primary or secondary. *Primary centre* appears before birth, usually during 8th week of intrauterine life and gives rise to diaphysis. *Secondary centre* appears at or after birth and gives rise to epiphysis.

3. Most of the long bones have epiphysis at each end but the growth in length occurs mainly at one end. This end is called *growing end*. Here, the epiphysis usually appears earlier and fuses with the body later than that at the non-growing end.

GROWTH OF A LONG BONE

Bone grows in length by multiplication of cells in the epiphyseal plate. Bone grows in thickness by multiplication of cells in the periosteum. Excess bone is removed by osteoclasts, a process is called *remodelling*.

Clavicle

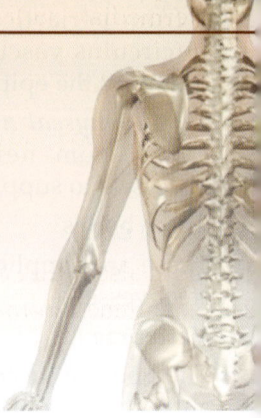

TERMINOLOGY

Clavicle is a Latin word means *little key*.

SIDE DETERMINATION

1. Curvatures lie in horizontal plane.
2. Flattened end is lateral.
3. Roughened areas near the ends and longitudinal groove in the middle 3rd, face inferiorly.
4. Medial 2/3rd of the clavicle shows convexity forwards.

ANATOMICAL POSITION

The clavicle extends laterally almost horizontally at the root of neck (Fig. 2.1).

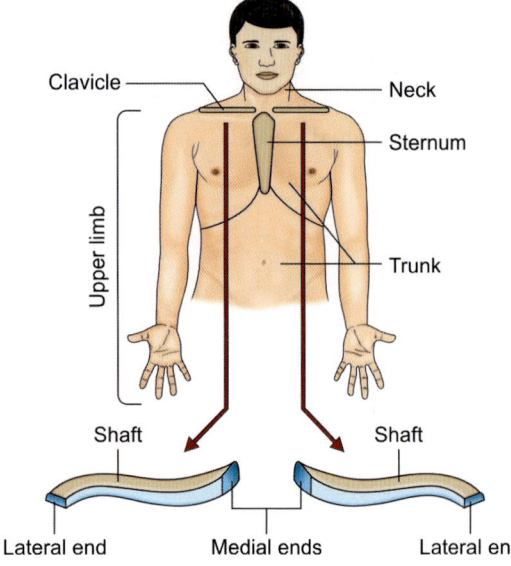

Fig. 2.1: Clavicle: Anatomical position.

FUNCTIONS

1. It acts as a strut for holding the upper limb free from the trunk.
2. It transmits weight of upper limb to axial skeleton (sternum).
3. It provides area for the attachment of muscles.

PECULIARITIES OF CLAVICLE

1. It is the only long bone lying horizontally in the body.

2. It has no medullary cavity.
3. The whole clavicle is almost visible through skin and can be easily palpated.
4. It is first bone to start ossification in the body (the second bone to ossify is mandible).
5. It is the only long bone which ossifies by two primary centres.
6. It is the only long bone which ossifies in membrane (long bones ossify in cartilage).

7. It may be pierced by a cutaneous nerve (intermediate supraclavicular nerve).

FEATURES AND ATTACHMENTS

Clavicle has two ends and a shaft (Fig. 2.2).

I. ENDS

A. Lateral end
1. This is also called *acromial end*.
2. It is flattened from above downwards.

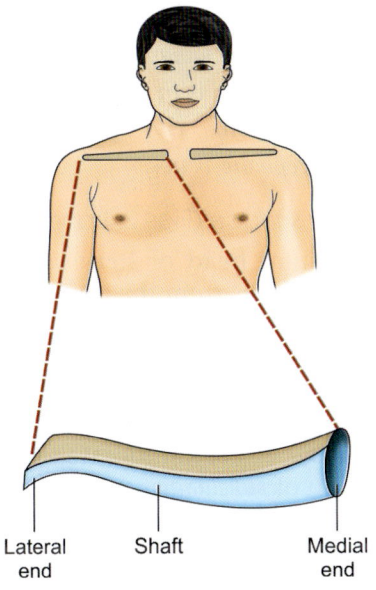

Lateral   Shaft   Medial
end   end

Fig. 2.2: Parts of right clavicle

3. It meets with acromion process to form *acromio-clavicular joint*.

B. Medial end
1. This is also called *sternal end*.
2. It meets with sternum to form *sterno-clavicular joint*.
3. It receives following attachments (Fig. 2.3):
      i. *Fibrous capsule*
      ii. *Articular disc*
      iii. *Interclavicular ligament*

II. SHAFT
A. Lateral 1/3rd of clavicle
It is flattened from above downwards. It has two surfaces (superior and inferior) and two borders (anterior and posterior).

a. Superior surface (Figs 2.4 and 2.5)
It is subcutaneous.

b. Inferior surface
It has a *conoid tubercle* and a *trapezoid ridge* which provide attachments to conoid and trapezoid parts of *coraco-clavicular ligament* respectively (Fig. 2.6).

c. Anterior border
It is concave forwards and provides origin to *deltoid* muscle.

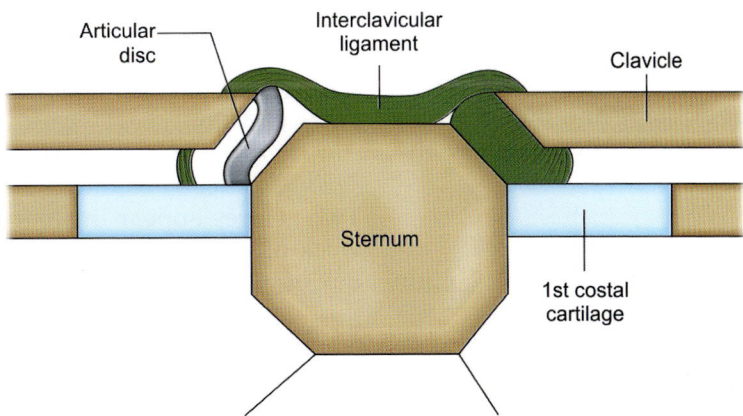

Fig. 2.3: Attachments to the medial end of clavicle

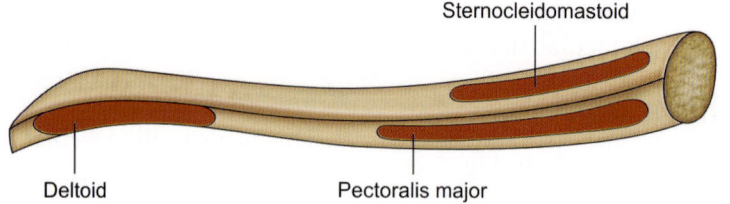

Fig. 2.4: Right clavicle: Anterosuperior aspect

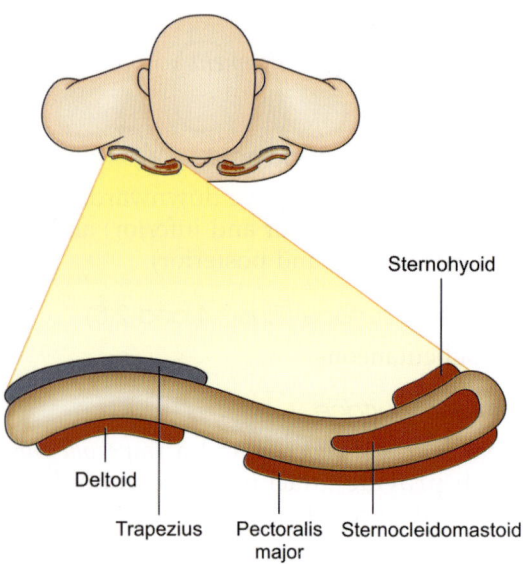

Fig. 2.5: Right clavicle: Superior aspect

d. Posterior border

It shows convexity backwards and provides insertion to *trapezius* muscle.

B. Medial 2/3rd of clavicle

It is quadrilateral in shape and thus has four surfaces, i.e., anterior, posterior, superior and inferior.

a. Anterior surface

It shows convexity forwards. It gives origin to clavicular head of *pectoralis major*.

b. Posterior surface

It exhibits concavity backwards. The origin of *sternohyoid* muscle extends on this surface medially. It is related to the following structures:

  i. *Divisions of trunks of brachial plexus*
 ii. *3rd Part of subclavian artery*
iii. *Internal jugular vein*
 iv. *Subclavian vein*
  v. *Brachiocephalic vein*

c. Superior surface (Figs 2.4 and 2.5)

The clavicular head of *sternocleido-mastoid* muscle originates from this surface medially.

d. Inferior surface (Fig. 2.6)

1. *Costoclavicular ligament* is attached to a rough oval impression at its medial end.
2. *Subclavian groove* on its lateral half is for insertion of *subclavius*.
3. *Clavipectoral fascia* is attached to the margins of subclavian groove.
4. *Nutrient foramen* is on the lateral end of subclavian groove. *Nutrient artery* of clavicle arises from suprascapular artery.

OSSIFICATION

It has two primary and one secondary centres for ossification.

A. Primary centres

Two centres appear in shaft during 5th–6th week of intrauterine life. They fuse on 45th day of intrauterine life.

B. Secondary centre

Appearance: One centre at the medial end appears at puberty.
Fusion: 20 years.

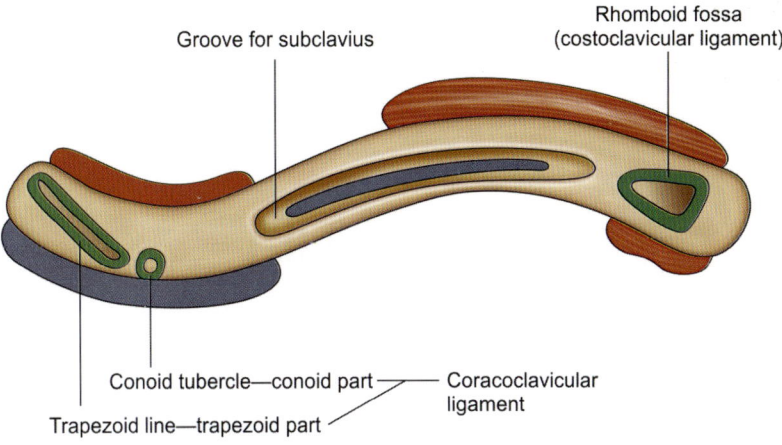

Fig. 2.6: Right clavicle: Inferior aspect

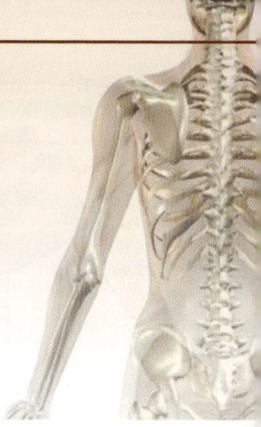

Scapula

TERMINOLOGY

Scapula is also called *shoulder blade*.

SITUATION

Scapula is located on the posterolateral aspect of thorax against the 2nd to 7th ribs (Fig. 3.1).

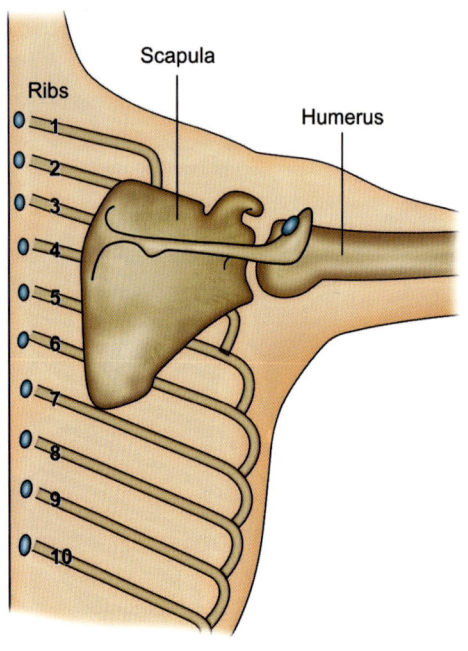

Fig. 3.1: Situation of scapula

SIDE DETERMINATION (Fig. 3.2)

1. The truncated angle (*glenoid cavity*) or triangular scapula faces laterally.
2. A bracket like projection (*spine*) from surface of scapula, is directed posteriorly.
3. Scapula's upper border is marked by a hook like projection (*coracoid process*) adjacent to glenoid cavity and a notch (*suprascapular notch*) near the root of coracoid process.

ANATOMICAL POSITION

Keep the scapula on the back of thorax in such a way that,
1. Glenoid cavity looks laterally, forwards and slightly upwards.
2. Coracoid process is directed forwards.

FEATURES AND ATTACHMENTS

Scapula has two surfaces (costal and dorsal), three borders (superior, medial and lateral), three angles (superior, inferior and lateral) and three processes (spine, acromion and coracoid).

I. Surfaces

A. Costal surface (subscapular fossa)

1. It is concave.
2. It is directed medially and ventrally.

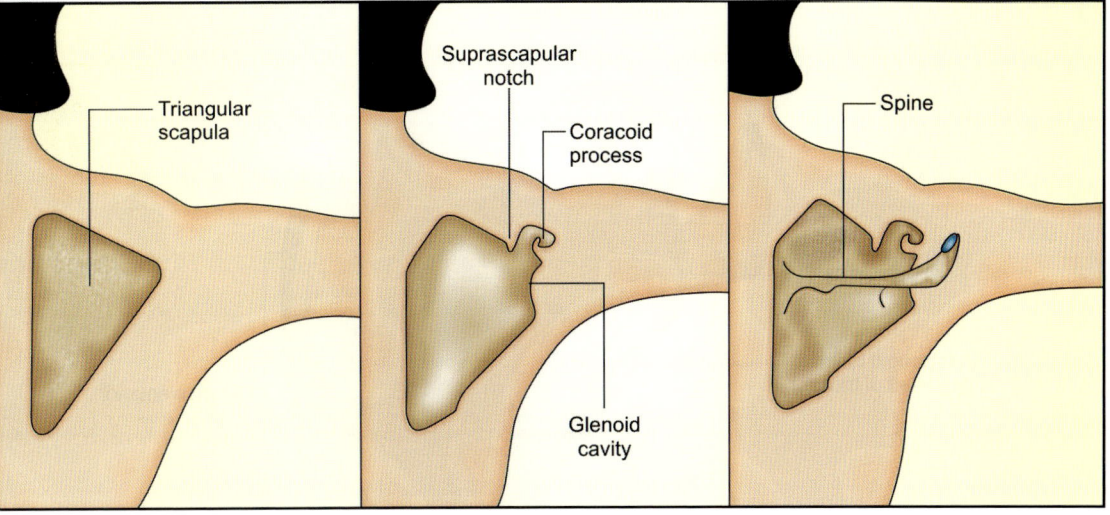

Fig. 3.2: Determination of side of scapula

3. It is subdivided by 3 longitudinal ridges into smooth areas. These ridges provide attachments to *intramuscular tendons of subscapularis* (Fig. 3.3).

4. *Subscapularis*, a multipennate muscle, is attached to the medial 2/3rd of subscapular fossa including the vertical grooved area near the lateral border (Fig. 3.4).

5. *Subscapular bursa* is related to scapula near the glenoid cavity.

B. Dorsal surface (Figs 3.5 and 3.6)

1. It is convex.
2. Spine divides it into *supraspinous* and *infraspinous fossae.*
3. *Spinoglenoid notch* is the connection between two fossae on the back of glenoid cavity.

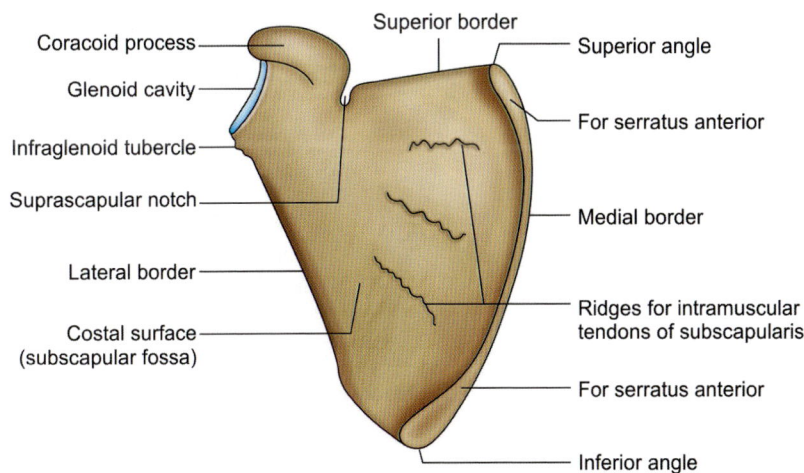

Fig. 3.3: Right scapula: Ventral aspect

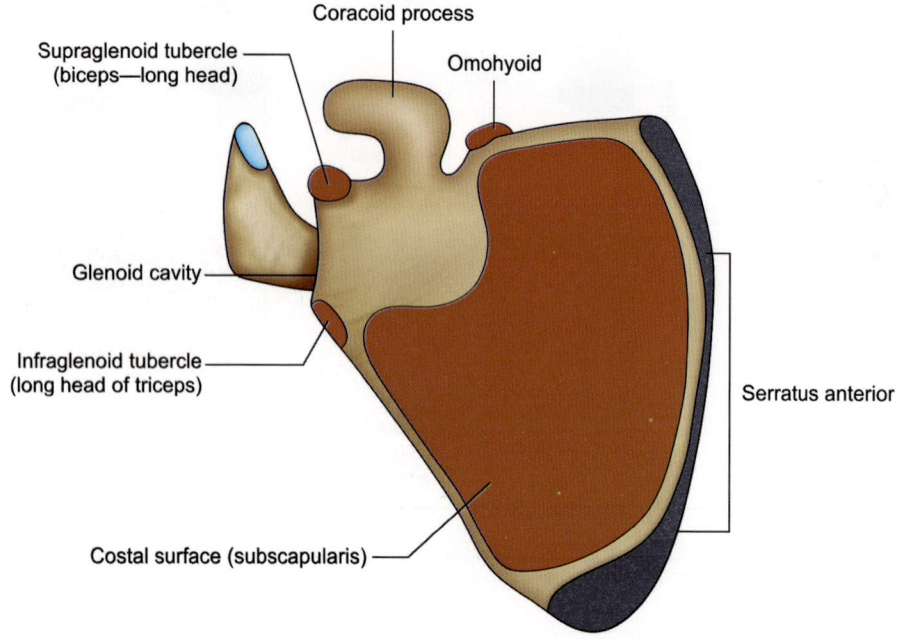

Fig. 3.4: Right scapula: Ventral aspect

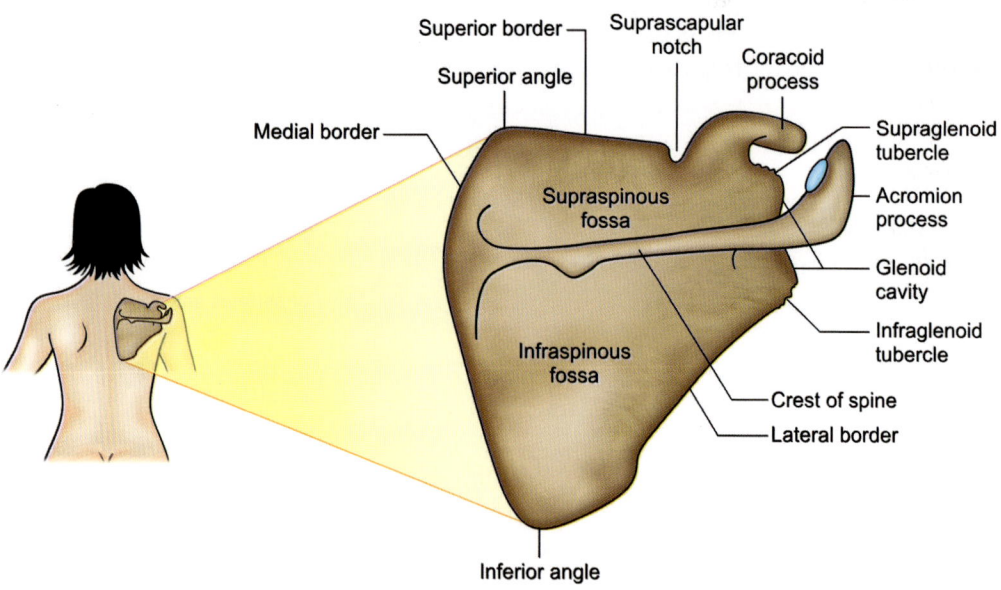

Fig. 3.5: Right scapula: Dorsal aspect

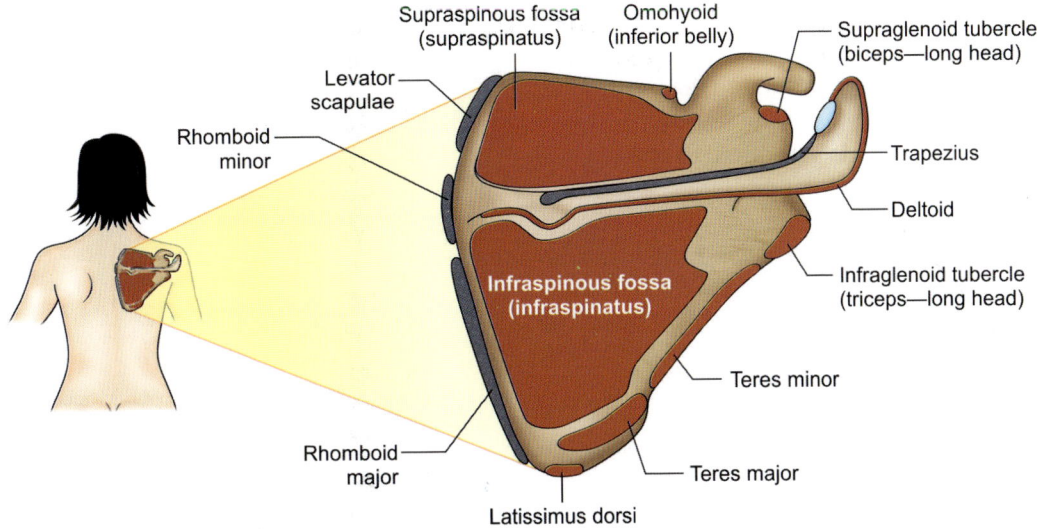

Fig. 3.6: Right scapula: Dorsal aspect

4. *Supraspinatus* is attached to medial 2/3rd of supraspinous fossa.

5. *Infraspinatus* is attached to medial 2/3rd of infraspinous fossa.

6. *Teres minor* is attached to the upper 2/3rd of the dorsal surface of lateral border. This origin is interrupted by the circumflex scapular artery.

7. *Teres major* is attached to the lower 1/3rd of the dorsal surface of lateral border and inferior angle.

Note: *Remember that child is always carried by adults in their arms, therefore, minor is above major*

8. *Latissimus dorsi* also originates from dorsal surface of the inferior angle by a small slip.

II. Borders

A. Superior border

1. It is the shortest border.

   Note: Superior begins with 'S' and 'Shortest' also begins with 'S'

2. *Suprascapular notch* is present near the root of coracoid process.

3. *Superior transverse (suprascapular) ligament* converts the suprascapular notch into *suprascapular foramen.*

4. *Suprascapular artery* passes above the ligament and *suprascapular nerve* passes below the ligament, through foramen.

Note: *To remember this fact think that Air Force flies above the Navy, i.e. A: Artery is above and N: Nerve is below*

5. *Inferior belly of omohyoid* is attached to the superior border near the suprascapular notch.

B. Lateral border

1. It is the thickest border.

2. *Infraglenoid tubercle* is present at its upper end, just below the glenoid cavity.

3. *Long head of triceps* originates from infraglenoid tubercle.

C. Medial border (vertebral border)

1. It extends from superior angle to inferior angle.

2. *Serratus anterior* is inserted to the costal surface of the medial border and the inferior angle.

3. *Levator scapulae* is attached to the medial border above the root of spine.
4. *Rhomboid minor* is attached to the medial border opposite the root of spine.
5. *Rhomboid major* is attached to the medial border below the root of spine.

Note: *Levator scapulae has to elevate the scapula and, therefore, is always superior most, rhomboid minor has to be superior to rhomboid major as the baby is carried by adults in their arms, i.e. minor is above the major.*

III. Angles

A. Superior angle

It is covered by trapezius.

B. Inferior angle

It is covered by latissimus dorsi.

C. Lateral angle (glenoid angle)

1. It bears the *glenoid cavity*, a pear shaped concave articular surface.
2. It is also known as the *head of scapula*.
3. *Labrum glenoidale* is attached to the margins of glenoid cavity deepening its concavity which receives the convexity of humerus to make shoulder joint.
4. *Capsule of shoulder joint* is attached to labrum and bone beyond it.
5. Long head of biceps originates from the *supraglenoid tubercle* (a small tubercle just above the glenoid cavity) which is intra-capsular (Fig. 3.7).

Note: *Glenoid tubercles are always meant for long heads, since 2 comes before 3, i.e. 2 is above 3 therefore biceps is attached to supraglenoid tubercle and triceps to infraglenoid tubercle.*

IV. Processes

A. Spinous process

1. It is a bracket like projection from upper part of dorsal aspect of scapula, also called *spine of scapula*

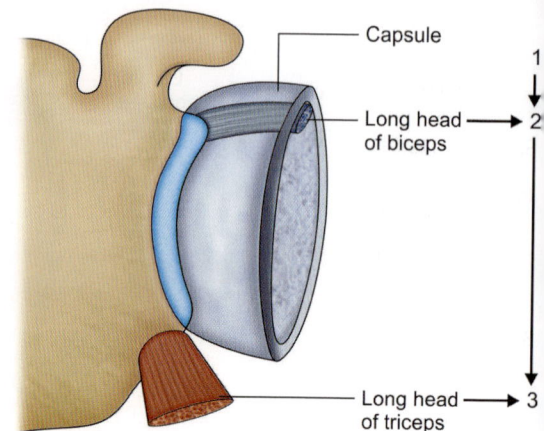

Fig. 3.7: Attachments of long heads of biceps (2) and triceps (3)

2. It divides the dorsal surface of scapula into *supraspinous* and *infraspinous fossae* (Figs 3.8 and 3.9).
3. Spine has 2 surfaces (superior and inferior) and 3 borders (anterior, posterior and lateral).

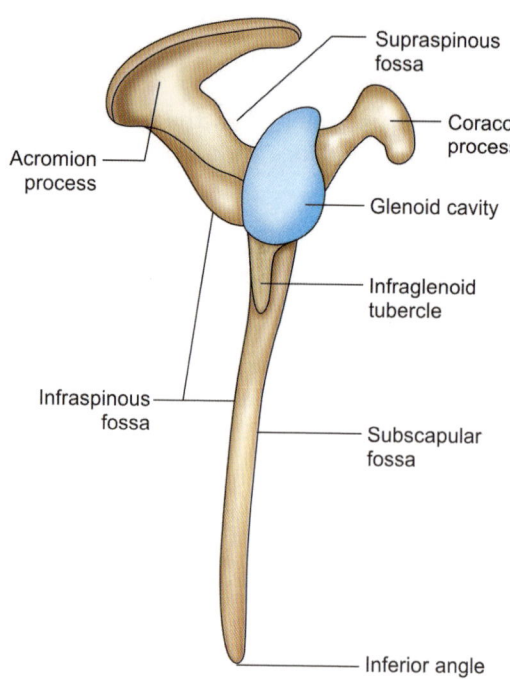

Fig. 3.8: Right scapula: Lateral view

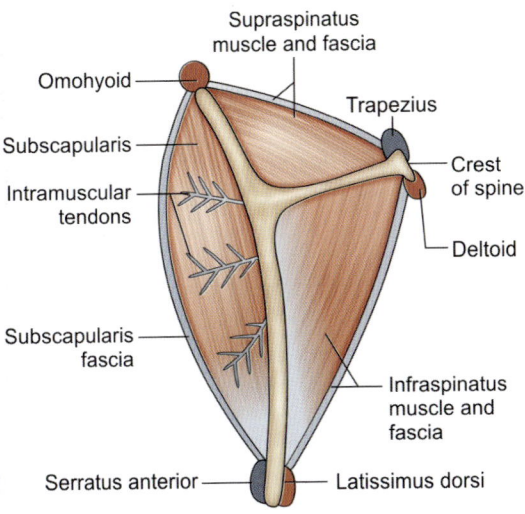

Omohyoid

Subscapularis

Intramuscular tendons

Subscapularis fascia

Serratus anterior

Suprasinatus muscle and fascia

Trapezius

Crest of spine

Deltoid

Infraspinatus muscle and fascia

Latissimus dorsi

Fig. 3.9: Vertical sectional view of scapula

4. Its superior surface contributes to *supra-spinous fossa* whose medial 2/3rd provides attachment to *supraspinatus* while lateral 1/3rd is related to *suprascapular nerve and vessels* (Fig. 3.10).

5. Inferior surface of spine contributes to *infraspinous fossa* whose medial 2/3rd gives attachment to *infraspinatus*.

6. Anterior border of spine is attached to dorsal surface of scapula.

7. Lateral border of spine bounds *spinoglenoid notch* meant for the passage of *suprascapular nerve and vessels*.

8. Posterior border of spine is also called *crest of spine*. *Trapezius* is attached to the upper lip of crest of spine while posterior fibres of *deltoid* are attached to its lower lip.

B. Acromion (acromial process)

1. It projects forwards from lateral end of spine.

2. It overhangs the glenoid cavity.

3. It is subcutaneous.

4. It has 2 borders (medial and lateral), 2 surfaces (superior and inferior) and a tip.

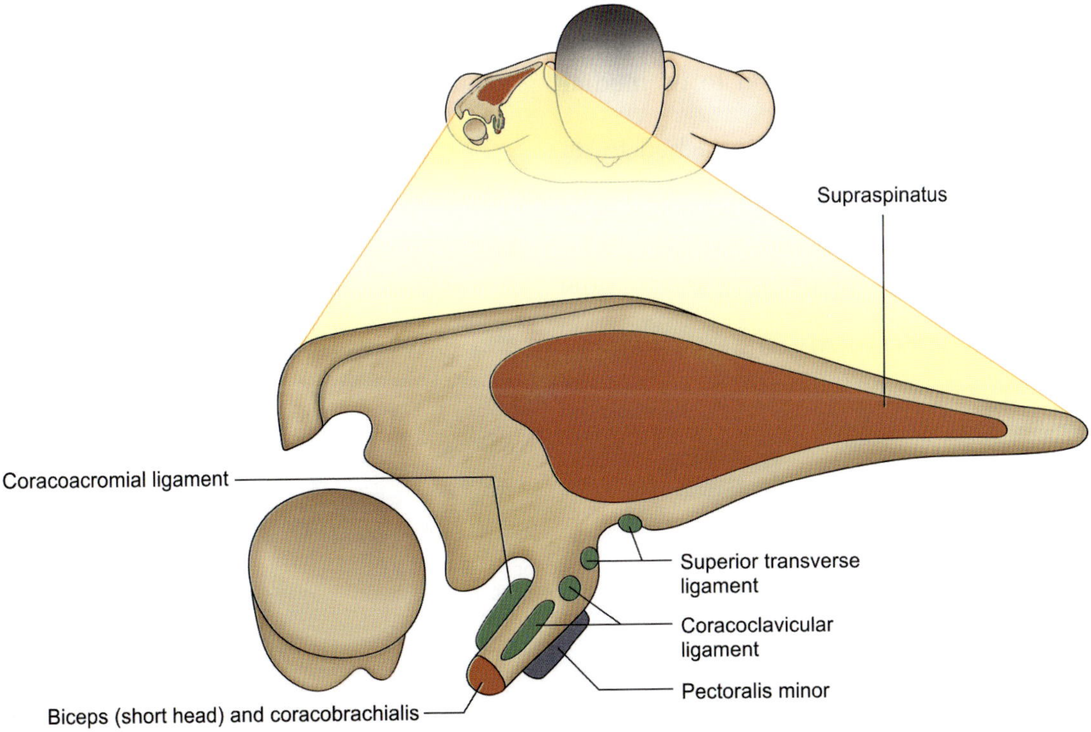

Coracoacromial ligament

Supraspinatus

Superior transverse ligament

Coracoclavicular ligament

Pectoralis minor

Biceps (short head) and coracobrachialis

Fig. 3.10: Right scapula: Superior aspect

5. Medial and lateral borders continue with the upper and lower lips of the crest of spine respectively.
6. Superior surface is subcutaneous.
7. Inferior surface is related to *subacromial bursa*.
8. *Trapezius* is attached to the medial border in continuation of its attachment to the upper lip of crest of spine.
9. *Deltoid's middle fibres* are attached to the lateral border in continuation of its attachment to the lower lip of crest of spine.
10. *Coracoacromial ligament* is attached to the medial side of tip.
11. *A small articular facet on its medial border* just behind the tip meets with lateral end of clavicle to form *acromioclavicular joint*.

C. Coracoid process (Fig. 3.11)

1. It lies below the junction of lateral 1/4th with the rest of clavicle.
2. It is directed forwards and slightly laterally.
3. It arises from upper part of glenoid cavity.
4. *Short head of biceps* and *coracobrachialis* arise from its tip by a common tendon.
5. *Pectoralis minor* is inserted to its medial border.
6. *Coracoacromial ligament* is attached to its lateral border.
7. *Conoid part of coracoclavicular ligament* is attached to its knuckle.

8. *Trapezoid part of coracoclavicular ligament* is attached to a ridge on its superior aspect between the attachments of pectoralis minor and coracoacromial ligament.
9. *Coracohumeral ligament* is attached to its root adjacent to glenoid cavity.

OSSIFICATION

A. Primary centre

One centre appears in the body during 8th week of intrauterine life.

B. Secondary centres: 7 in all

Appearance: 1st secondary centre appears in the middle of coracoid process during 1st year.

Following 6 centres appear at puberty:

1 for root of coracoid process (subcoracoid centre),

2 for acromion process,

1 for medial border,

1 for inferior angle,

1 for lower 2/3rd of rim of glenoid cavity.

Fusion: Subcoracoid centre fuses with rest of bone by 15th year. All other centres fuse by 20th year.

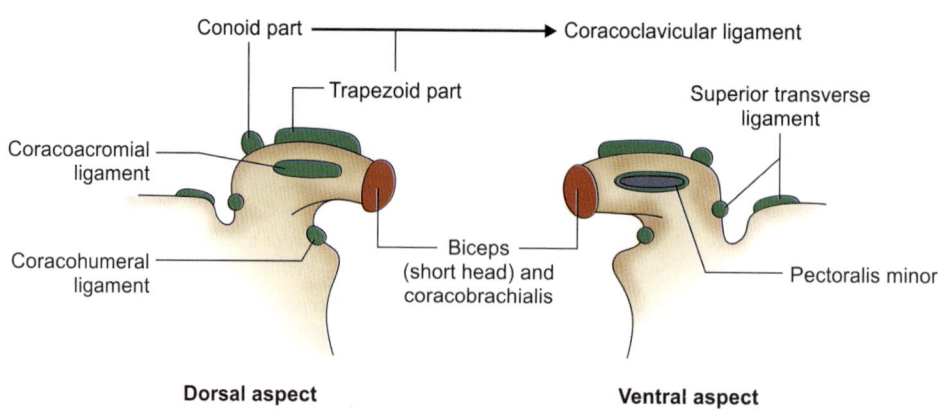

Dorsal aspect   Ventral aspect

Fig. 3.11: Coracoid process of right scapula

Humerus

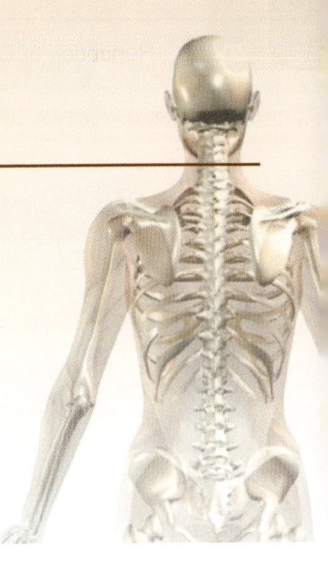

Humerus is the vertical bone located in the arm. It is said to be largest and longest bone of upper limb.

SIDE DETERMINATION (Fig. 4.1)

1. The rounded end (the end with head) is superior.
2. The head is directed medially.
3. Lesser tuberosity at the upper end faces forwards.

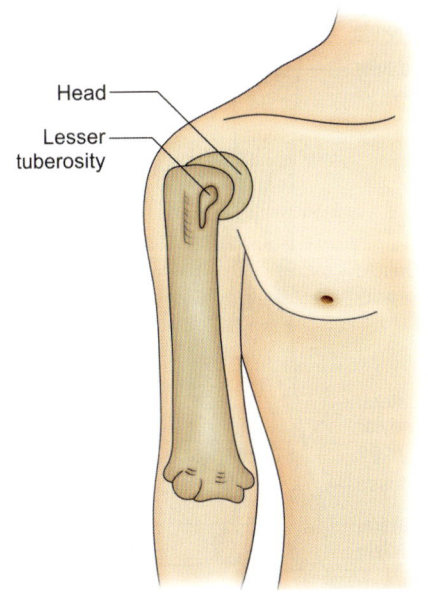

Head
Lesser tuberosity

Fig. 4.1: Determination of side of humerus

ANATOMICAL POSITION

Humerus is placed vertically in such a way that the head at its upper end faces medially, backwards and upwards.

FEATURES AND ATTACHMENTS

Humerus has two ends (upper and lower) and a shaft.

I. Upper end

It includes head, neck, greater and lesser tubercles and intertubercular sulcus.

A. Head

1. It is 1/3rd of a sphere.
2. It is covered by articular cartilage.

B. Neck

Three necks are described.

a. Anatomical neck

1. It is adjacent to head.
2. Capsular ligament of shoulder joint is attached to anatomical neck. Capsular attachment is deficient at the upper end of intertubercular sulcus for the passage of tendon of long head of biceps. Medially the capsule extends for about 2 cm on the shaft thus enclosing the medial part of epiphyseal line (Fig. 4.2).

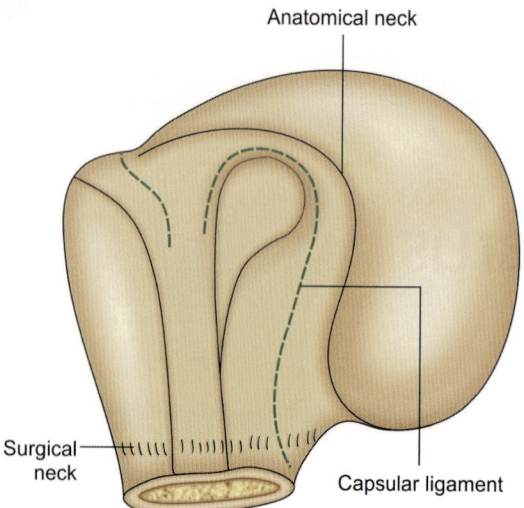

Fig. 4.2: Upper end of right humerus: Anterior aspect

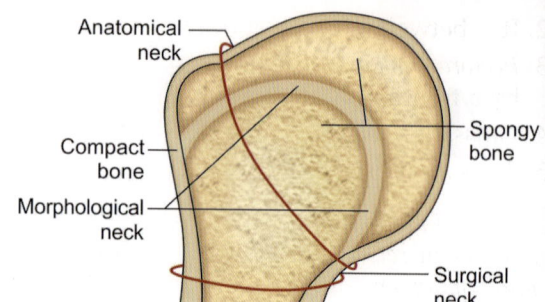

Fig. 4.3: Longitudinal section through upper end of humerus

3. It is covered by *subacromial bursa*.

D. Lesser tubercle

1. *Subscapularis* is inserted on it.
2. *Transverse humeral ligament* is attached to it.

E. Intertubercular sulcus (Fig. 4.4)

1. It is also called bicipital groove due to its relation with the long head of biceps.

b. Surgical neck

1. It is the junction of upper end and the shaft.
2. It is related to axillary nerve and posterior circumflex humeral vessels.

Note: *Remember, it is the anatomy which is taught 1st and surgery is taught afterwards in medical curriculum, therefore the 1st constriction from head is the anatomical neck and the next constriction is surgical neck.*

c. Morphological neck

The upper convex end of diaphysis is received by concavity of the epiphysis at the upper end of humerus. This junction is called morphological neck which can be appreciated only in vertical sectional view (Fig. 4.3).

C. Greater tubercle

1. It is the lateral most point in the shoulder region.
2. There are three impressions on the greater tubercle-upper, middle and lower. These impressions provide attachments to *supraspinatus, infraspinatus* and *teres minor* respectively.

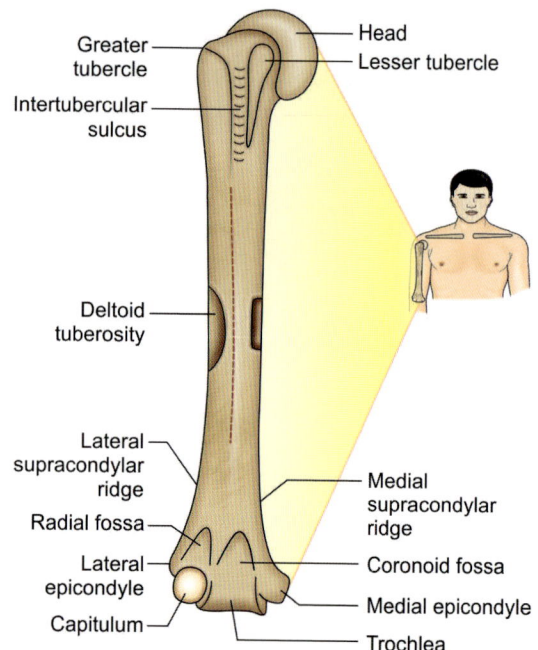

Fig. 4.4: Right humerus: Anterior aspect

2. It is between greater and lesser tubercles.
3. *Pectoralis major* is attached to its lateral lip by a trilaminar tendon.
4. *Latissimus dorsi* is attached to its floor.
5. *Teres major* is inserted on the medial lip.

> **Note:** *For remembering the attachments of muscles in relation to bicipital groove, keep in mind the axiom "LADY between two MAJORS." LADY stands for Latissimus dorsi while Majors are Pectoralis Major and Teres Major.*

6. Contents of bicipital groove:
   i. *Long head of biceps.*
   ii. *Synovial sheath of this tendon.*
   iii. *Ascending branch of anterior circumflex humeral artery.*

II. Shaft

1. It is rounded in upper half.
2. It is triangular in lower half.
3. It has 3 borders, anterior, medial and lateral.
4. It has 3 surfaces, anterolateral, anteromedial and posterior (Fig. 4.5).

A. Borders

a. Anterior border

1. It continues with lateral lip of bicipital groove.
2. *Brachialis muscle* arises from its lower half.

b. Lateral border

1. It is prominent only in the lower part where it forms the *lateral supracondylar ridge.*
2. *Radial groove* crosses its middle.
3. *Lateral intermuscular septum* is attached to the whole extent of lateral supracondylar ridge.
4. *Brachioradialis* originates from the upper 2/3rd of lateral supracondylar ridge.
5. *Extensor carpi radialis longus* arises from lower 1/3rd of lateral supracondylar ridge.

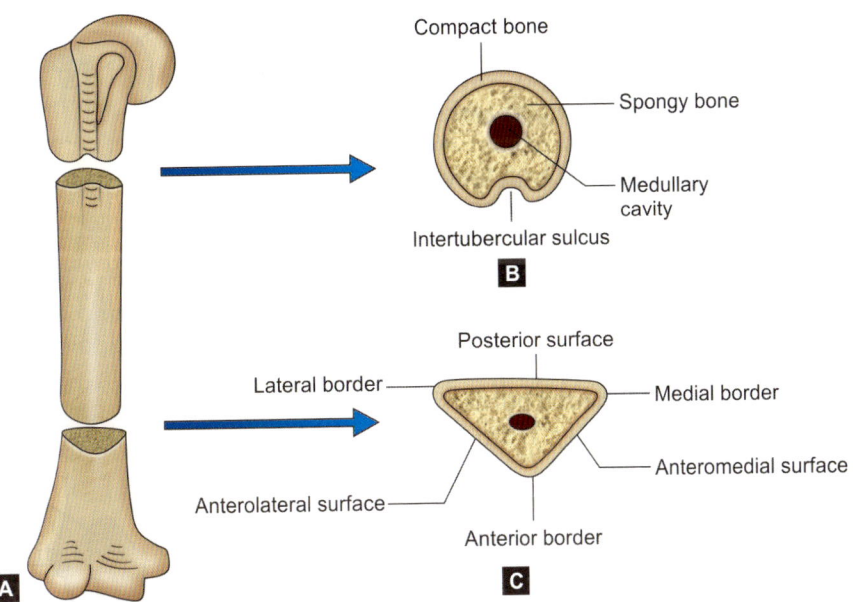

Compact bone
Spongy bone
Medullary cavity
Intertubercular sulcus
B

Posterior surface
Lateral border
Medial border
Anterolateral surface
Anteromedial surface
Anterior border
A   **C**

Fig. 4.5: Right humerus: (A) Anterior view; (B) Upper cross-section; (C) Lower cross-section

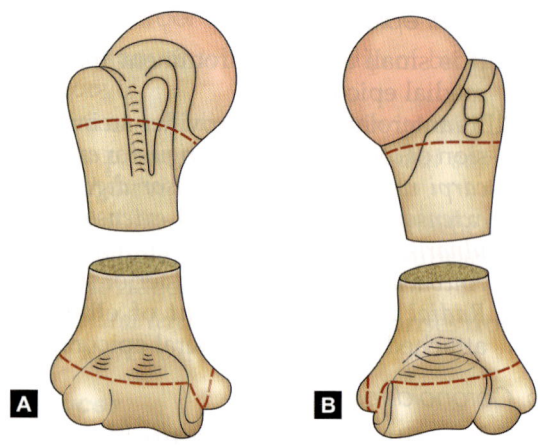

Fig. 4.8: Epiphyseal lines and capsular attachments of right humerus. (A) Anterior view; (B) Posterior view. Continuous lines, capsular attachments; Dotted lines, epiphyseal lines

ANGLES

I. Carrying angle (Fig. 4.9)

1. It is an angle observed between long axis of arm and long axis of forearm.
2. It is seen in fully extended and fully supinated forearm.
3. It is due to the downward projection of the medial part of trochlea.
4. It is about 15°.
5. It is more in female than male.

II. Angle of humeral torsion (Fig. 4.9)

1. It is the angle between the long axes of upper and lower ends of humerus.
2. In quadrupeds it is 90°, while in human being it is about 164°.
3. It is more in males than females.

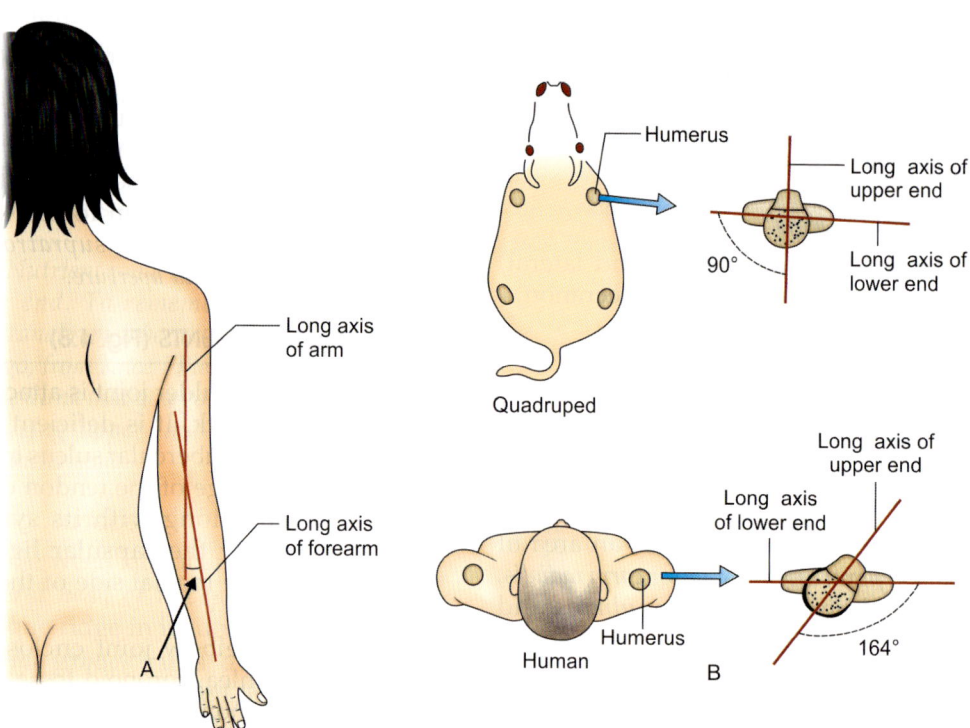

Fig. 4.9: Angles: (A) Carrying angle (posterior view of right upper limb); (B) Angle of humeral torsion (superior view of right humerus)

OSSIFICATION

A. Primary centre

One centre appears for the shaft during 8th week of intrauterine life.

B. Secondary centres

Seven secondary centres appear in all, of which three appear for the upper end and four for the lower end.

Note: *For remembering the ossification, keep in mind that a part which is larger requires more time to ossify in comparison to a part which is smaller, therefore, the centre for the larger parts appear early as compared to the centres for smaller parts, in other words remember, bigger the size, earlier the appearance.)*

a. Upper end

Three secondary centres,

Appearance

Head   – 1st year
Greater tubercle – 3rd year
Lesser tubercle – 5th year

Fusion

All three centres at the upper end fuse together at 7 years to form conjoint epiphysis which itself fuses with the shaft by 20th year.

Note: *To remember the appearance of secondary centres at the upper end of humerus, start from '1' and go on adding '2', i.e. 1^{+2} 3^{+2} $5^{+2}7$.*

b. Lower end

Four secondary centres,

Appearance

Medial epicondyle   – 5th year
Lateral epicondyle   – 12th year
Capitulum and lateral
   flange of trochlea   – 2nd year
Medial part of trochlea – 12th year

Fusion

Two epiphyses are formed at the lower end, one for medial epicondyle and other for the rest. The centres for lateral epicondyle, capitulum and trochlea fuse with each other during the 14th year, the epiphysis thus formed fuses with the shaft at 16th year. Medial epicondyle fuses with shaft at 18th year.

Note: *'Medial epicondyle is located below lesser tubercle therefore centre appears at the same time, i.e. 5th year. There is one centre for TWO parts, i.e. capitulum and lateral part of trochlea and therefore the time of appearance is TWO years.*

For the secondary centres at lower end and their fusions, formula of '2' can be applied which is as follows:

Centre for medial part of trochlea
Centre for lateral epicondyle
                                    12 years
Fusion of lateral 3 centres to form big lateral epiphysis at lower end
                              12 + 2 = 14 years
Fusion of lateral epiphysis with shaft
                              14 + 2 = 16 years
Fusion of medial epiphysis or epicondyle with shaft
                              16 + 2 = 18 years

For remembering the time of fusion of epiphysis of long bones with the shaft in cases of the limbs, following formula (Fig. 4.10) can be remembered:

Table 4.1: Time of fusion of epiphyses with shaft of long bones of limbs

Region	Time of fusion
Shoulder	20 years
Elbow	18 years
Wrist	20 years
Hip	18 years
Knee	20 years
Ankle	18 years

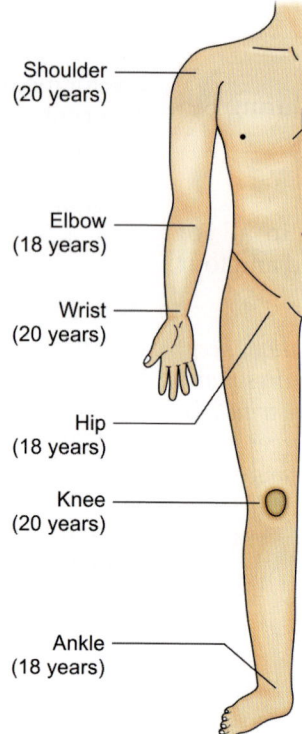

Shoulder
(20 years)

Elbow
(18 years)

Wrist
(20 years)

Hip
(18 years)

Knee
(20 years)

Ankle
(18 years)

Fig. 4.10: Time of fusion of epiphyses with shaft of long bones of limbs

Radius

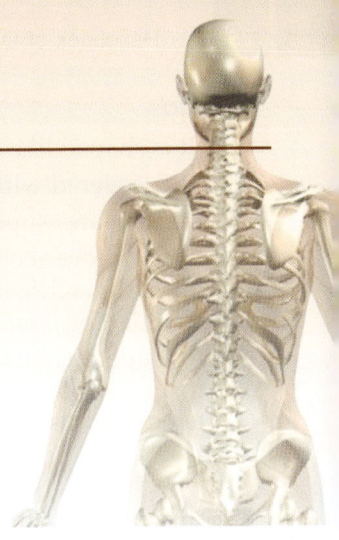

It is the lateral bone of forearm and is homologous with tibia of leg.

SIDE DETERMINATION (Fig. 5.1)

1. Keep the bone vertically in such a way that the narrow end is superior while the wider end is inferior.
2. Keep the lower end in such a manner that the *styloid process* is directed laterally and prominent tubercle (*Lister's tubercle*) faces dorsally.
3. Keep the sharpest border (*interosseous border*) of shaft medially.

ANATOMICAL POSITION

Radius is vertically placed with the *head* superior, *radial tuberosity* and *interosseous border* medial, *styloid process* lateral and *Lister's tubercle* posterior.

FEATURES AND ATTACHMENTS

It has two ends (upper and lower) and a shaft.

I. Upper end

It has head, neck and tuberosity.

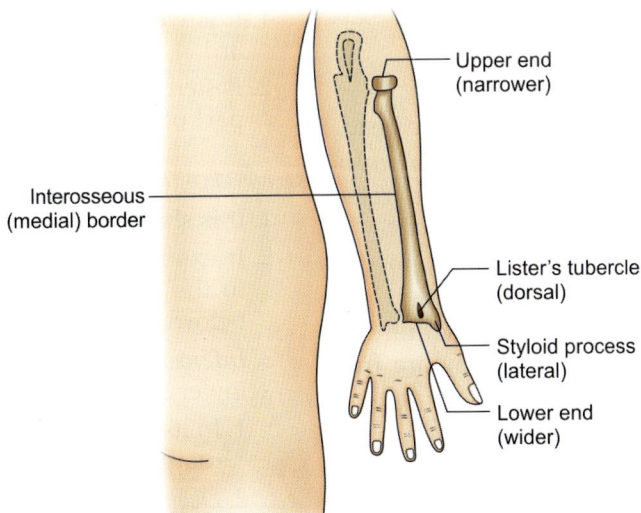

Fig. 5.1: Determination of side of radius

A. Head

1. It is shaped like disc.
2. It is covered with *hyaline cartilage.*
3. It articulates superiorly with capitulum.
4. Circumference of head articulates medially with ulna, rest of it is surrounded by *annular ligament* (Fig. 5.2).
5. Its superior surface participates in the formation of elbow while the circumference forms *superior radio-ulnar joint.*

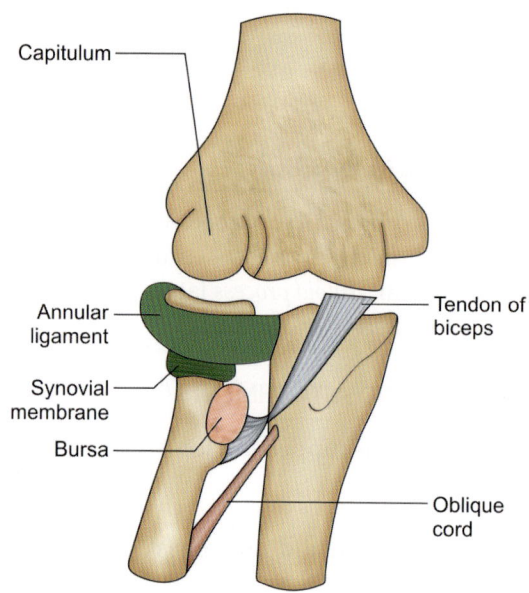

Fig. 5.2: Relations of head of radius

Capitulum

Annular ligament

Synovial membrane

Bursa

Tendon of biceps

Oblique cord

B. Neck

1. It is the constricted part below the head.
2. It is covered by the lower part of *annular ligament.* The *synovial membrane* separates the neck from the annular ligament.
3. *Quadrate ligament* is attached to the medial part of the neck.
4. Head and neck rotate freely within the annular ligament because they are free from capsular ligament.

C. Tuberosity

1. It is situated just below the medial part of neck.

2. *Biceps tendon* is attached to the rough posterior part of radial tuberosity.
3. A *bursa* covers the smooth anterior part of tuberosity.

Note: *Remember that attachment of muscular tendon to bone produces roughness while the part of bone covered by bursa or cartilage is smooth.*

4. *Oblique cord* is attached just below the radial tuberosity.

II. Shaft

It has 3 borders and 3 surfaces.

A. Borders

a. Anterior border

1. It extends from anterior margin of radial tuberosity to the styloid process of radius.
2. *Anterior oblique line* is the oblique upper half of the anterior border (Fig. 5.3.)
3. *Radial head of flexor digitorum superficialis* originates from the anterior oblique line (Fig. 5.4).
4. *Extensor retinaculum* is attached to the lower crest like part of anterior border.

b. Posterior border (Fig. 5.5)

1. It is well demarcated only in its middle 3rd.
2. *Posterior oblique line* is the upper oblique part of posterior border.

c. Medial (interosseous) border

1. It is sharpest amongst all the borders.
2. It extends from radial tuberosity above to the posterior margin of ulnar notch below.
3. *Interosseous membrane* is attached to its lower 3/4th.
   1. In its lower part, it forms the posterior margin of a triangular area.
   2. *Deep fibres of pronator quadratus* are inserted on this triangular area.

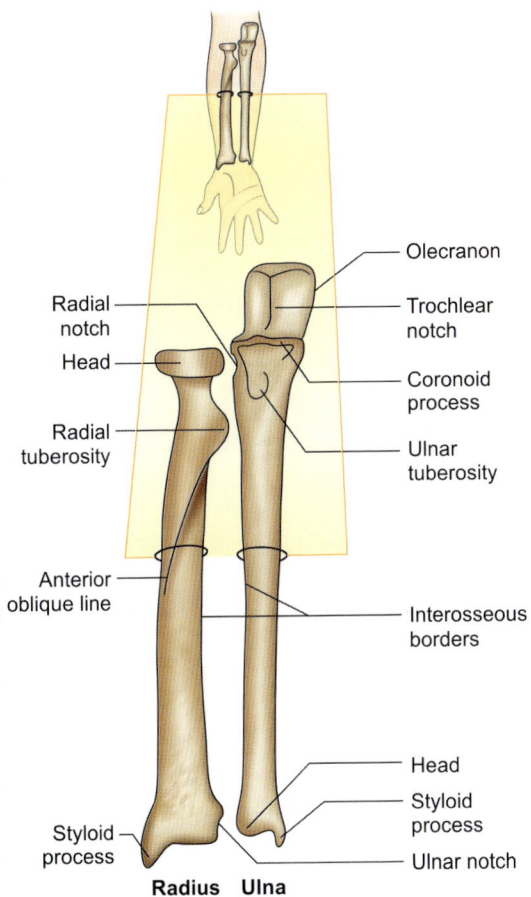

Fig. 5.3: The bones of right forearm: Anterior aspect

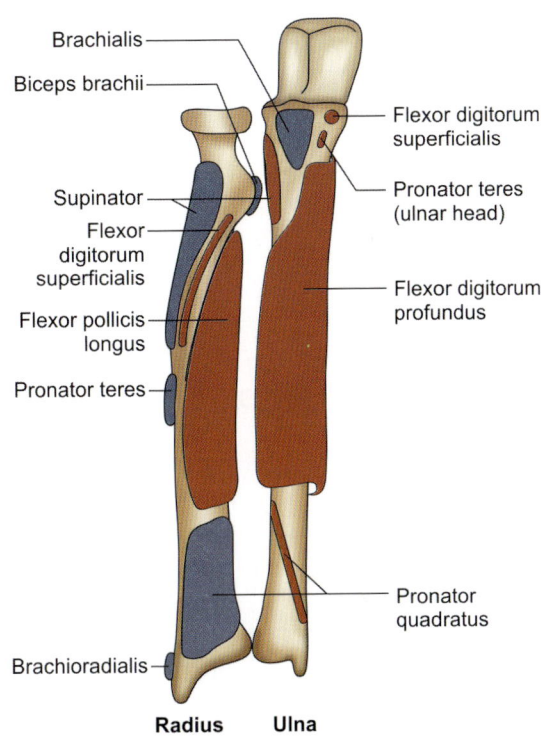

Fig. 5.4: Bones of right forearm: Anterior aspect

B. Surfaces

a. Anterior surface

1. *Flexor pollicis longus* originates from its upper 3/4th.
2. *Pronator quadratus* is inserted on its lower 1/4th.
3. *Nutrient foramen* is situated in its upper part. Nutrient foramen leads into nutrient canal which is directed upwards.

Note: *Remember the axiom "Towards Elbow I go, and from Knee I flee".*

1. *Nutrient artery* for radius is a branch from anterior interosseous artery.

b. Posterior surface (Fig. 5.6)

1. *Abductor pollicis longus* arises from the middle 1/3rd of this surface.
2. *Extensor pollicis brevis* originates from posterior surface just distal to the attachment of abductor pollicis longus.
3. Extensor muscles of thumb cover the lower part of posterior surface.

c. Lateral surface

1. *Supinator* is inserted on its upper 1/3rd.
2. *Pronator teres* is inserted on its middle 1/3rd.
3. Extensor tendons cover its lower 1/3rd.

III. Lower end

1. It is the widest part of the bone.
2. It has 5 surfaces (anterior, posterior, medial, lateral and inferior):
   i. **Anterior surface** is in the form of a thick ridge and provides attachment to

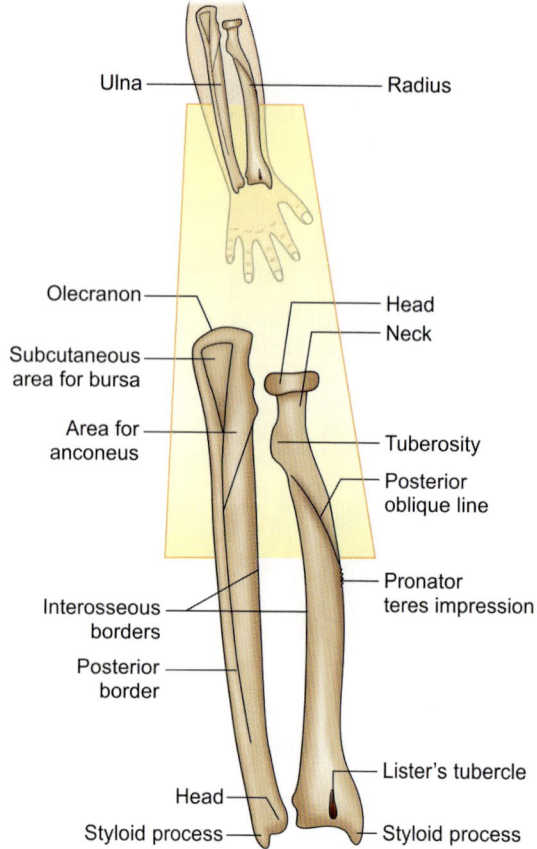

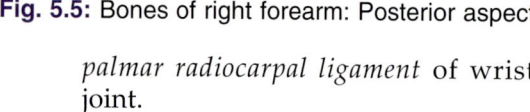

Fig. 5.5: Bones of right forearm: Posterior aspect

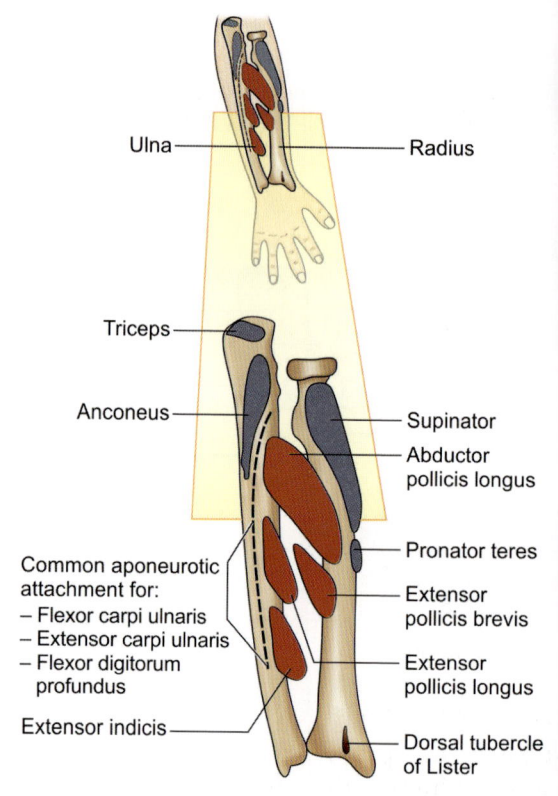

Fig. 5.6: Bones of right forearm: Posterior aspect

palmar radiocarpal ligament of wrist joint.

ii. **Posterior surface** presents four grooves for extensor tendons. *Dorsal tubercle of Lister* is a prominent tubercle on the posterior surface, lateral to the *groove for extensor pollicis longus*.

Note: *Remember both 'Lister' and 'Longus' start with 'L' showing that 'Extensor pollicis longus grooves Lister's tubercle.*

Groove lateral to Lister's tubercle is traversed by *extensor carpi radalis longus* and *extensor carpi radialis brevis*. The groove medial to groove for extensor pollicis longus, is meant for *extensor digitorum* and *extensor indicis* (Fig. 5.7).

iii. **Medial surface** is occupied by the *ulnar notch* for the head of ulna. *Articular disc of inferior radioulnar joint is attached to the lower margin of ulnar notch.*

iv. **Lateral surface** is related to tendons of *abductor pollicis longus* and *extensor pollicis brevis*. The lateral surface is prolonged downwards as the *styloid process. Brachioradialis* is inserted on this surface just proximal to the base of styloid process. *Radial collateral ligament* of wrist joint is attached to the tip of styloid process.

v. **Inferior surface** presents a lateral triangular area for scaphoid and a medial quadrangular area for lunate.

Note: *Remember MLA, i.e. Medial is Lunate Area.*

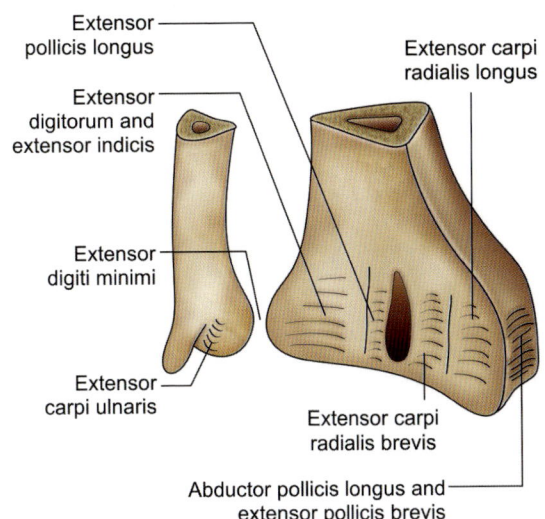

Extensor pollicis longus

Extensor carpi radialis longus

Extensor digitorum and extensor indicis

Extensor digiti minimi

Extensor carpi ulnaris

Extensor carpi radialis brevis

Abductor pollicis longus and extensor pollicis brevis

Fig. 5.7: Lower ends of right radius and ulna: Dorsal aspect

OSSIFICATION

A. Primary centre

One centre appears for the shaft during 8th week of intrauterine life.

B. Secondary centres

Two in all, one for upper end and one for lower end.

a. Upper end

Appearance: 4 years

Fusion: 18 years

b. Lower end

Appearance: 2 years

Fusion: 20 years

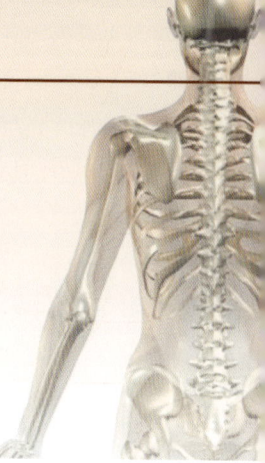

Ulna

It is the medial bone of forearm and is homologous with fibula of lower limb.

SIDE DETERMINATION (Fig. 6.1)

1. Keep the bone vertically in such a way that the hook-like end is upwards.
2. The concavity of hook and the *coronoid process* are looking forwards.
3. Sharp crest like border of shaft is directed laterally.

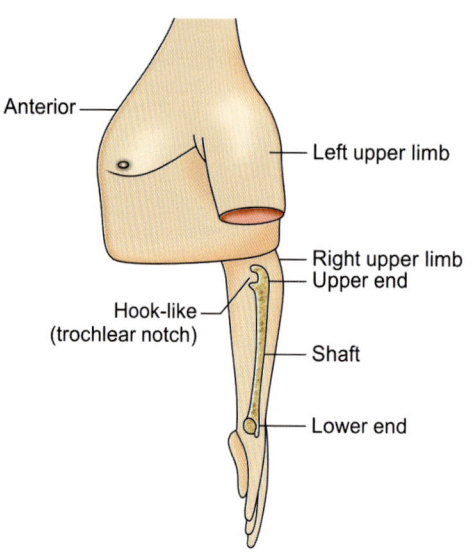

Anterior

Left upper limb

Right upper limb
Upper end

Hook-like
(trochlear notch)

Shaft

Lower end

Fig. 6.1: Determination of side of ulna

ANATOMICAL POSITION

Ulna is the medial bone of forearm lying vertically in such a way that the concavity at the upper end faces forwards and interosseous border is directed towards lateral bone of forearm i.e., radius.

FEATURES AND ATTACHMENTS

It has two ends (upper and lower) and a shaft.

I. Upper end

It has two processes (olecranon and coronoid) and two notches (trochlear and radial).

A. Processes

a. Olecranon process (Figs 6.2 and 6.4)

It projects upwards from shaft. It has 5 surfaces:
  i. *Superior surface*
    1. *Triceps* is attached to its rough posterior 2/3rd.
    2. *Capsular ligament* is attached anteriorly to the margins.
    3. A *bursa* is located between tendon of triceps and capsule.
  ii. *Anterior surface*
    It forms the upper part of trochlear notch.

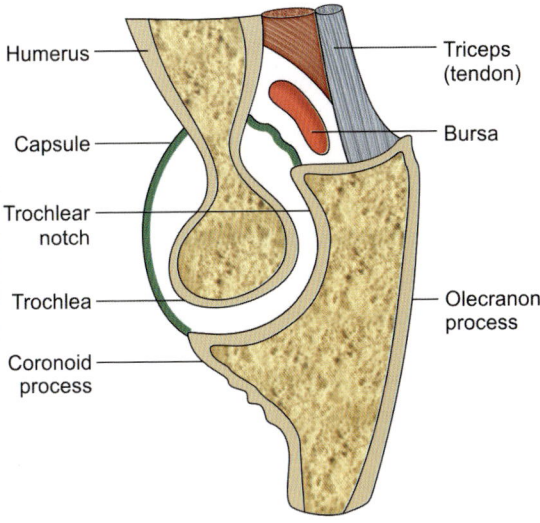

Fig. 6.2: Relations of olecranon process

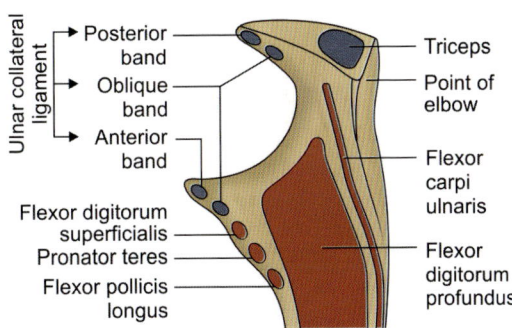

Fig. 6.4: Medial aspect of upper end of right ulna

iii. *Posterior surface*

1. It forms a triangular subcutaneous area (Fig. 6.3).

2. A *bursa* separates the posterior surface of the olecranon from the skin.

3. Its upper part forms the *point of elbow*.

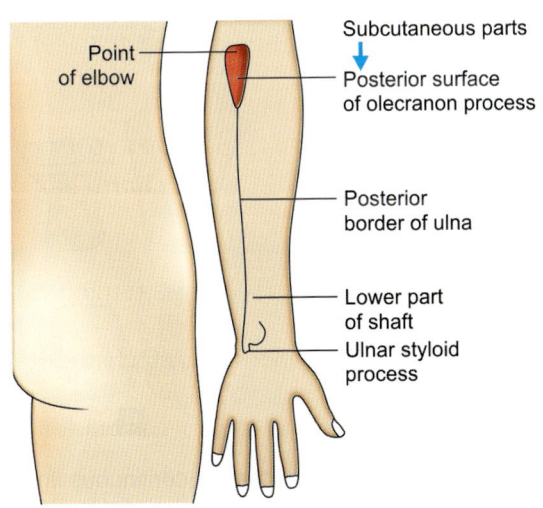

Fig. 6.3: Subcutaneous parts of right ulna

iv. *Medial surface*

1. *Flexor carpi ulnaris* originates from its upper part.

2. *Flexor digitorum profundus* (upper fibres) arises from its lower part.

3. *Ulnar collateral ligament* (posterior and oblique bands) is attached to its upper part.

v. *Lateral surface*

Anconeus is inserted on this surface.

b. *Coronoid process*

It projects forwards from the shaft just below the olecranon process. It has 4 surfaces:

i. *Superior surface*

It forms the lower part of *trochlear notch*.

ii. *Anterior surface*

1. At the lower corner of this surface there is *ulnar tuberosity* (Fig. 6.5).

2. *Brachialis* is attached to the whole of the anterior surface including ulnar tuberosity.

3. The medial margin of the anterior surface is sharp and provides attachments to following from proximal to distal:

   – *Anterior band of ulnar collateral ligament.*

   – *Oblique band of ulnar collateral ligament.*

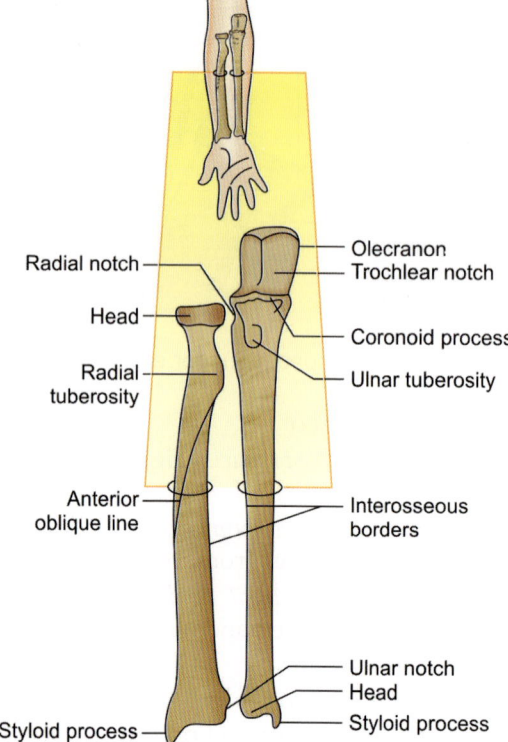

Radial notch

Head

Radial tuberosity

Anterior oblique line

Styloid process

Olecranon

Trochlear notch

Coronoid process

Ulnar tuberosity

Interosseous borders

Ulnar notch

Head

Styloid process

Fig. 6.5: The bones of right forearm: Anterior aspect

– *Lower part of humero-ulnar head of flexor digitorum superficialis.*
– *Ulnar head of pronator teres.*
– Very rarely the *ulnar head of flexor pollicis longus.*

iii. Medial surface

It receives attachment of *flexor digitorum profundus.*

iv. Lateral surface

1. The upper part of this surface is articular for the circumference of head of radius and, therefore, called *radial notch.*

2. *Annular ligament* is attached to the anterior and posterior margins of the radial notch.

3. The lower part of the lateral surface forms a depressed area called *supinator*

fossa. The supinator fossa accommodates radial tuberosity.

4. Supinator fossa is limited posteriorly by *supinator crest.* Supinator crest and posterior part of fossa are meant for the origin of deep part of supinator.

B. Notches (articular surfaces)

a. Trochlear notch

1. It articulates with the trochlea of humerus.

2. The capsule of elbow joint is attached to the margins of trochlear notch except laterally where trochlear notch is continuous with the radial notch.

b. Radial notch

1. It articulates with the head of radius to form the superior radio-ulnar joint.

2. *Annular ligament* is attached to the anterior and posterior margins of the notch.

II. Shaft

It has 3 borders (lateral, anterior and posterior) and 3 surfaces (anterior, medial and posterior).

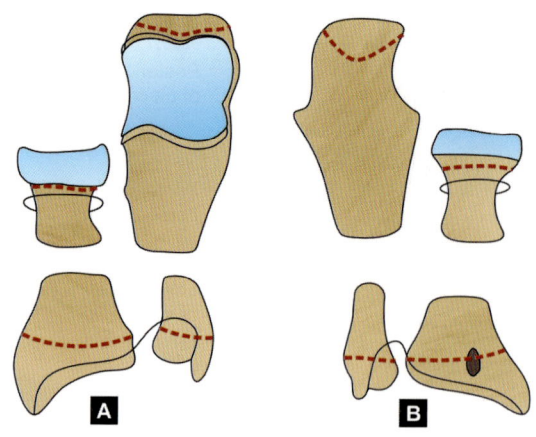

Fig. 6.6: Capsular attachments (continuous lines) and epiphyseal lines (dotted lines) of the radius and ulna. (A) Anterior view; (B) Posterior view

A. Borders

a. Lateral border

1. This is also called *interosseous border*.
2. It is sharpest in its middle 2/4th.
3. *Interosseous membrane* is attached to it, except at its upper end (Fig. 6.7). The

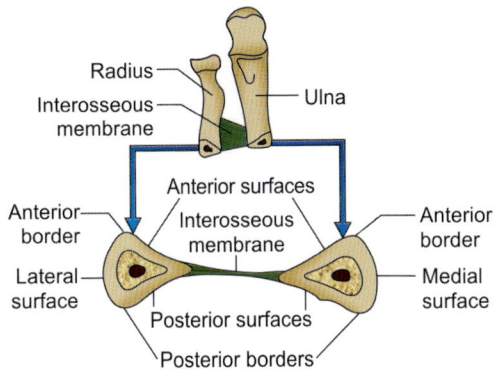

Fig. 6.7: Borders and surfaces of radius and ulna

direction of fibres in interosseous membrane is downwards and medial.

b. Anterior border

1. It is thick and round.
2. Its upper 3/4th is covered by the originating fibres of the *flexor digitorum profundus*.

c. Posterior border (Figs 6.3 and 6.8)

1. It is subcutaneous.
2. The deep fascia of forearm is attached to it. The deep fascia acts as common aponeurosis for the attachment of following 3 muscles:
   - i. *Flexor digitorum profundus* from its upper 3/4th.
   - ii. *Flexor carpi ulnaris* from its upper 3/5th.
   - iii. *Extensor carpi ulnaris* from its middle 1/3rd.

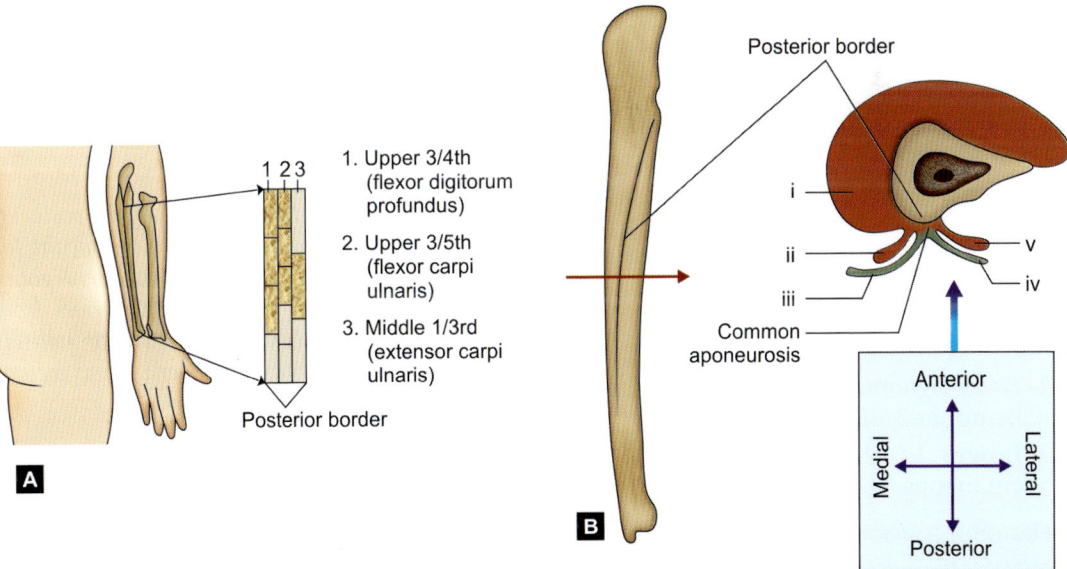

Fig. 6.8: Common aponeurotic attachment to the posterior border of right ulna. (A) Muscles attached; (B) Attachments from medial to lateral; (i) flexor digitorum profundus; (ii) flexor carpi ulnaris; (iii and iv) deep fascia; (v) extensor carpi ulnaris

B. Surfaces

a. Anterior surface (Fig. 6.9)

1. *Flexor digitorum profundus* arises from its upper 3/4th.
2. *Pronator quadratus* originates from an oblique ridge in its lower 1/4th.
3. *Nutrient foramen* is located in its upper part which leads into nutrient canal directed upwards.

> **Note:** *Nutrient canal is directed opposite to the growing end therefore upwards in ulna because lower end is growing end.*

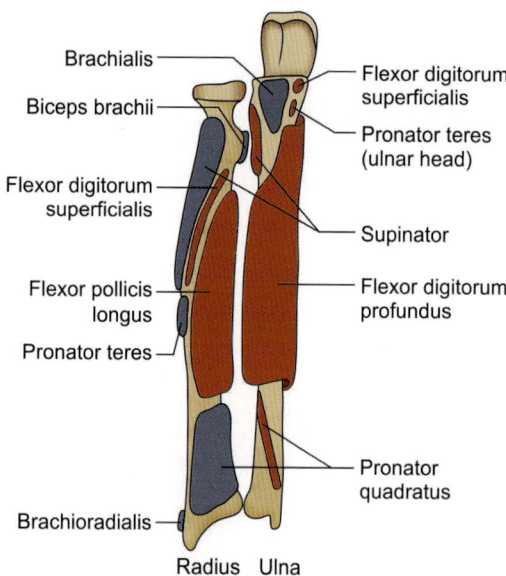

Fig. 6.9: The bones of right forearm: Anterior aspect

b. Medial surface

1. *Flexor digitorum profundus* originates from its upper 3/4th.
2. Lower 1/4th of this surface is subcutaneous.

c. Posterior surface (Figs 6.10 and 6.11)

1. It lies between posterior and interosseous borders.
2. It is divided into smaller upper and larger lower part by an oblique line.

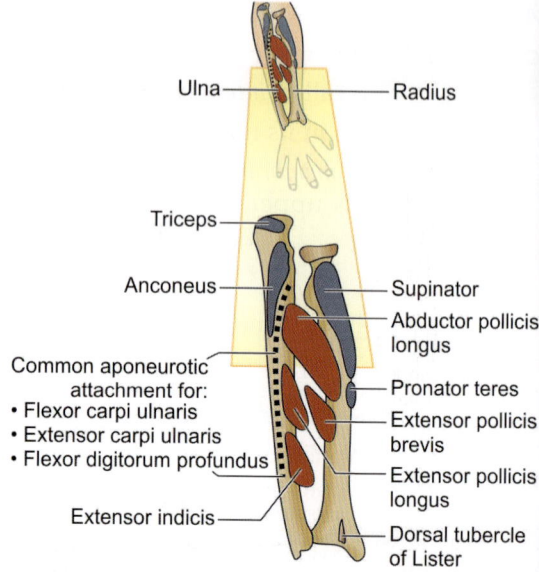

Fig. 6.10: The bones of right forearm: Posterior aspect

3. Area above the oblique line receives insertion of *anconeus*.
4. The posterior surface below the oblique line is divided into medial and lateral areas by a vertical line. The lateral one provides attachments to 3 muscles from proximal to distal:
   – *Abductor pollicis longus*
   – *Extensor pollicis longus*
   – *Extensor indicis*

> **Note:** *Remember the middle 3rd of the posterior surfaces of both radius and ulna are meant for longus tendons of extensor compartment going to thumb. Extensor pollicis longus arises from middle 1/3rd of ulna only. Abductor pollicis longus originates from the upper ulna as well as middle 1/3rd of radius.*

III. Lower end

It includes the head and styloid process.

A. Head

1. It articulates with the ulnar notch of radius and forms the inferior *radio-ulnar joint*.

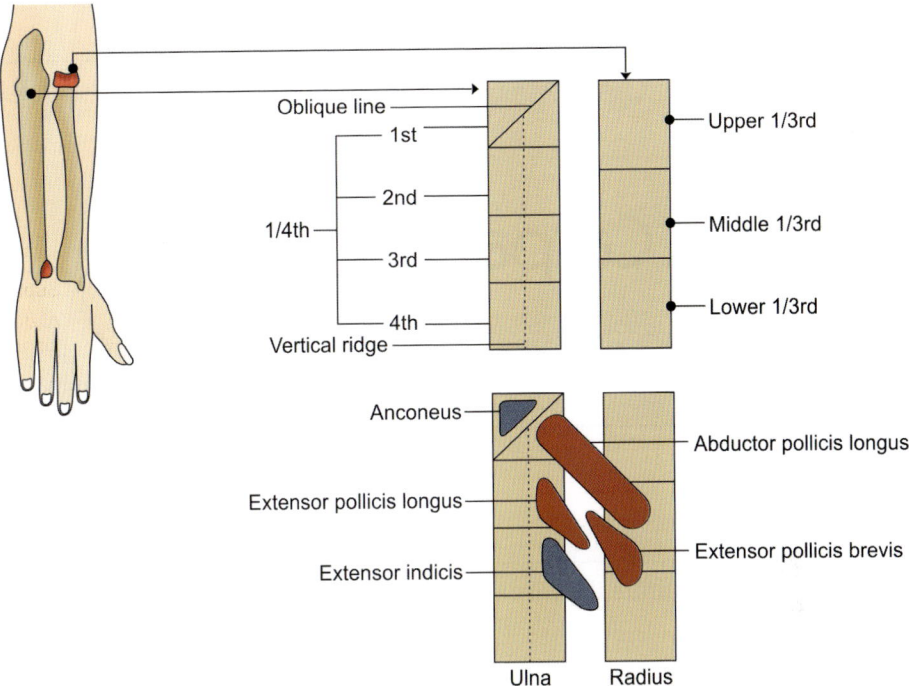

Fig. 6.11: Attachments to the posterior surfaces of radius and ulna

2. Articular disc separates the head from wrist joint.

B. Styloid process

1. It projects downwards from the postero-medial aspect of lower end of ulna.
2. *Medial (ulnar) collateral ligament of wrist joint* is attached to its apex.
3. The *apex of triangular articular disc is* attached to the depression between the head and styloid process.
4. *Tendon of extensor carpi ulnaris* grooves the area between the head and styloid process posteriorly (Fig. 6.12).

OSSIFICATION

A. Primary centre

One centre appears for the shaft during 8th week of intrauterine life.

B. Secondary centres

Two in all, one for upper end and one for lower end.

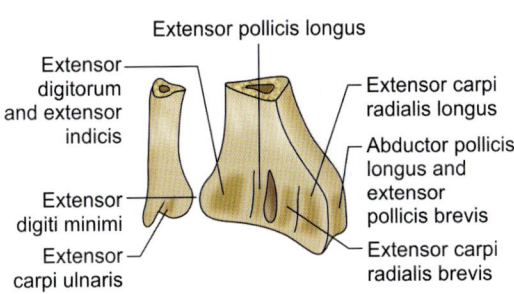

Fig. 6.12: Lower ends of the right radius and ulna: Dorsal aspect

a. Upper end

Appearance: 8 years

Fusion: 18 years

b. Lower end

Appearance: 6 years

Fusion: 20 years.

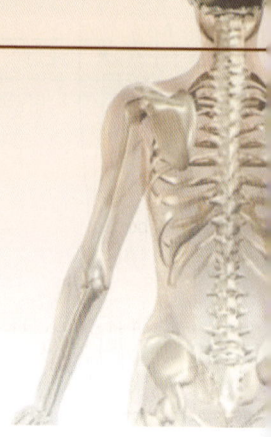

Carpal Bones

CARPUS

8 carpal bones together constitute the carpus.

NAMES

The carpal bones are arranged in two rows, proximal and distal. They are named from lateral to medial (Fig. 7.1) as follows:

In proximal row – *Scaphoid*
Lunate
Triquetral
Pisiform
In distal row – *Trapezium*
Trapezoid
Capitate
Hamate

Note: *To remember the names and the sequences, remember the following; "She Looks Too Pretty, Try To Catch Her".*

ARTICULATED CARPAL BONES (Fig. 7.2)

When all the carpal bones articulate with each other, the carpus in general shows following features:

1. It is semicircular in shape.
2. The circumference of semicircle meets with radius proximally to form wrist joint.

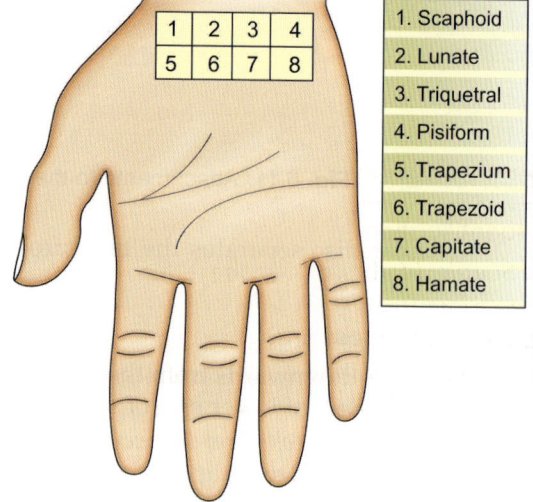

| 1 | 2 | 3 | 4 |
| 5 | 6 | 7 | 8 |

1. Scaphoid
2. Lunate
3. Triquetral
4. Pisiform
5. Trapezium
6. Trapezoid
7. Capitate
8. Hamate

Fig. 7.1: Naming the carpal bones

3. The diameter of semicircle is distal and articulates with bases of 5 metacarpals (I–V).
4. The carpus shows overall concavity on the palmar aspect than the dorsal aspect. This concavity forms fibro-osseous tunnel (*carpal tunnel*) with flexor retinaculum.
5. The proximal row is convex proximally and concave distally.
6. The distal row is convex proximally but flat distally.

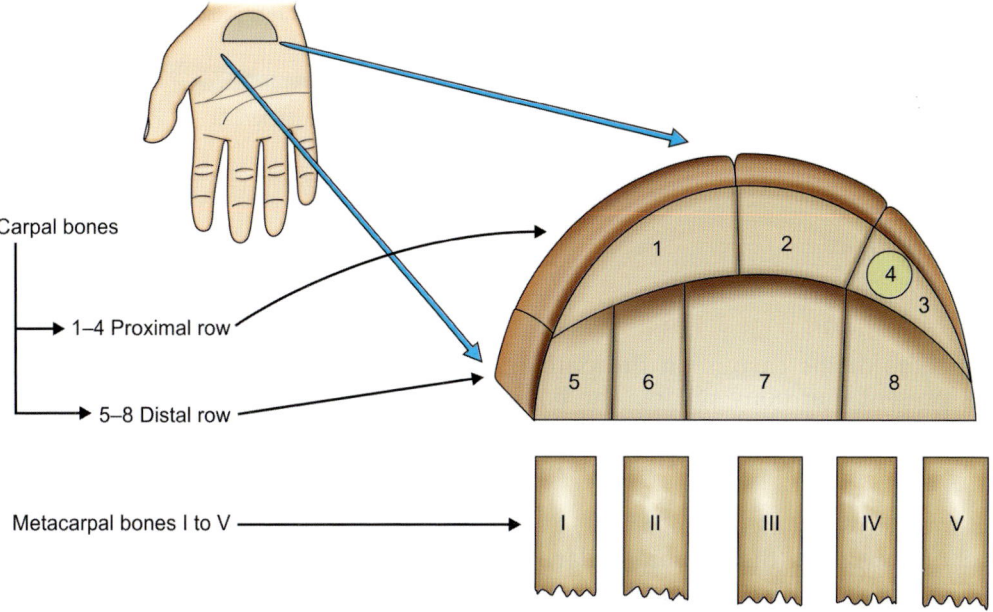

Fig. 7.2: Right carpus: Anterior view

INDIVIDUAL CARPAL BONE

. Identification

1. Scaphoid: It is boat shaped, has a *con-striction* (neck) and *tubercle*.

2. Lunate: It is half moon shaped.

3. Triquetral: It is pyramidal in shape. It has an *oval articular facet* for pisiform.

4. Pisiform: It is pea like.

5. Trapezium: It is quadrilateral and possesses a *groove* and *crest*.

6. Trapezoid: It is shaped like a baby's foot.

7. Capitate: It is largest among carpal bones and has a rounded *head*.

8. Hamate: It is wedge shaped and has a *hook* like process.

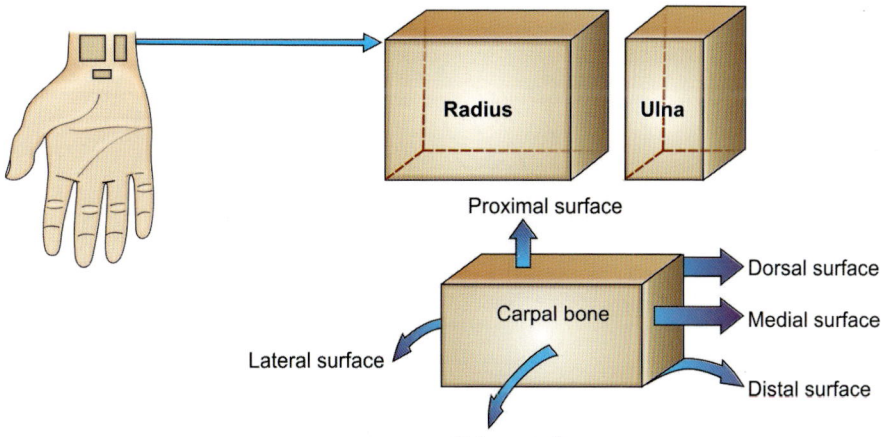

Fig. 7.3: Surfaces of a carpal bone

II. Surfaces (Fig. 7.3)

All the carpal bones in general may be considered to have following 6 surfaces:

1 – Proximal
2 – Distal
3 – Medial
4 – Lateral
5 – Palmar
6 – Dorsal

III. Four bony pillars (Figs 7.4 and 7.5)

Four corners of the carpus on the palmar aspects present four bony pillars. The bony pillars are formed by:

1. Tubercle of scaphoid (proximal, lateral pillar)
2. Pisiform (proximal medial pillar)
3. Crest of trapezium (distal lateral pillar)
4. Hook of hamate (distal medial pillar)

These pillars increase the concavity of the carpus on palmar aspect and provide attachments to *flexor retinaculum* to form *carpal tunnel*.

IV. Articulations

1. *Radiocarpal articulation:* Proximal surfaces of scaphoid, lunate and triquetral form

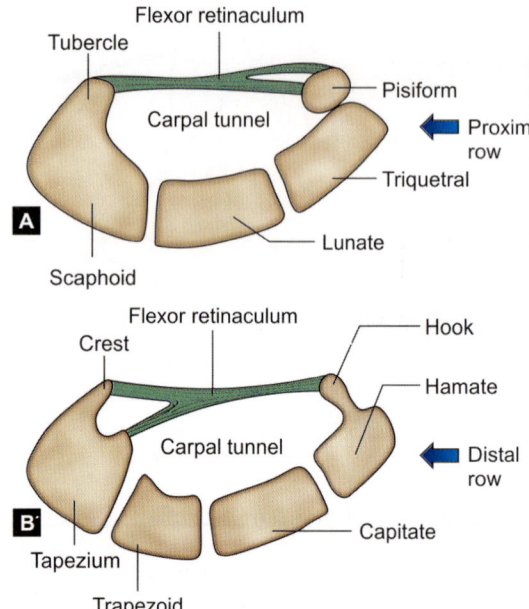

Fig. 7.5: Transverse sections through carpus (A) Proximal row; (B) Distal row

wrist joint with lower end of radius and articular disc. In normal anatomical position, scaphoid is related to radius and

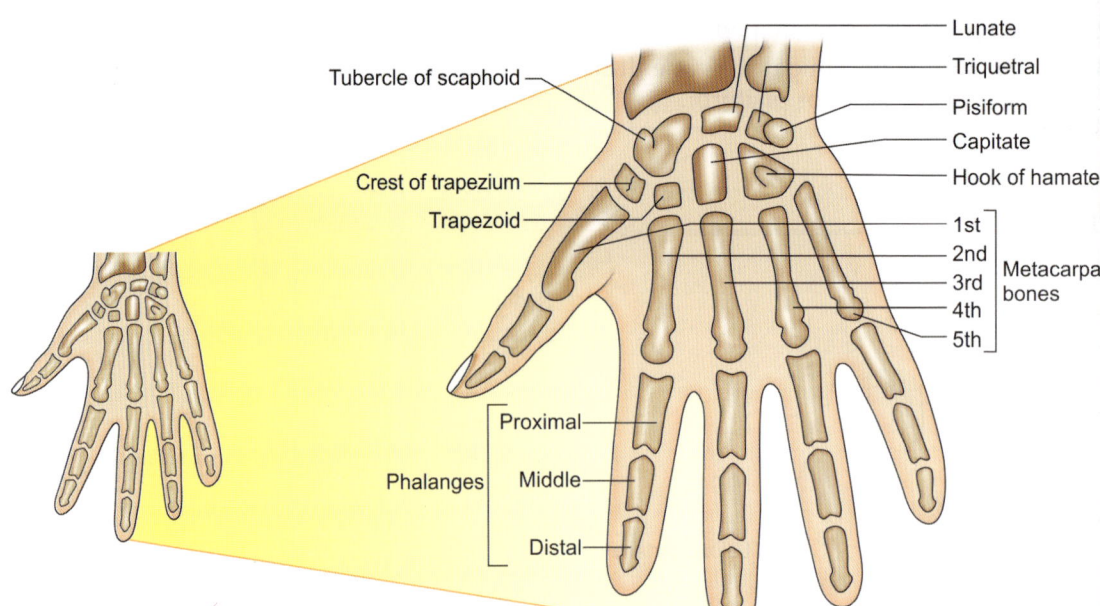

Fig. 7.4: Skeleton of right hand : Palmar aspect

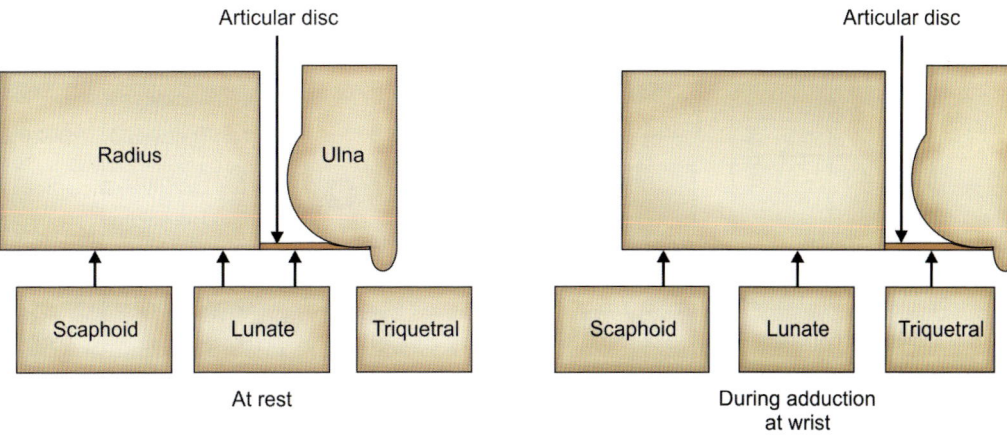

Fig. 7.6: Relations of proximal row of carpal bones to radius and articular disc

lunate to radius and articular disc. During adduction at wrist scaphoid and lunate come to lie under radius while articular disc is related to triquetral (Fig. 7.6).

2. Intercarpal articulations (Table 7.1 and Fig. 7.7)

Table 7.1: Intercarpal articulations

Carpal bones	Surfaces	Adjacent bones
Scaphoid	Medial	Lunate
	Distal	Trapezium, trapezoid, capitate
Lunate	Lateral	Scaphoid
	Medial	Triquetral
	Distal	Capitate
Triquetral	Lateral	Lunate
	Palmar	Pisiform
	Distal	Hamate
Pisiform	Dorsal	Triquetral
Trapezium	Medial	Trapezoid
	Proximal	Scaphoid
Trapezoid	Lateral	Trapezium
	Medial	Capitate
	Proximal	Scaphoid
Capitate	Lateral	Trapezoid
	Proximal	Scaphoid, lunate
	Medial	Hamate
Hamate	Lateral	Capitate
	Proximal	Triquetral

3. Carpometacarpal articulations (Table 7.2): Distal surfaces of carpal bones of distal row articulate with bases of metacarpals as follows.

Table 7.2: Carpometacarpal articulations

Carpal bones	Metacarpal number
Trapezium	1st
Trapezoid	2nd
Capitate	3rd
Hamate	4th and 5th

4. Non-articular surfaces of carpal bones: These surface provide attachments to palmar, dorsal, interosseous and collateral ligaments (Fig. 7.8).

V. Attachments to bony pillars

A. Tubercle of scaphoid

1. *Flexor retinaculum.*
2. *Abductor pollicis brevis.*

B. Pisiform

1. *Flexor retinaculum.*
2. *Extensor retinaculum.*
3. *Flexor carpi ulnaris.*
4. *Abductor digiti minimi.*
5. *Pisohamate ligament.*
6. *Pisometacarpal ligament.*

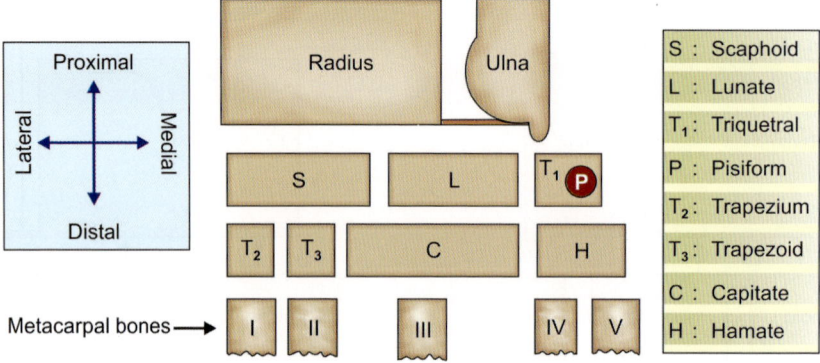

Fig. 7.7: Carpal articulations

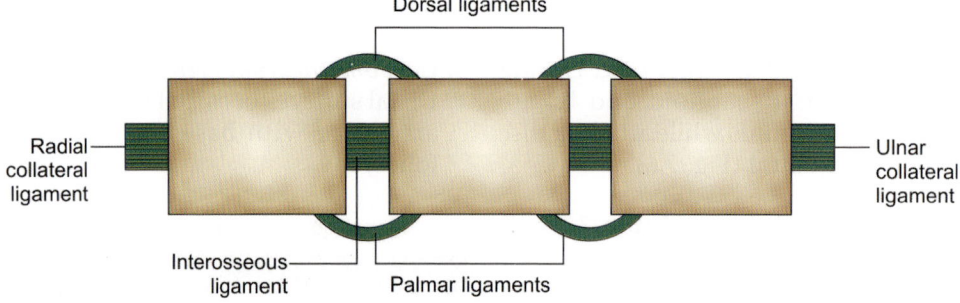

Fig. 7.8: Attachments to nonarticular surfaces of carpal bones

C. Crest of trapezium

1. *Flexor retinaculum.*
2. *Abductor pollicis brevis.*
3. *Flexor pollicis brevis.*
4. *Opponens pollicis.*

Note: *There is a groove on the palmar aspect of trapezium just medial to its crest. The layers of flexor retinaculum are attached to the margins of groove which itself lodges the tendon of flexor carpi radialis.*

D. Hook of hamate

1. *Flexor retinaculum.*
2. *Flexor digiti minimi.*
3. *Opponens digiti minimi.*

Note: *Deep branch of ulnar nerve grooves it on the medial side)*

OSSIFICATION

Each carpal bone ossifies by single centre. All these centres appear after birth (Table 7.3).

Table 7.3: Ossification of carpal bones

Carpal bones	Time of appearance
Capitate	3rd month
Hamate	4th month
Triquetral	3rd year
Lunate	4th year
Scaphoid and trapezoid	5th year
Trapezium	6th year
Pisiform	12th year

Note: *You can remember like this—Capitate and Hamate are First to ossify therefore in First Year. Triquetral is 3rd bone, TRI—3, therefore during 3rd year. Lunate is 4th bone to ossify therefore in 4th year. Except Pisiform all the rest (i.e. Scaphoid, Trapezoid and Trapezium) ossify during 5–6 years. Pisiform is the smallest bone, therefore, last to ossify. Count the number of alphabets in Pisiform Bone. It is 12 and therefore centre appears at 12th year.*

Metacarpal Bones

METACARPUS

Five metacarpal bones together constitute the metacarpus.

NAMING THE METACARPAL BONES

Metacarpal bones are named by numbering them. They are numbered from lateral to medial, i.e. the metacarpal bone along thumb is called 1st metacarpal bone and the metacarpal bone along little finger is known as 5th metacarpal bone.

IDENTIFICATION OF METACARPAL BONES (Fig. 8.1)

I. **First metacarpal bone**

1. It is smallest.
2. Facet on the proximal surface of base is concavo-convex.

II. **Second metacarpal bone**
Its base is grooved.

III. **Third metacarpal bone**
Its base has a styloid process.

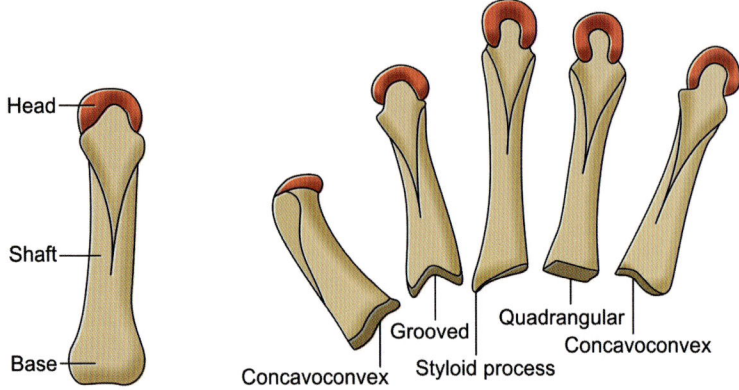

Fig. 8.1: Right metacarpal bones: Dorsal view

IV. Fourth metacarpal bone

The proximal surface of its base has large quadrilateral surface.

V. Fifth metacarpal bone

The base shows concavoconvex facet on its proximal surface and an elongated facet on one side of it.

FEATURES AND ATTACHMENTS

Metacarpal bones are miniature long bones. Each metacarpal bone has got a distal end (head), a proximal end (base) and a shaft.

I. Head

1. It is covered with *articular area* which is more extensive on palmar aspect.

2. It articulates with the base of proximal phalanx.

3. The heads of medial four metacarpal bones form knuckles of hand.

4. On the dorsal surface on each side there is a small *tubercle for collateral ligament.*

II. Shaft (body)

1. It is concave on the palmar aspect contributing to the hollow of palm.

2. It is also concave on its sides for the attachments of *interossei.*

3. The dorsal surface presents a triangular area distally.

4. *Transverse head of adductor pollicis* arises from the anterior surface of shaft of 3rd metacarpal bone.

5. *Opponens pollicis* is inserted on the shaft of 1st metacarpal bone.

6. *Opponens digiti minimi* is inserted on the shaft of 5th metacarpal bone.

III. Base

1. Its proximal surface articulates with the adjacent carpal bone as follows:
   1st metacarpal bone with trapezium
   2nd metacarpal bone with trapezoid
   3rd metacarpal bone with capitate
   4th metacarpal bone with hamate
   5th metacarpal bone with hamate

2. Except the base of 1st metacarpal bone, adjacent sides of bases of rest of the metacarpal bones articulate with each other (Fig. 8.2).

3. *Oblique head of adductor pollicis* arises from bases of 2nd and 3rd metacarpal bones.

4. *Abductor pollicis longus* is attached to the base of 1st metacarpal bone.

5. *Flexor carpi radialis* gets attached to the bases of 2nd and 3rd metacarpal bones on their palmar aspects.

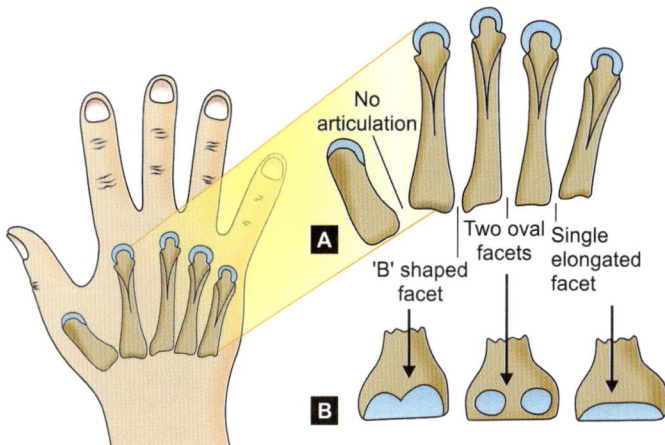

Fig. 8.2: Right metacarpal bones: (A) Dorsal aspect; (B) Adjacent bases

6. *Extensor carpi radialis longus* is attached to base of 2nd metacarpal bone on its dorsal aspect.

7. *Extensor carpi radialis brevis* is attached to the base of 3rd metacarpal bone on its dorsal aspect.

8. Both *flexor carpi ulnaris* (indirectly via pisometacarpal ligament) and *extensor carpi ulnaris* (directly) are attached to the base of 5th metacarpal bone on its palmar and dorsal aspects respectively.

PECULIARITIES OF 1ST METACARPAL BONE

1. It is placed more anteriorly than the rest of the metacarpal bones.

2. It is rotated medially through 90°. This facilitates the opposition of thumb.

3. Its base does not articulate with adjacent metacarpal bone making it free to move.

OSSIFICATION

A. Primary centre

One centre appears for shaft during 9th week of intracterine life.

B. Secondary centres

Only one secondary centre appears for each metacarpal bone. This is located in the base of the 1st metacarpal bone and heads of rest of the metacarpal bones.

Appearance : 2 years

Fusion   : 1st metacarpal bone—16 years

Rest of the metacarpal bones—18 years

Phalanges of the Hand

The total number of phalanges in each hand is 14. Thumb has got only two phalanges, i.e. proximal and distal. Rest of the fingers have got three phalanges each, i.e. proximal, middle and distal (Fig. 9.1).

CHARACTERISTICS (Figs 9.2 and 9.3)

1. Each phalanx has:
   a. A proximal end—*base*
   b. An intervening part—*shaft*
   c. A distal end—*head*

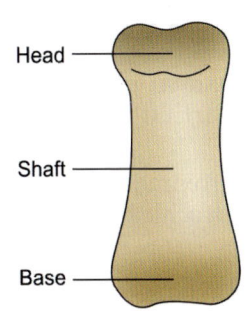

Fig. 9.2: Parts of phalanx

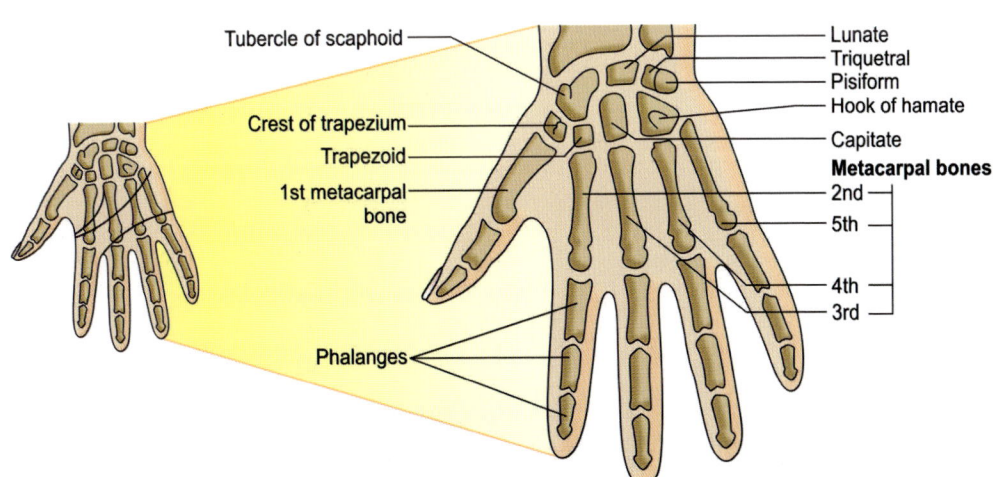

Fig. 9.1: Skeleton of right hand: Palmar aspect

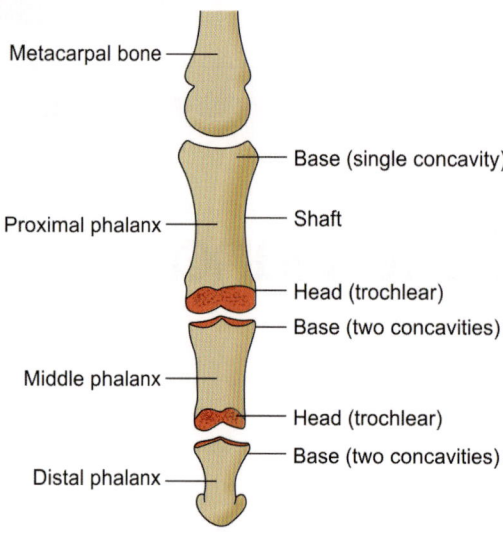

Metacarpal bone

Base (single concavity)

Proximal phalanx — Shaft

Head (trochlear)

Base (two concavities)

Middle phalanx

Head (trochlear)

Base (two concavities)

Distal phalanx

Fig. 9.3: Phalanges

2. Base of proximal phalanx has a concave surface to articulate with the head of metacarpal.

3. Heads of proximal phalanx and middle phalanx are trochlear (pulley like) in nature.

4. Bases of middle and distal phalanges are concave and divided into two parts by a ridge.

5. The distal end of distal phalanx is non-articular and rough.

OSSIFICATION

A. Primary centre

One centre appears for the shaft as follows:

Proximal phalanx: 10th week of intrauterine life.

Middle phalanx: 12th week of intrauterine life.

Distal phalanx: 8th week of intrauterine life.

B. Secondary centre

Only one centre appears for the base of each phalanx

Appearance: 2 years

Fusion: 16 years

Hip Bone

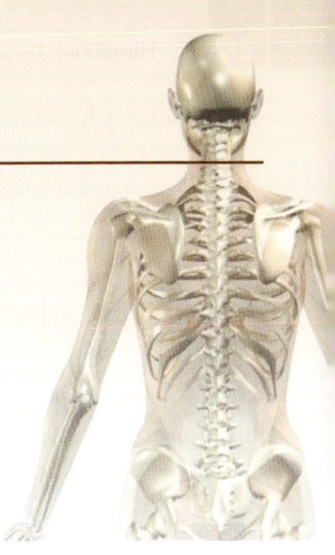

OS INNOMINATUM

Hip bone is also called os innominatum because of its irregular shape and no definite name.

SIDE DETERMINATION (Fig. 10.1)

1. The upper and lower parts of hip bone are expanded while the middle part is constricted.
2. The expanded part with a foramen (*obturator foramen*) is inferior. The other expanded part called *ilium*, is superior.

3. The constriction is marked by a deep hollow (*acetabulum*) which faces laterally.
4. The lower part of hip bone has a thin part (*pubis*) and a thick part (*ischium*). The ischium is relatively posterior while pubis is directed anteriorly.

NORMAL ANATOMICAL POSITION (Fig. 10.2)

1. Pubic tubercle and anterior superior iliac spine lie in the same coronal plane

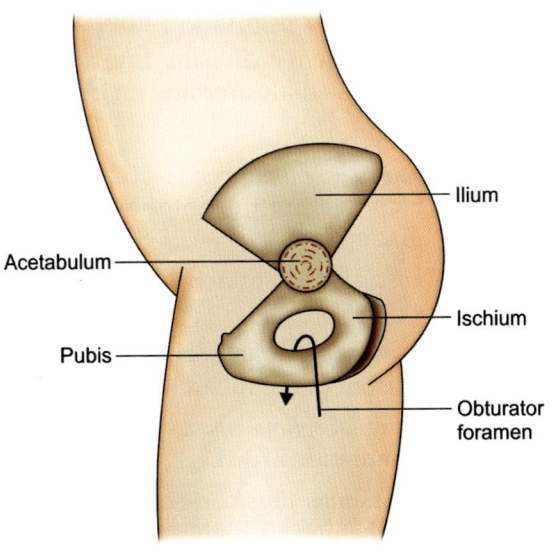

Fig. 10.1: Side determination: Left hip bone

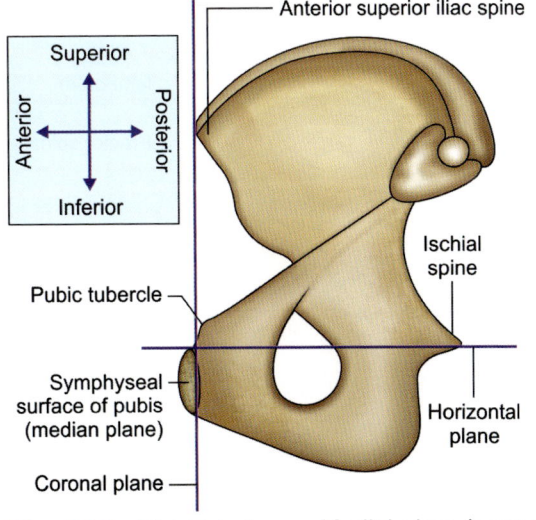

Fig. 10.2: Right hip bone: Medial view (normal anatomical position)

2. The symphyseal surface of pubis lies anteriorly in the median plane.

3. Upper border of pubic symphysis and ischial spine lie in the same horizontal plane.

FEATURES AND ATTACHMENTS
(Figs 10.3, 10.4, 10.6 and 10.7)

Hip bone is made up of three parts known as ilium, ischium and pubis.

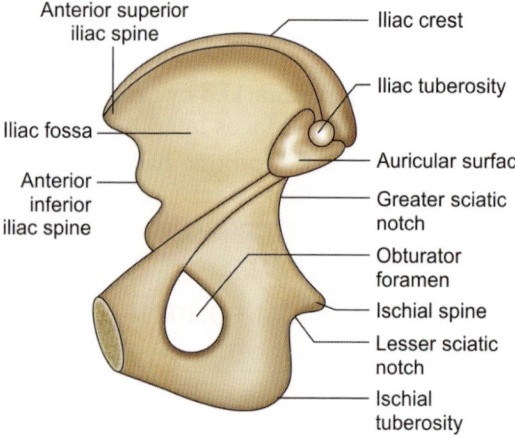

Fig. 10.3: Right hip bone: Medial aspect

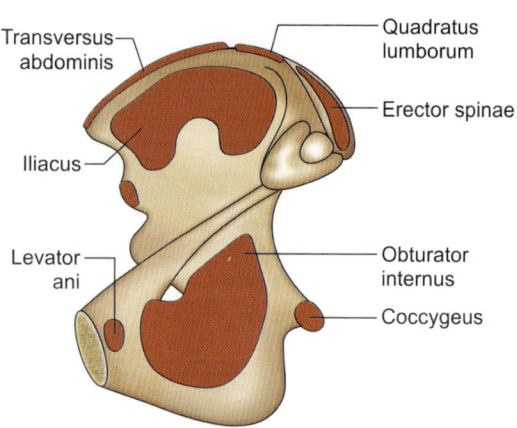

Fig. 10.4: Right hip bone: Medial aspect

I. ILIUM

It forms the upper fan shaped expanded part of the hip bone. It has 2 ends (upper and lower), 3 borders (anterior, posterior and medial) and 2 surfaces (lateral and medial).

A. Ends of ilium

a. Upper end (Fig. 10.5)

1. It is also called *iliac crest*.

2. It is convex upwards in a vertical plane.

3. In the horizontal plane, it is concave inwards anteriorly and convex inwards posteriorly.

4. *Highest point of the iliac crest* is at the level of the interval between 3rd and 4th lumbar spines.

5. *Anterior superior iliac spine* is the anterior end of iliac crest. It receives attachments of *lateral end of inguinal ligament* and *sartorius* which also arises from the upper half of notch below it.

6. *Posterior superior iliac spine* is the posterior end of iliac crest. A dimple 4 cm lateral to the second sacral spine marks the posterior superior iliac spine on the body.

7. Morphologically the iliac crest is divided into a *ventral segment* or anterior 2/3rd and a *dorsal segment* or posterior 1/3rd.

8. Ventral segment is divisible into an outer lip an intermediate area and an inner lip.

   i. *Outer lip*

      – *Tubercle of iliac crest* is situated on it 5 cm behind the anterior superior iliac spine.

      – *Fascia lata* is attached to its entire extent.

      – *Tensor fasciae latae* originates from it in front of the tubercle of iliac crest.

      – *External oblique muscle* is inserted to its anterior 2/3rd.

      – *Latissimus dorsi* originates from it just behind its highest point.

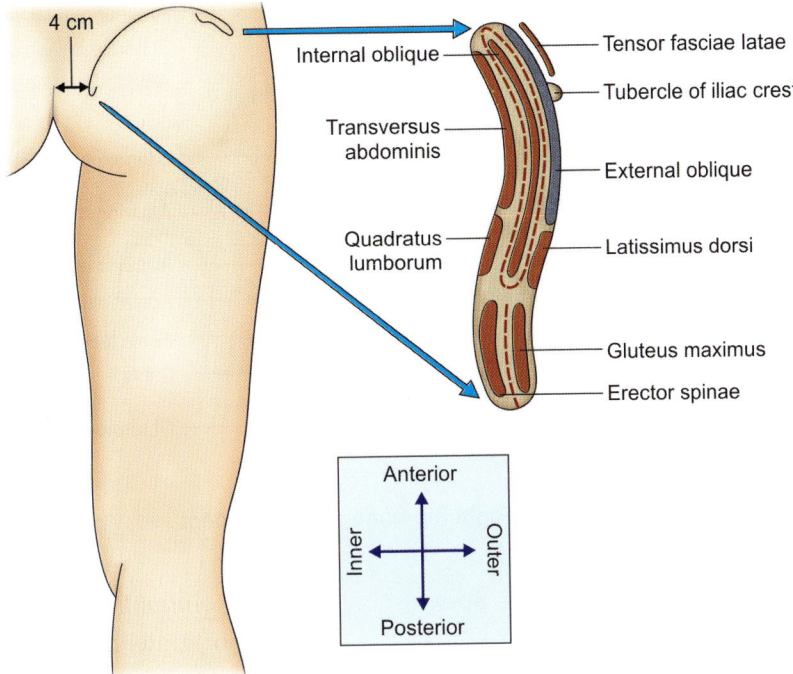

Fig. 10.5: Right iliac crest: Superior view

ii. *Intermediate area*
  – *Internal oblique muscle* arises from its whole extent.

iii. *Inner lip*
  – Its anterior 2/3rd provides attachments to *transversus abdominis, fascia transversalis* and *fascia iliaca*.
  – Its posterior 1/3rd provides attachments to *quadratus lumborum* and *thoracolumbar fascia*.

9. Dorsal segment is divisible into medial (inner) and lateral (outer) slopes.

  i. *Lateral slope: Gluteus maximus* originates from the lateral slope.

  ii. *Medial slope: Erector spinae muscle* originates from its medial slope.

  iii. *Interosseous and dorsal sacroiliac ligaments* are attached to the medial margin of the dorsal segment deep to erector spinae.

b. Lower end

Lower end of ilium reaches acetabulum and forms its upper 2/5th.

B. Borders of ilium

a. Anterior border

1. It extends from anterior superior iliac spine to acetabulum.
2. Its upper half is concave forming a notch. *Sartorius* originates from upper half of this notch.
3. Its lower half is convex and is called *anterior inferior iliac spine. Straight head of rectus femoris* originates from the upper half of this spine. *Iliofemoral ligament* is attached to the lower half of anterior inferior iliac spine.

b. Posterior border

1. It extends from the posterior superior iliac spine to the upper end of the posterior border of ischium.

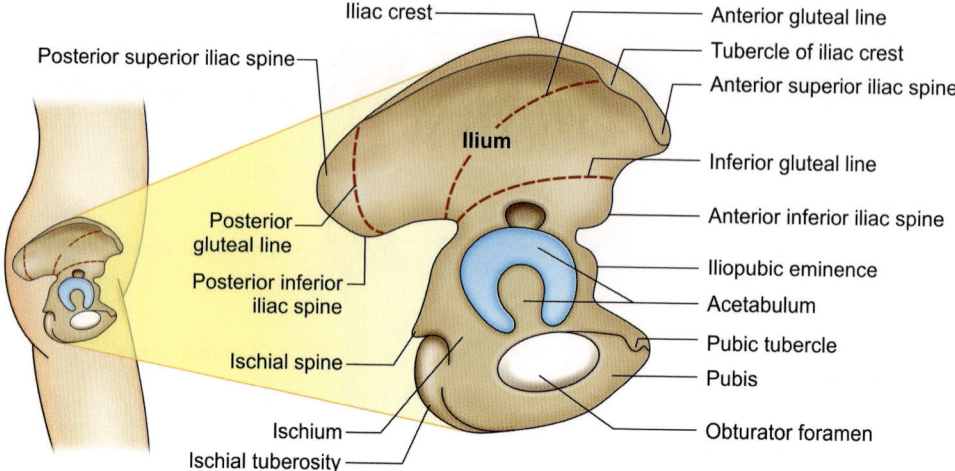

Fig. 10.6: Right hip bone: Lateral aspect

2. Its lower part contributes to the apex, upper margin and upper half of the lower margin of *greater sciatic notch*.

3. Some fibres of *piriformis* originate from upper margin of greater sciatic notch.

4. The junction of greater sciatic notch and upper part of posterior border is marked by *posterior inferior iliac spine*.

5. Posterior border between the two posterior iliac spines receives attachment of *sacrotuberous ligament*.

c. Medial border

1. It extends from the iliac crest to the iliopubic eminence on the inner surface of ilium.

2. This border intervenes between iliac fossa and sacropelvic surface of ilium.

3. Lower part of medial border forms *arcuate line* (*iliac part of linea terminalis*).

C. Surfaces of ilium

a. Gluteal surface

1. It is outer surface of ilium.

2. It is convex in front and concave behind.

3. It is divided into 4 areas by 3 gluteal lines from anterior to posterior:

i. *Inferior gluteal line*

ii. Anterior gluteal line

iii. Posterior gluteal line

Note: *It is important to note that the posterior most line is posterior gluteal line, the middle line is the anterior gluteal line and the anterior most line is inferior gluteal line.*

4. *Gluteus maximus muscle* arises from the area behind the posterior gluteal line.

5. *Gluteus medius muscle* arises from the area between anterior and posterior gluteal lines.

6. *Gluteus minimus muscle* arises from the area between anterior and inferior gluteal lines.

7. *Reflected head of rectus femoris* arises from a groove just above the acetabulum.

8. *Capsule of hip joint* is attached to the acetabular margins.

b. Medial surface

It is divided into iliac fossa and sacropelvic surface by the medial border.

i. *Iliac fossa*

1. It is situated on the inner aspect of ilium, in front of medial border.

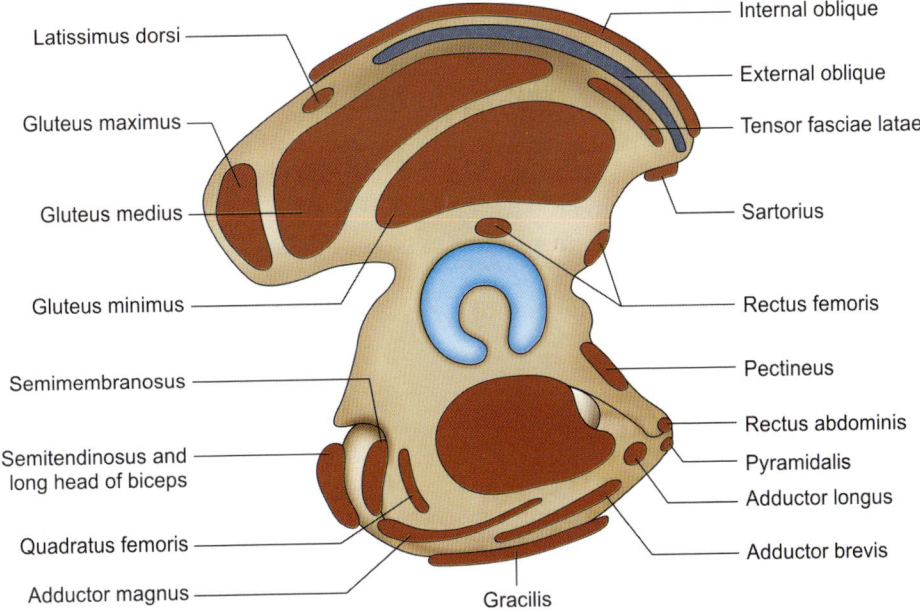

Internal oblique
External oblique
Tensor fasciae latae
Sartorius
Rectus femoris
Pectineus
Rectus abdominis
Pyramidalis
Adductor longus
Adductor brevis

Latissimus dorsi
Gluteus maximus
Gluteus medius
Gluteus minimus
Semimembranosus
Semitendinosus and long head of biceps
Quadratus femoris
Adductor magnus
Gracilis

Fig. 10.7: Right hip bone: Lateral aspect

2. It is concave in shape.
3. *Iliacus* arises from its upper 2/3rd

ii. *Sacropelvic surface*

It is situated behind the medial border, on the inner side of ilium. It has following 3 parts.

1. Iliac tuberosity
   - It is a rough area just below the dorsal segment of iliac crest.
   - *Interosseous sacroiliac ligament* is attached to the greater part of iliac tuberosity.
   - *Dorsal sacroiliac ligament* and *iliolumbar ligament* are also attached to iliac tuberosity.

2. Auricular surface
   - It is situated anteroinferior to iliac tuberosity. It is articular.
   - *Sacroiliac joint* is formed by the articulation of sacrum with the auricular surface.

3. Pelvic surface
   - It is situated anteroinferior to auricular surface.

   - Major part of this surface provides attachment to *obturator internus*.
   - A few fibres of *piriformis* also arise from it.
   - *Preauricular sulcus* is seen on this surface along the upper border of greater sciatic notch. It is deeper in females than males.

II. PUBIS

It is anteroinferior part of hip bone. It forms anterior 1/5th of acetabulum as well as anterior boundary of obturator foramen. Pubis has a body, a superior ramus and an inferior ramus.

A. Body of pubis

It is comprised of pubic crest, pubic tubercle and 3 surfaces (anterior, posterior and medial).

a. Pubic crest

1. It is superior border of body of pubis.
2. *Anterior wall of rectus sheath* and *conjoint tendon* get attached to its anterior margin.

3. *Lateral head of rectus abdominis* and *pyramidalis* arise from its lateral part.
4. Medial head of rectus abdominis is related to medial part of pubic crest.

b. Pubic tubercle

1. It is the lateral end of pubic crest.
2. It is an important land-mark in pubic region.
3. It gives attachment to the medial end of *inguinal ligament*.
4. *Spermatic cord* crosses it in males.

c. Surfaces

i. *Anterior surface*
   1. *Adductor longus* originates from the angle between pubic crest and pubic symphysis.
   2. *Gracilis* originates from its lower part and also extends over inferior ramus.
   3. *Adductor brevis* is attached to it lateral to gracilis.
   4. *Obturator externus* is attached to this surface adjacent to obturator foramen.
   5. Adjacent to pubic symphysis, it gives attachment to *ventral pubic ligament*.

ii. *Posterior surface*
   1. This is also called *pelvic surface*.
   2. It is directed upwards and backwards.
   3. It is related to *urinary bladder*.
   4. *Levator ani* and *obturator internus* originate from this surface.

iii. *Symphyseal surface*
   1. This is also called *medial surface*.
   2. Two symphyseal surfaces articulate to form secondary cartilaginous joint called *pubic symphysis*.

B. Superior ramus of pubis

It extends from body of pubis to acetabulum. It is located just above the obturator foramen. It has 3 borders (pectineal line, obturator crest and inferior border) and 3 surfaces (pectineal, pelvic and obturator).

a. Borders

i. *Pectineal line*
   1. This is also called *pecten pubis*.
   2. It extends from pubic tubercle to posterior part of iliopubic eminence.
   3. It receives attachment of *conjoint tendon* near its medial end.
   4. *Lacunar ligament* is attached to its medial end just in front of conjoint tendon.
   5. *Pectineal ligament* is attached to its whole length lateral to lacunar ligament.
   6. *Fascia covering pectineus* is attached to its whole extent.
   7. *Psoas minor muscle*, when present, is attached to pectineal line.

ii. *Obturator crest*
   1. This is also called *anterior border*.
   2. It extends from pubic tubercle to the acetabular notch.

iii. *Inferior border*
   It forms the upper border of *obturator foramen*.

b. Surfaces

i. *Pectineal surface*
   1. It is situated between obturator crest and pectineal line.
   2. It is triangular in shape.
   3. It extends from pubic tubercle to iliopubic eminence.
   4. *Pectineus* arises from the upper part of this surface.

ii. *Pelvic surface*
   1. It is between pectineal line and inferior border of superior ramus.
   2. It is continuous medially with the pelvic surface of the body of pubis.
   3. *Ductus deferens* in males and *round ligament of uterus* in females are related to this surface.

iii. *Obturator surface*
   1. It is situated between obturator crest and inferior border.
   2. *Obturator nerve and vessels* traverse the *obturator groove* seen on this surface.

C. Inferior ramus of pubis

   1. It extends from body of pubis to ramus of ischium.
   2. It joins the ramus of ischium to form conjoint *ischiopubic ramus*.
      (Attachments to inferior ramus are discussed with ischiopubic ramsus)

III. ISCHIUM

It is the posteroinferior part of hip bone. It contributes to 2/5th of acetabulum. It comprises a body and a ramus.

A. Body of ischium

It is very thick. It lies below and posterior to the acetabulum. It has 2 ends (upper and lower), 3 borders (anterior, posterior and lateral) and 3 surfaces (femoral, dorsal and pelvic).

a. Ends

   i. *Upper end*
      It forms posteroinferior 2/5th of acetabulum.
   ii. *Lower end* (Fig. 10.9)
      1. It forms *ischial tuberosity*.

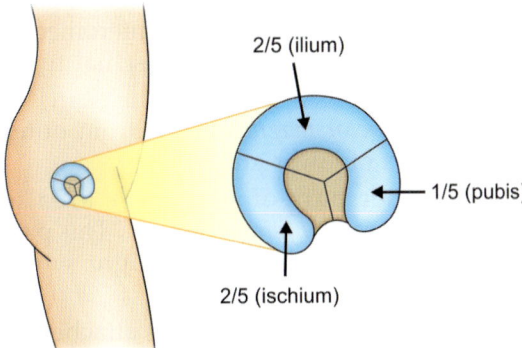

Fig. 10.8: Right acetabulum: Lateral view

   2. Inferior ramus arises from lower end.
   3. Ischial tuberosity is divided by a horizontal ridge into an upper quadrilateral and lower triangular areas.
   4. The upper area of ischial tuberosity is divided by a diagonal line into upper lateral and lower medial areas.
   5. A longitudinal ridge subdivides the lower triangular area of ischial tuberosity into outer and inner areas.
   6. *Semimembranosus* arises from the superolateral part of upper area of ischial tuberosity.

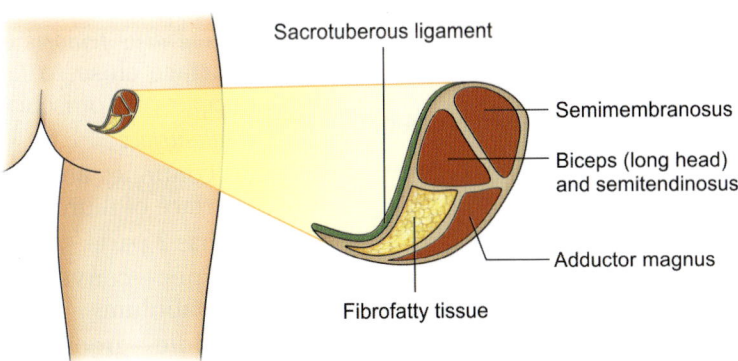

Fig. 10.9: Right ischial tuberosity: Posterior aspect

7. *Semitendinosus* and the *long head of biceps femoris* arise from inferomedial part of upper area of ischial tuberosity.

8. *Adductor magnus* arises from outer part of lower area.

9. Inner part of the lower area is covered by *fibrofatty tissue*. This part supports the body weight while sitting.

10. *Sacrotuberous ligament* is attached to the medial margin of ischial tuberosity.

b. Borders

i. *Anterior border*

It forms posterior part of *obturator foramen*.

ii. *Posterior border*

1. It is continuous with the posterior border of ilium.

2. It ends below at the upper end of ischial tuberosity.

3. It presents a spine called *ischial spine*. *Sacrospinous ligament* is attached to the margins of ischial spine. *Coccygeus and levator ani* also arise from this spine.

4. Ischial spine forms lower boundary of *greater sciatic notch*.

5. Below the ischial spine is *lesser sciatic notch*.

6. Both greater and lesser sciatic notches are converted into foramina by sacrotuberous and sacrospinous ligaments.

7. Structures passing through greater sciatic foramen are:

   – *Piriformis*

   – Superior and inferior gluteal nerves and vessels

   – Nerve to obturator internus

   – Pudendal nerve

   – Internal pudendal vessels

   – Sciatic nerve

   – Posterior cutaneous nerve of thigh

   – Nerve to quadratus femoris

8. Structures related to lesser sciatic foramen are:

   – *Tendon of obturator internus* passes through it.

   – *Superior and inferior gemelli* arise from corresponding margins.

   – *Nerve to obturator internus* enters through it to supply obturator internus.

   – *Pudendal nerve* and *internal pudendal vessels* enter the perineum by passing through it.

Note: *To remember structures passing through lesser sciatic foramen you can remember, Never Tell Indian Police,*

N—Nerve to obturator internus

T—Tendon of obturator internus

I—Internal pudendal vessels

P—Pudendal nerve

iii. *Lateral border*

It continues with lateral border of ischial tuberosity.

c. Surfaces

i. *Femoral surface*

1. It is situated between anterior and lateral borders.

2. *Obturator externus* orginates from this surface along the obturator foramen.

3. *Quadratus femoris* arises from this surface close to lateral border of upper part of ischial tuberosity.

ii. *Dorsal surface*

1. It continues above with the gluteal surface of ilium.

2. It has 3 parts:

   Upper—convex area adjacent to acetabulum

   Middle—grooved area

   Lower—upper part of ischial tuberosity

3. *Piriformis, sciatic nerve* and *nerve to quadratus femoris* are related to upper convex area.

4. *Obturator internus tendon* along with *two gemelli* traverses the middle grooved area.

5. *Semitendinosus, long head of biceps* and *semimembranosus* arise from the lower part of dorsal surface.

iii. *Pelvic surface*

1. It is between anterior and posterior borders.

2. *Obturator internus* arises from the greater part of pelvic surface.

B. Ramus of ischium

It arises from the lower part of body and runs forwards, upwards and medially. It meets with the inferior pubic ramus to form ischiopubic ramus.

IV. ISCHIOPUBIC RAMUS

It has 2 borders (upper and lower) and 2 surfaces (outer and inner).

A. Borders

a. Upper border

1. It forms lower margin of *obturator foramen*.

2. *Obturator membrane* is attached to it.

b. Lower border

1. It is everted. This feature is more marked in males than females.

2. *Fascia lata* and *membranous layer of superficial fascia (Colles' fascia)* are attached to it.

B. Surfaces

a. Outer surface

1. It is concave

2. Following muscles are attached to it from above downwards:

    i. *Obturator externus*

ii. Adductor magnus

iii. Gracilis

b. Inner surface (Fig. 10.10)

It is convex. It has 2 ridges (upper and lower) and 3 areas (upper, middle and lower) which are meant for following structures:

1. Upper ridge receives attachments of *obturator fascia* and *superior fascia of urogenital diaphragm.*

2. Lower ridge provides attachments to *perineal membrane* and *falciform process of sacrotuberous ligament.*

3. Upper area is meant for attachment of *obturator internus.*

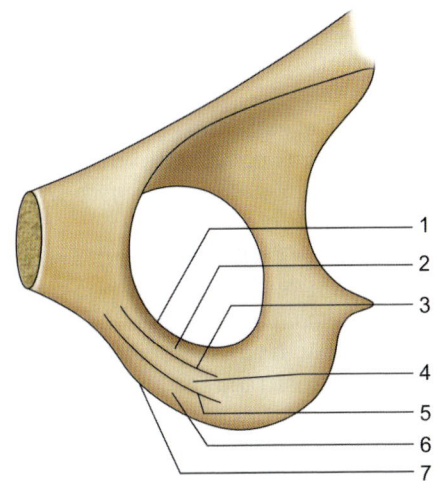

1. Upper border (obturator membrane)
2. Upper area (obturator internus)
3. Upper ridge (obturator fascia and superior fascia of urogenital diaphragm)
4. Middle area (sphincter urethrae and deep transversus perinei)
5. Lower ridge (perineal membrane and falciform process of sacrotuberous ligament)
6. Lower area (crus penis, ischiocavernosus and superficial transversus perinei)
7. Lower border (Colles' fascia and fascia lata)

Fig. 10.10: Inschiopubic ramus of right hip. Inner aspect

4. Middle area receives attachments of *sphincter urethrae* and *deep transversus perinei* muscles.
5. Lower area provides attachments to *crus penis, ischiocavernosus* and *superficial transversus perinei.*

V. ACETABULUM (Fig. 10.8)

1. Literal meaning of acetabulum is vinegar cup.
2. It is a cup shaped deep concavity facing laterally and anteroinferiorly.
3. All the three parts of hip bone contribute to it as follows:
   Pubis—its anterior 1/5th
   Ischium—little more than its posterior 2/5th
   Ilium—little less than its superior 2/5th.
4. Its margin is deficient inferiorly to form *acetabular notch. Transverse acetabular ligament* bridges this gap to form *acetabular foramen.*
5. Margin of acetabulum provides attachment to *labrum acetabulare* which bridges the acetabular notch as *transverse acetabular ligament.*
6. It has a horseshoe shaped articular surface (*lunate surface*) and nonarticular central *acetabular fossa.* Lunate surface is covered by hyaline cartilage while acetabular fossa lodges a pad of fat.

VI. OBTURATOR FORAMEN

1. It is the gap in the lower part of hip bone.
2. It is situated between pubis and ischium.
3. *Obturator membrane* is attached to its margins. The membrane bridges the *obturator groove* to convert it into *obturator canal* which transmits *obturator nerve and vessels.*

OSSIFICATION

A. Primary centres

3 primary centres appear:

1 for ilium—appears during 2nd month of intrauterine life.

1 for ischium—appears during 3rd month of intrauterine life.

1 for pubis—appears during 4th month of intrauterine life.

The ramus of ischium and inferior ramus of pubis fuse during 7th year.

At birth most of the bone is ossified except for 3 cartilaginous parts which are:
   a. Whole of iliac crest.
   b. 'Y' shaped cartilage of acetabulum.
   c. A strip along inferior margin of hip bone.

B. Secondary centres

There are 5 secondary centres:
   2 for iliac crest
   2 for 'Y' shaped acetabular cartilage
   1 for ischial tuberosity

Appearance: Puberty

Fusion

1. Ossification of acetabulum is completed by 17 years.
2. Ossification of rest of the bone is completed by 20–25 years.

SEXUAL DIMORPHISM

Sexual dimorphism in hip bone is given in Table 10.1.

Table 10.1: Sexual dimorphism in hip bone

Features	Female	Male
1. Greater sciatic notch	Wider (90º)	Narrower (<90º)
2. Ischial spine	Not inverted	Inverted
3. Ischiopubic ramus	Not everted	Everted
4. Obturator foramen	Triangular	Oval
5. Acetabular diameter	Less than 5cm	More than 5cm.
6. Distance between pubic tubercle and acetabular margin.	Greater than acetabular diameter.	Equal or less than acetabular diameter.

Bony Pelvis

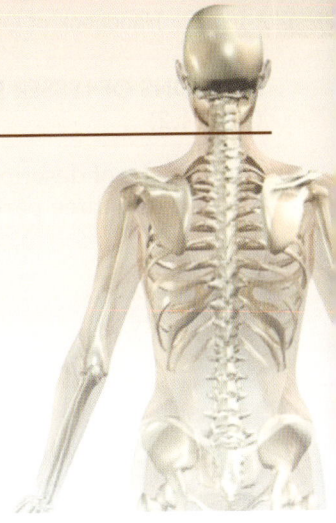

TERMINOLOGY

Pelvis is a Latin word which means 'a basin'. Following are the similarities between the pelvis and basin (Fig. 11.1).

1. Back or posterior wall is wide
2. Front or anterior wall is narrow
3. Walls are sloping
4. Inlet is above
5. Outlet is below

PELVIC GIRDLE

It is a bony ring below the fifth lumbar vertebra and between femoral heads. Four bones participate in the formation of pelvic girdle. These are two hip bones, one sacrum and one coccyx.

These four bones articulate with each other to form two synovial (sacroiliac) and two symphyseal (pubic and sacrococcygeal) joints.

DIVISIONS OF PELVIS

The plane of pelvic inlet divides the bony pelvis into two parts:

I. Part above the pelvic inlet is called pelvis major or greater pelvis or false pelvis.
II. Part below the pelvic inlet is called pelvis minor or lesser pelvis or true pelvis or obstetric pelvis.

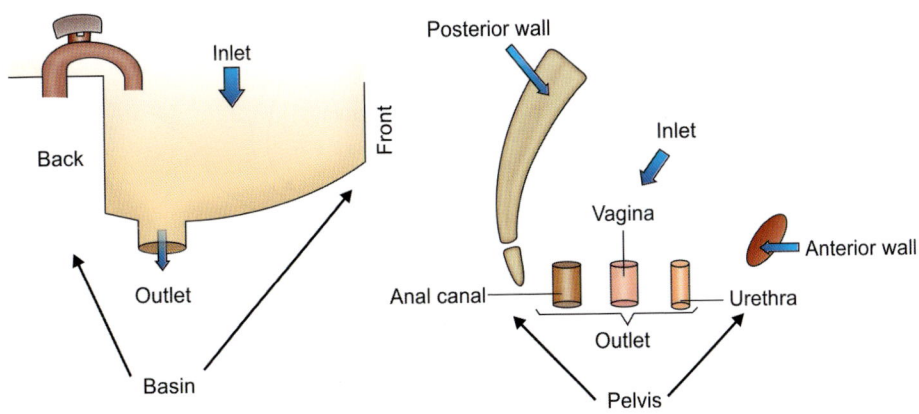

Fig. 11.1: Comparing pelvis with basin

DIVISIONS OF LESSER PELVIS (Fig. 11.2)

For the sake of description the lesser pelvis is divided into three parts:

   I. Inlet

  II. Outlet

 III. Cavity

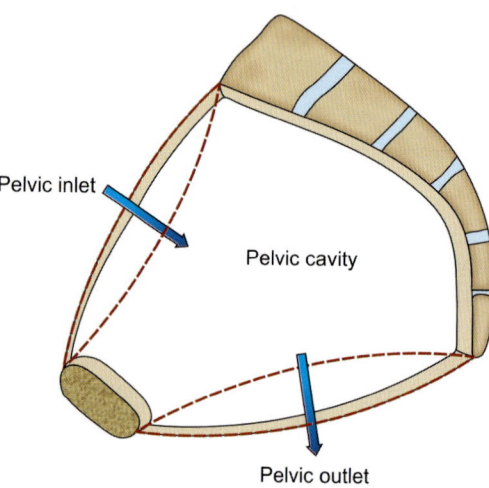

Fig. 11.2: Subdivisions of lesser pelvis

ANATOMICAL POSITION

1. Pubic symphysis lies in midsagittal plane.
2. Anterior superior iliac spines and pubic tubercles lie in the same coronal plane.

BOUNDARIES OF PELVIC INLET (Fig. 11.3)

I. Bony contributions (pelvic brim)

   A. Sacral contributions

     a. Sacral promontory

     b. Ala of sacrum

   B. Contributions by hip bone (*linea terminalis*)

     a. Iliac part: *Arcuate line*

     b. Pubic part: (i) *Pecten pubis*; (ii) *Pubic crest*

> **Note:** *Pelvic brim and pelvic inlet are synonyms for obstetricians.*

II. Articular contributions

   A. Anteriorly in the midline: *Pubic symphysis*

   B. Posterolateral: *Sacroiliac joints*

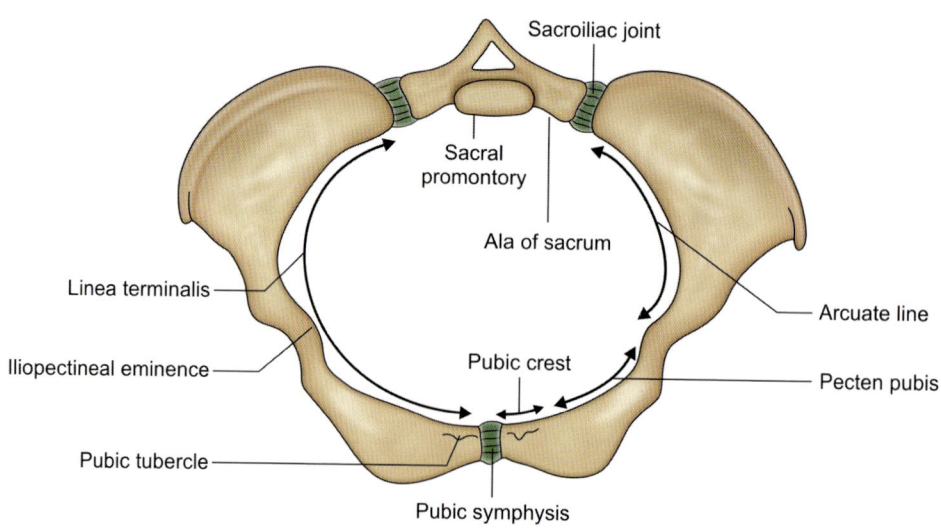

Fig. 11.3: Boundaries of pelvic inlet

BOUNDARIES OF PELVIC OUTLET (Fig. 11.4)

Anteriorly   – *Lower border of pubic symphysis*

Posteriorly   – *Tip of coccyx*

On each side – *Half of the pubic arch*

                – *Ischiopubic ramus*

                – *Ischial tuberosity*

                – *Sacrotuberous ligament*

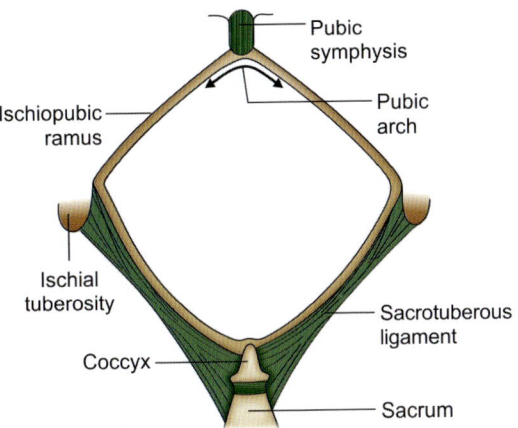

Fig. 11.4: Boundaries of pelvic outlet

Note: *Obstetricians ignore coccyx due to its mobility. Therefore 'obstetrical outlet' is bounded posteriorly by tip of sacrum. Tip of coccyx forms the posterior boundary of 'anatomical outlet'.*

BOUNDARIES OF PELVIC CAVITY (Fig. 11.5)

Anteriorly: Pelvic surfaces of

                - *Pubic symphysis*

                - *Body of pubis*

                - *Pubic rami*

Posteriorly: Pelvic surfaces of

                - *Sacrum*

                - *Coccyx*

Laterally: Pelvic surfaces of - *Ilium*

                - *Ischium*

Note: *To simplify the boundaries, one can remember that pelvic cavity is bounded by pelvic surfaces of all the three components of hip bone i.e. ilium, pubis and ischium and pelvic surfaces of sacrum and coccyx.*

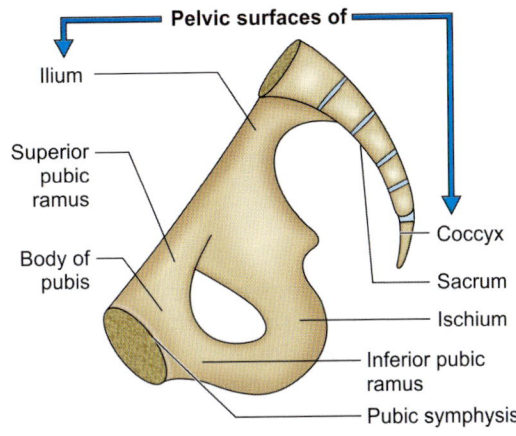

Fig. 11.5: Boundaries of pelvic cavity

PUBIC ARCH AND SUBPUBIC ANGLE (Fig. 11.6)

The inferior margins of pubic symphysis and adjacent inferior pubic rami together form pubic arch. Angulation between margins of pubic arch is called subpubic angle. In gynecoid pelvis the subpubic angle is more than 90° and is called Norman type. In android pelvis this angle is acute, i.e. less than 90° and is also called Gothic type.

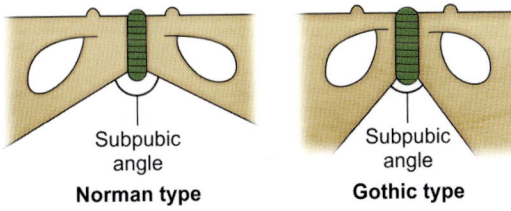

Fig. 11.6: Pubic arch and subpubic angle

FUNCTIONS OF PELVIS

1. Locomotion.
2. Weight transmission.

3. Provides areas for the attachments of muscles.

4. Protection of pelvic viscera.

5. Plays important role in parturition (birth of baby).

AXES OF PELVIS (Fig. 11.7)

I. Axis of inlet

It is perpendicular to the plane of pelvic inlet and passes through its centre. On projection it passes through umbilicus and middle of coccyx.

II. Axis of outlet

It passes through centre of anteroposterior axis of outlet. It is also perpendicular to this axis and is directed downwards and slightly backwards. When projected upwards, it reaches the sacral promontory.

III. Axis of pelvic cavity

It is a curved line following the curvature of pelvic surfaces of sacrum and coccyx. It is perpendicular to innumerable planes of pelvis between planes of inlet and outlet.

PELVIC SEGMENTS (Fig. 11.8)

The widest transverse diameter divides the pelvic brim into anterior segment (forepelvis) and posterior segment (hindpelvis). The hindpelvis is important clinically because of being more variable in shape and capacity.

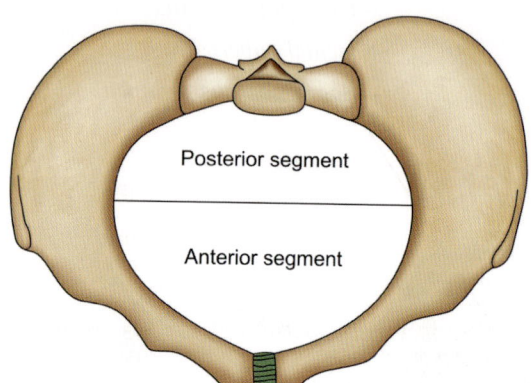

Fig. 11.8: Pelvic segments

POSTERIOR SAGITTAL DIAMETER OF KLEIN (Fig. 11.9)

It extends from middle of bituberous diameter to the tip of sacrum. The diameter is of clinical significance. In cases of android pelvic, the foetal head is pushed backwards. If the said diameter is inadequate, there will be difficulty in delivery.

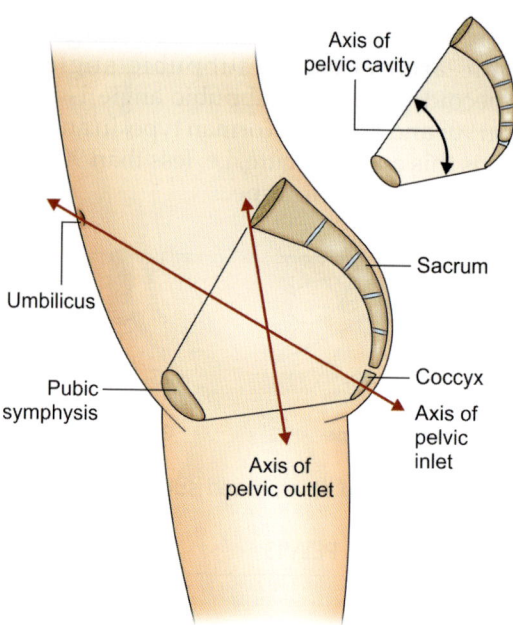

Fig. 11.7: Axes of pelvis

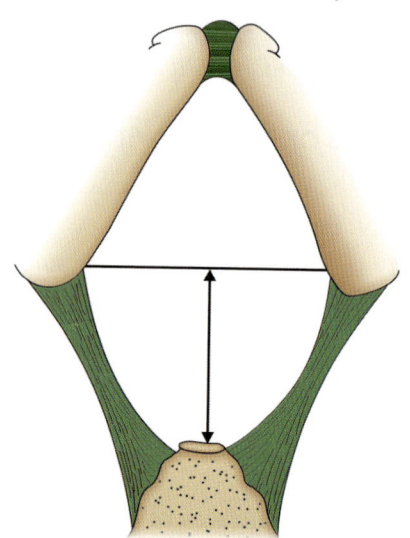

Fig. 11.9: Posterior sagittal diameter of Klein

PELVIC INCLINATION (Fig. 11.10)

The plane of pelvic inlet forms an angle of 55° with the horizontal plane. The plane of pelvic outlet forms an angle of approximately 15° with the same.

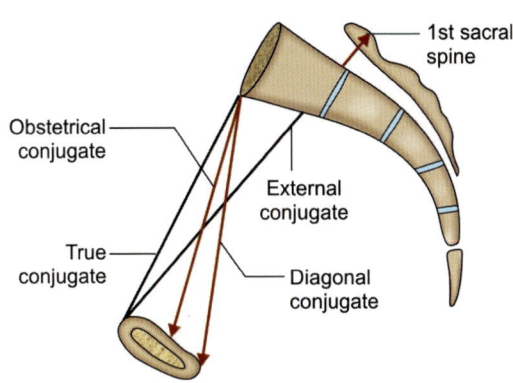

Fig. 11.11: Conjugate diameters

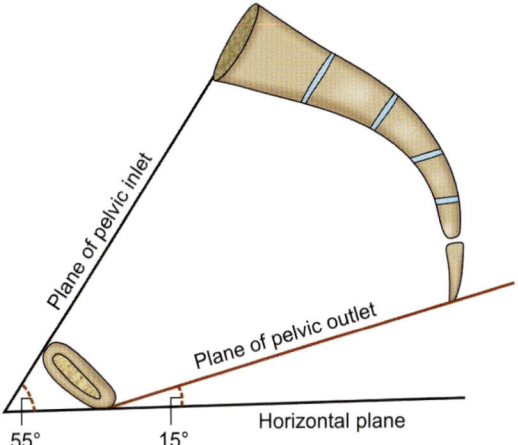

Fig. 11.10: Pelvic inclination

PLANES OF PELVIC DIMENSIONS

I. Plane of greatest pelvic dimensions

It is an imaginary plane passing through middle of pubic symphysis and junction of 2nd and 3rd sacral vertebrae.

II. Plane of least pelvic dimensions or narrow pelvic plane

It is an imaginary plane passing through the lower border of pubic symphysis, the ischial spines and the tip of sacrum.

CONJUGATE DIAMETERS (Fig. 11.11)

I. External conjugate

It is the distance between upper border of pubic symphysis and tip of 1st sacral spine.

II. True conjugate

This is also called anteroposterior diameter of inlet. It is the distance between middle of sacral promontory and superior border of pubic symphysis.

III. Diagonal conjugate

It is the distance between middle of sacral promontory and inferior border of pubic symphysis. It is important clinically because it is an indirect assessment of anteroposterior diameter of pelvic inlet and can be roughly measured by per vaginal (P/V) examination.

IV. Obstetrical conjugate

It is the shortest distance between the pelvic surface of pubic symphysis and sacral promontory.

LEAST DIAMETER OF PELVIS

It is the distance between two ischial spines.

TYPES OF PELVIS (Fig. 11.12)

Four types of female pelvis have been described.

I. Gynaecoid/gynecoid type

1. It is typical female pelvis.
2. It is observed in 42% females.
3. It is spacious and roomy and, therefore, suitable for easy passage of baby during delivery.

II. Android type

1. It is typical male type of pelvis found in females.
2. It is observed in 32% females.
3. Its inlet is heart shaped.
4. It may result into obstructed labour.

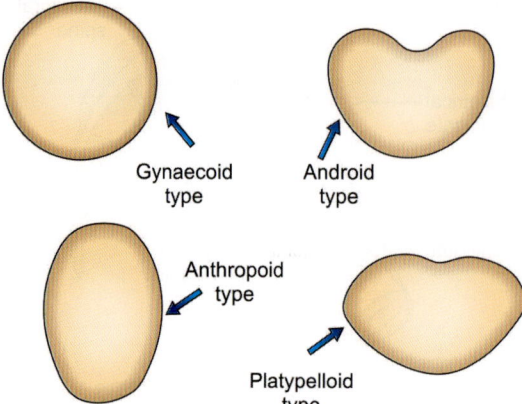

Fig. 11.12: Shapes of inlets in four types of female bony pelvis

III. Anthropoid type

1. Its inlet is compressed from sides.
2. It is found in 23% females.
3. Such pelvis will obstruct the smooth delivery of foetus.

IV. Platypelloid type

1. Its inlet is anteroposteriorly compressed.
2. It is rare type of pelvis observed in 2% females only.
3. This type of pelvis also poses difficulty in delivery.

DIAMETERS OF PELVIS
(Figs 11.13 and 11.14)

Three diameters, i.e. anteroposterior, oblique and transverse (Table 11.1), are considered at each of the three levels, i.e. inlet, cavity and outlet. The details are as follows:

I. Inlet of pelvis

A. Anteroposterior diameter

It extends from middle of sacral promontory to upper margin of pubic symphysis.

B. Oblique diameter

It extends from upper end of sacroiliac joint of one side to iliopectineal eminence of the opposite side.

C. Transverse diameter

It is the greatest width of inlet, i.e. maximum transverse diameter.

II. Cavity of pelvis

A. Anteroposterior diameter

It extends from middle of pubic symphysis to middle of body of 3rd sacral vertebra.

B. Oblique diameter

It is the distance between the lower end of sacroiliac joint of one side to the middle of obturator membrane of opposite side.

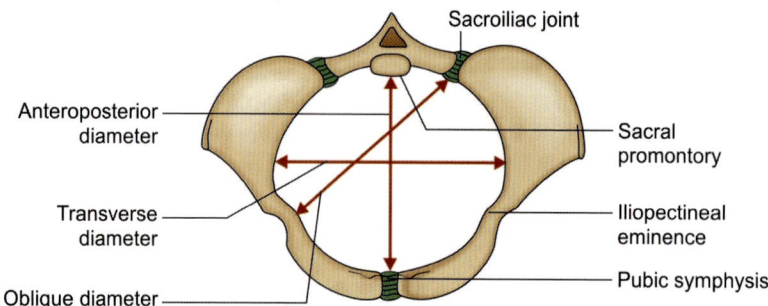

Fig. 11.13: Diameters of inlet of pelvis

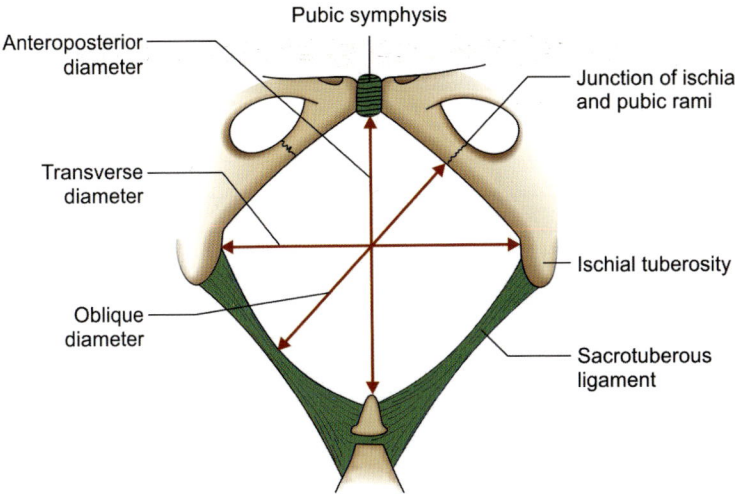

Fig. 11.14: Diameters of outlet of pelvis

C. Transverse diameter

It is the greatest width of the cavity.

III. Outlet of pelvis

A. Anteroposterior diameter

It extends between tip of coccyx to the lower border of pubic symphsysis.

B. Oblique diameter

It is the distance between the middle of sacro-tuberous ligament of one side and junction of ischial and pubic rami of opposite side.

C. Transverse diameter

It is the distance between inner margins of two ischial tuberosities.

Table. 11.1: Approximate measurements (cm) of different pelvic diameters

Diameters	Inlet	Cavity	Outlet
Anteroposterior diameter	11	12	13
Oblique diameter	12	12	12
Transverse diameter	13	12	11

SEX DIFFERENCES IN ADULT PELVIS

For details given in Table 11.2

Table. 11.2: Sex differences in adult pelvis

Features	Male	Female
1. General structure	Thick and heavy	Thin and light
2. Markings for muscular attachments	Very prominent	Less prominent
3. False pelvis	Deep	Shallow
4. Pelvic inlet	Heart shaped	Circular or oval
5. Sacral promontory	More prominent	More flat
6. Pubic tubercles	Closer	Wider apart
7. Cavity	Narrower and deeper	Wider and shallower
8. Sacrum evenly curved	Narrower, longer and sharply forwards in its lower part	Wider, shorter and bends

Contd.

Table. 11.2: Sex differences in adult pelvis (Contd.)

Features	Male	Female
9. Sciatic notch	Narrower	Wider
10. Ischial spine	Projected inwards	Projected outwards
11. Ischial tuberosity	Inverted	Everted
12. Subpupic angle	More acute (angle, <90º)	Wider (angle, 90º or >90º)
13. Ischiopubic rami	More everted	Less everted
14. Obturator foramen	Oval	Triangular
15. Preauricular sulcus	Less prominent	More prominent
16. At the sacral base, ratio between transverse width of facet for 5th lumbar vertebra and that of entire base	1 or <1:2	>1 : 2
17. Acetabulum	Larger	Smaller
18. If the distance between anterior rim of acetabulum and pubic symphysis is '1', then the diameter of acetabulum is	1	> 1
19. Sacral index, i.e. Breadth of sacrum × 100/ Length of sacrum	Lesser	Greater
20. Pelvic outlet	Comparatively smaller	Comparatively larger

Femur

TERMINOLOGY

Femur is a Latin word means thigh. It is named so because it belongs to thigh.

PECULIARITIES

1. Femur is the strongest and longest bone of the body.
2. Femur constitutes more than one-quarter of the height of the individual.

SIDE DETERMINATION

1. Femur is a vertical bone.
2. Rounded head is located at the upper end.
3. Head is directed medially.
4. Convexity of shaft is directed forwards.

ANATOMICAL POSITION
(Figs 12.1 and 12.2)

1. Keep the bone vertically in such a way so that head faces upwards, medially and slightly forwards.

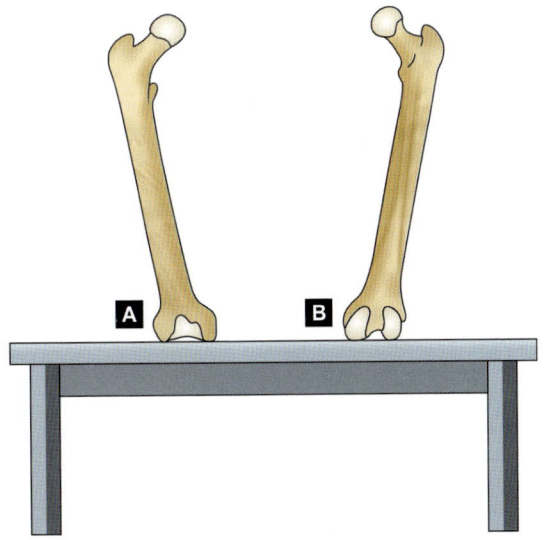

Fig. 12.1: Right femur held vertically on a table. (A) Front view; (B) Posterior view

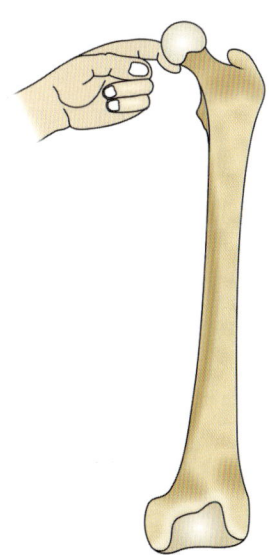

Fig. 12.2: Balancing the femur with index finger

FEATURES AND ATTACHMENTS
(Figs 12.4 and 12.6 to 12.8)

Note: *Remember the femur helps the body in pushing forwards, i.e. propulsion, therefore, the head is directed forwards.*

2. The long axis of shaft is directed downwards and medially.

Note: *To achieve this keep the lower end of femur on a table in such a way that the inferior surfaces of both the condyles touch the table. This can also be achieved by balancing the neck on your index finger.*

ANGLE OF FEMORAL TORSION
(Fig. 12.3)

The vertical plane passing through the long axis of head and neck does not lie in coronal plane due to forward bending of head and neck in normal anatomical position. The long axis of the lower end of femur runs transversely in coronal plane. The angle between aforementioned planes at the two ends of femur is called torsion of femur. It is approximately 15°.

Femur has an upper end, a shaft and a lower end.

I. UPPER END

It includes head, neck, greater trochanter and lesser trochanter. The junction of neck with the shaft is marked anteriorly by intertrochanteric line and posteriorly by intertrochanteric crest.

A. Head

1. It forms more than half of a sphere.
2. It articulates with hip bone at acetabulum to form *hip joint*.
3. *Fovea capitis* is a roughened pit just below and behind the centre of head. *Ligament of head of femur (ligamentum teres)* is attached to fovea and carries acetabular

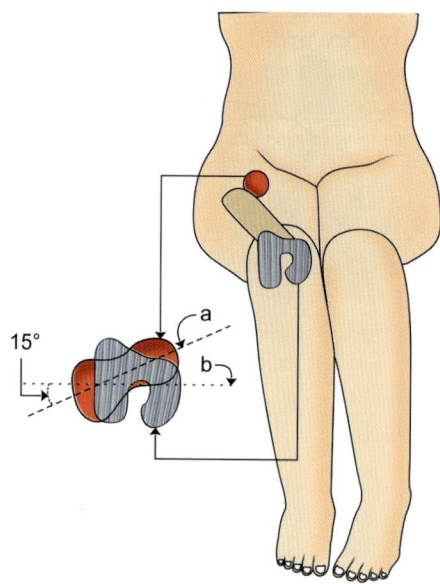

Fig. 12.3: Torsion of femur: (a) Long axis of upper end, (b) long axis of lower end

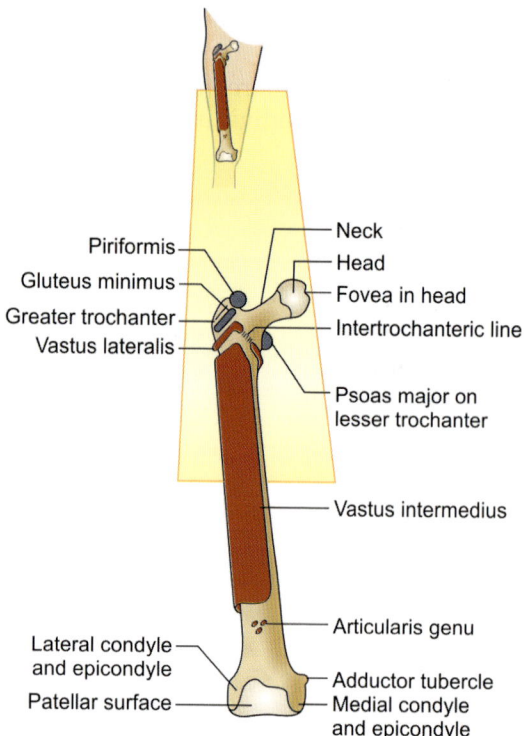

Piriformis
Gluteus minimus
Greater trochanter
Vastus lateralis

Neck
Head
Fovea in head
Intertrochanteric line

Psoas major on lesser trochanter

Vastus intermedius

Lateral condyle and epicondyle
Patellar surface

Articularis genu

Adductor tubercle
Medial condyle and epicondyle

Fig. 12.4: Right femur: Anterior aspect

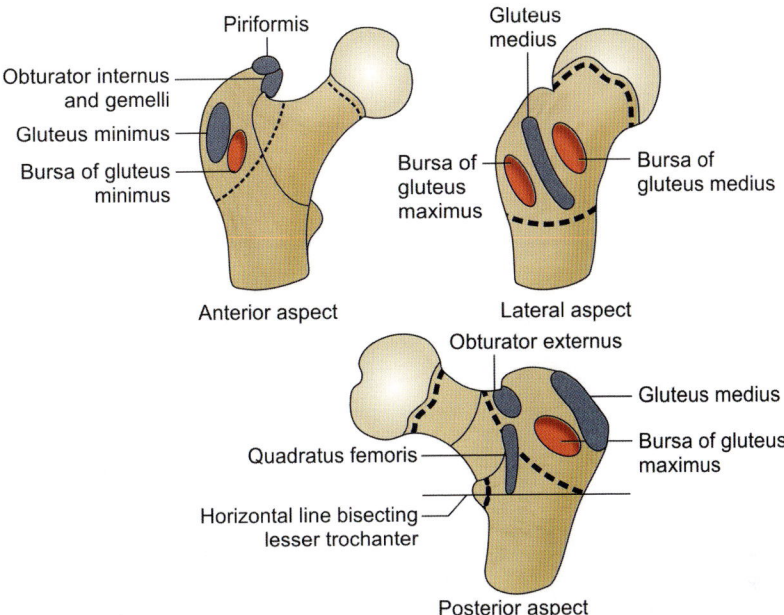

Fig. 12.5: Relations and attachments of greater trochanter of right side. Continuous lines, capsular attachments; Dotted lines, epiphyseal lines

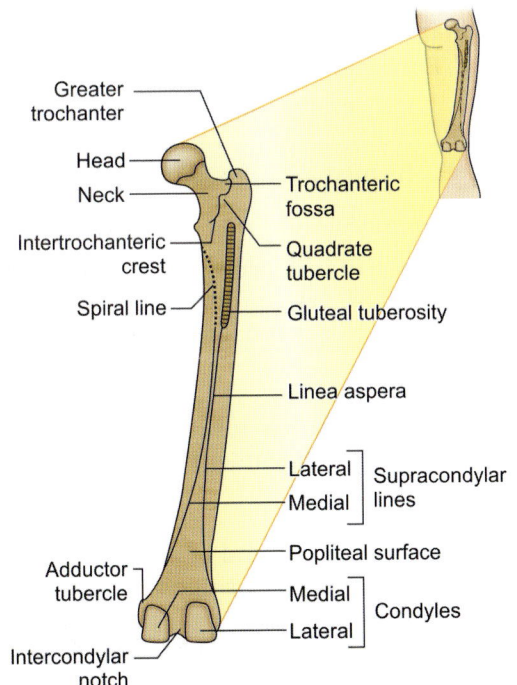

Fig. 12.6: Right femur: Posterior aspect

branches of obturator and medial circumflex femoral arteries.

B. Neck

1. It connects head with shaft.
2. It is 5 cm long.
3. Neck-shaft angle is the angle between lower border of neck and medial border of shaft. It is about 125° in adult male. It is less in female and short femora.
4. Neck has two borders (upper and lower) and two surfaces (anterior and posterior).

   a. Upper border

   It meets the shaft near greater trochanter.

   b. Lower border

   It meets the shaft near lesser trochanter.

   c. Anterior surface

   1. It is completely intracapsular.
   2. It meets the shaft at intertrochanteric line.
   3. *Cervical fossa of Allen*

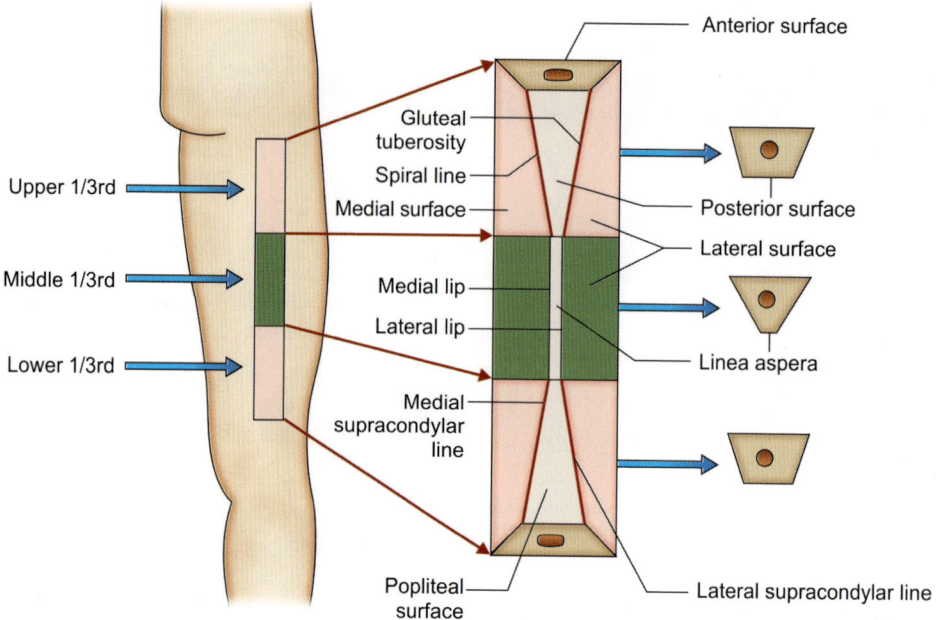

Fig. 12.7: General features of right femoral shaft: Posterior aspect

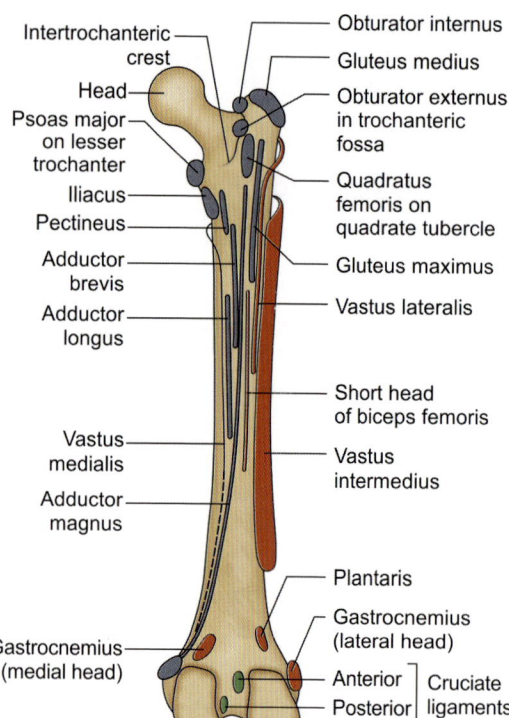

Fig. 12.8: Right femur: Posterior aspect

It is a small depression on the anterior surface of femoral neck near articular margin.

d. Posterior surface

1. It meets the shaft at intertrochanteric crest.
2. Its medial half is intracapsular.

C. Greater trochanter (Fig. 12.5)

Lateral aspect of femur continues up as greater trochanter. It has one border (upper) and three surfaces (anterior, medial and lateral).

a. Upper border

Its posterior part is inturned called *apex*. Apex receives attachment of *piriformis*.

b. Anterior surface

It is divided into lateral and medial areas.
  i. Lateral area has a ridge for attachment of *gluteus minimus*.
  ii. Medial area is related to a bursa under cover of gluteus minimus called *trochanteric bursa* of *gluteus minimus*.

c. Medial surface

It is divided into lower and upper parts.

i. Lower part is marked by a depression (*trochanteric fossa*) for *obturator externus.*

ii. Upper part is marked by an impression for insertion of *obturator internus, superior gemellus* and *inferior gemellus.*

Note: *Remember people of international fame need GUARDS for protection, i.e. INTER or Obturator Internus is accompanied by G or Gemelli. Also remember that trochanteric fossa is like guest house and it is the external examiner, i.e. Obturator Externus, who is kept inside the guest house.*

d. Lateral surface

It has a ridge, which runs downwards and forwards and two areas in relation to it.

i. *Ridge*

This is meant for the attachment of *gluteus medius.*

ii. *Area anterior to ridge*

It is covered by gluteus medius. A bursa between this muscle and area is called *trochanteric bursa of gluteus medius.*

iii. *Area posterior to ridge*

This is related to another bursa. Since this area is covered by gluteus maximus, the bursa is named as *bursa of gluteus maximus.*

D. Lesser trochanter

1. It is a conical projection directed medially.

2. It has an apex for the attachment of *psoas major.*

3. *Iliacus* is attached to its front.

Note: *Because of close association of iliacus and psoas major the two are considered together as iliopsoas getting attached to lesser trochanter.*

4. Its posterior surface is separated from upper horizontal fibres of *adductor magnus* by a *bursa.*

E. Intertrochanteric line

1. It marks the junction of neck and shaft anteriorly.

2. It continues downwards below the lesser trochanter and on the posterior aspect of femur as *spiral line.*

3. Following structures are attached to it:
   i. *Capsule of hip joint.*
   ii. *Iliofemoral ligament*
   iii. *Vastus lateralis* to its upper end
   iv. *Vastus medialis* to its lower end

F. Intertrochanteric crest

1. It marks the junction of neck with the shaft posteriorly.

2. It connects greater trochanter with the lesser trochanter.

3. *Quadrate tubercle*

It is a rounded tubercle above the middle of this crest. *Quadratus femoris* is attached to this tubercle and further downwards up to a line which bisects the lesser trochanter.

II. SHAFT

It is cylindrical in shape, convex forwards and narrowest in the middle.

A. General features of shaft

For describing borders and surfaces, the shaft is divided into upper 3rd, middle 3rd and lower 3rd.

a. Middle 1/3rd of shaft

It has 3 borders and 3 surfaces.

i. *Borders*
   1. *Medial border*
   2. *Lateral border*
   3. *Posterior border*

It is most prominent. It is also called *linea aspera.* It has distinct medial and lateral lips.

ii. *Surfaces*
   1. *Anterior surface*
   2. *Medial surface*
   3. *Lateral surface*

b. Upper 1/3rd of shaft

Medial lip of linea aspera continues upwards as *spiral line*. The lateral lip of linea aspera continues upwards as *gluteal tuberosity*. *Spiral line* and *gluteal tuberosity* diverge from each other to enclose a triangular posterior surface. Upper 1/3rd of shaft therefore has got four borders and four surfaces.

i. Borders

1. *Medial border*
2. *Lateral border*
3. *Spiral line*
4. *Gluteal tuberosity*

It is a broad rough ridge along the lateral limit of posterior surface. Some time there is a linear elevation along the gluteal tuberosity called *crista glutei*. If a conical projection is present in the gluteal tuberosity, it is called *third trochanter*. Third trochanter is present in 20% of Indian femora and is twice more common in females.

ii. Surfaces

1. *Anterior surface*
2. *Medial surface*
3. *Lateral surface*
4. *Posterior surface*.

c. Lower 1/3rd of shaft

Medial lip of linea aspera continues downwards as *medial supracondylar line*. Lateral lip of linea aspera continues downwards as *lateral supracondylar line*. Medial and lateral supracondylar lines diverge from each other to enclose an additional triangular surface called *popliteal surface*. Lower 1/3rd of shaft, therefore, has got four borders and four surfaces.

i. Borders

1. *Medial border*
2. *Lateral border*
3. *Medial supracondylar line*
4. *Lateral supracondylar line*

ii. Surfaces

1. *Anterior surface*
2. *Medial surface*
3. *Lateral surface*
4. *Popliteal surface*

Note: *Remember that the intertrochanteric line, spiral line, medial lip of linea aspera and medial supracondylar line form a continuous line from above downwards. Similarly the gluteal tuberosity, lateral lip of linea aspera and lateral supracondylar line form another continuous line.*

B. Attachments to the shaft

Shaft of femur receives attachments of muscle and intermuscular septa.

a. Attachments of muscles

i. *Gastrocnemius*

Medial head arises from popliteal surface just above the medial condyle. Lateral head arises mainly from the upper part of lateral surface of lateral condyle but also extends over the lower end of lateral supracondylar line.

ii. *Plantaris*

It originates from the lower end of lateral supracondylar line just above the lateral head of gastrocnemius.

iii. *Vastus intermedius*

It arises from the upper 3/4th of anterior and lateral surfaces.

iv. *Articularis genu*

It arises from lower 1/4th of anterior surface.

v. *Vastus lateralis*

It arises from:

1. Upper part of intertrochanteric line
2. Anterior and inferior borders of greater trochanter
3. Lateral lip of gluteal tuberosity
4. Upper half of lateral lip of linea aspera

vi. *Vastus medialis*

It arises from:

1. Lower part of intertrochanteric line
2. Spiral line
3. Medial lip of linea aspera
4. Upper 1/4th of medial supra-condylar line

vii. *Gluteus maximus*

Deeper part of its lower half is inserted into the gluteal tuberosity.

viii. *Adductor longus*

It is inserted into the medial lip of linea aspera.

ix. *Pectineus*

It is inserted into a line extending from lesser trochanter to upper end of linea aspera.

x. *Adductor brevis*

It is inserted into a line extending from the area lateral to lower part of pectineus to middle of linea aspera.

xi. *Adductor magnus*

It is attached to a line extending from the lower end of quadratus femoris to adductor tubercle. Specifically it is attached to:

1. Medial margin of gluteal tuberosity
2. Linea aspera
3. Medial supracondylar line
4. Adductor tubercle

xii. *Short head of biceps femoris*

It arises from:

1. Lateral lip of linea aspera
2. Upper 2/3rd of lateral supra-condylar line

b. Attachments of intermuscular septa (Fig. 12.9)

1. Medial intermuscular septum is attached to the medial lip of linea aspera.
2. Lateral intermuscular septum is attached to the lateral lip of linea aspera.

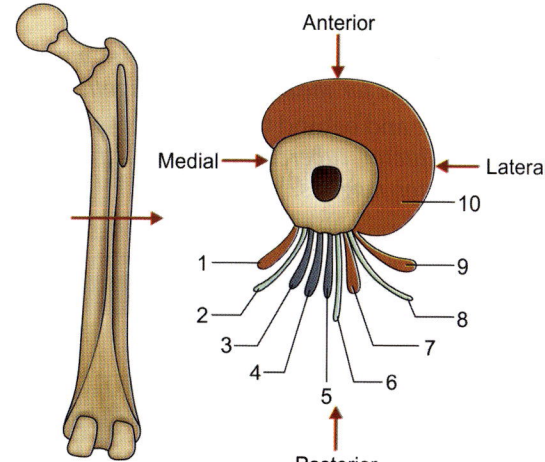

Fig. 12.9: Attachments to linea aspera (cross-sectional view): (1) Vastus medialis; (2) Medial intermuscular septum; (3) Adductor longus; (4) Adductor brevis; (5) Adductor magnus; (6) Posterior intermuscular septum; (7) Biceps femoris (short head); (8) Lateral intermuscular septum; (9) Vastus lateralis; (10) Vastus intermedius

3. Posterior intermuscular septum is attached to linea aspera just medial to attachment of short head of biceps femoris.

Note: *To remember the attachments of muscles to linea aspera remember the rhyme "I Love Bindu, Miss Bindu Loves Me, i.e. from lateral to medial these are I, L, B, M, B, L, M, which stand for vastus Intermedius, vastus Lateralis, short head of Biceps femoris, adductor Magnus, adductor Brevis, adductor Longus and vastus Medialis respectively.*

III. LOWER END

It includes two condyles (medial and lateral), a deep space between the two condyles posteriorly (intercondylar fossa or notch) and articular surfaces (patellar and tibial).

A. Medial condyle

It possesses 5 surfaces.

B. Secondary centres

Four in all, three for upper end and one for lower end.

a. Upper end

Appearance

- Head: 1 year
- Greater trochanter: 3 years
- Lesser trochanter: 13 years

Fusion

There will be three epiphyses which fuse with shaft separately at 18th year.

b. Lower end

Appearance

- 9 months of intrauterine life (i.e. day of birth)

Fusion

- 20 years

Patella

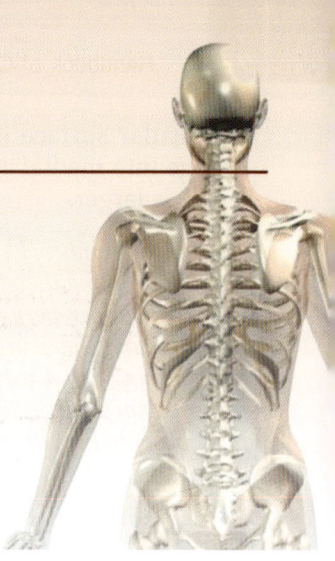

Patella is a Latin word which means *little plate*. It is also named as knee cap.

PECULIARITIES

1. Patella is a sesamoid bone developing in the tendon of quadriceps.
2. It is the largest sesamoid bone in the body.
3. It is situated in front of lower end of femur about 1 cm above the knee joint line.
4. It participates in the formation of knee joint.
5. It improves the leverage of quadriceps femoris by increasing the angulation of the line of pull of leg.

6. It lacks periosteum therefore patellectomy (removal of patella) is often a choice of treatment for fracture of patella as there is no chance for regeneration. Removal of patella does not hamper the movements at knee.

SIDE DETERMINATION (Fig. 13.1)

1. Patella is triangular in shape. Its base faces upwards while apex is downwards. Margins or borders are medial and lateral.
2. It has anterior and posterior surfaces. Posterior surface is marked by smooth articular surface.

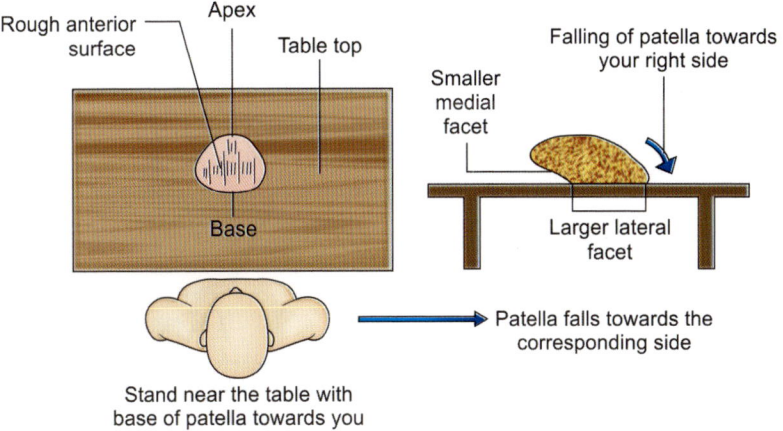

Fig. 13.1: Determination of side of patella by simple method

3. Articular surface is divided by a vertical ridge into medial and lateral parts. Lateral part is larger.

Note: *Remember 'L' stands for Lateral area as well as Large and therefore Lateral area is Larger. Observe another very interesting phenomenon. Keep the articular surface of patella on the flat table top in such a way that its base is directed towards you and apex is directed away from you. Now observe the tilt of patella. The patella will always tilt towards the side to which it belongs.*

FEATURES AND ATTACHMENTS

Patella has an apex, three borders (superior, lateral and medial) and two surfaces (anterior and posterior).

I. Apex

Ligamentum patellae is attached to the margins of apex and lower part of the rough portion of posterior surface.

II. Borders

A. Superior border

1. It is also called *base*.
2. *Rectus femoris* is attached to its anterior part.
3. *Vastus intermedius* is attached to its posterior part.

B. Lateral border

Expansion of tendon of vastus lateralis (*lateral patellar retinaculum*) is attached to it.

C. Medial border

1. Expansion of tendon of vastus medialis (*medial patellar retinaculum*) is attached to it.
2. *Muscular fibres of vastus medialis* get attached directly to the medial border behind the medial patellar retinaculum.

III. Surfaces

A. Anterior surface (Fig. 13.2)

1. It is rough and convex.

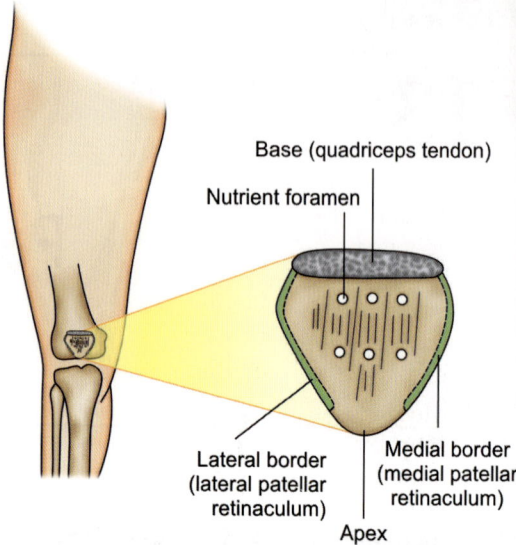

Fig. 13.2: Right patella: Anterior aspect

2. *Prepatellar bursa* intervenes between skin and anterior surface.
3. It is perforated by nutrient vessels.
4. It is covered by an *expansion from the quadriceps tendon.*

B. Posterior surface (Fig. 13.3)

1. Its lower 1/4th is rough and non-articular while upper 3/4th is smooth and articular.
2. Nonarticular part is divided into two areas:

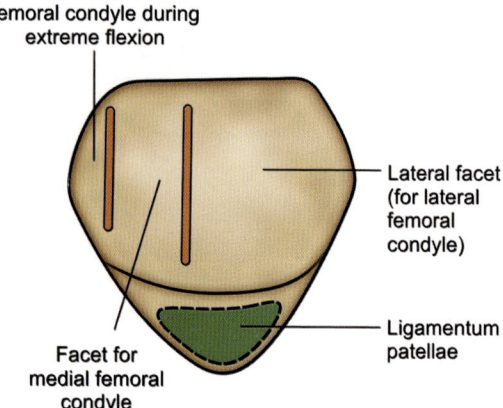

Fig. 13.3: Right patella: Posterior aspect

a. *Lower area* provides attachment to ligamentum patellae.

b. *Upper area* is related to *infrapatellar pad of fat*.

3. A vertical ridge divides the articular area into a larger lateral area and a smaller medial area. The ridge itself occupies the groove in the patellar surface of femoral lower end in the extended position of knee. The larger lateral area lies in contact with the lateral femoral condyle in all positions of knee.

4. Medial area is separated from medial strip by another vertical ridge. Medial femoral condyle is related to the medial area during extension of knee and the medial strip during full flexion at knee (Fig. 13.4).

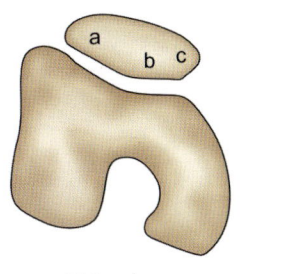 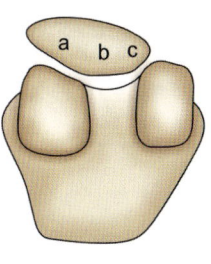

Extension Flexion

Fig. 13.4: Relations of right femoral condyles with patella in different positions at knee. (a) Lateral area; (b) Medial area; (c) Medial strip

OSSIFICATION

1. Several centres appear during 3–6 years.
2. Ossification of patella is completed at puberty.

Tibia

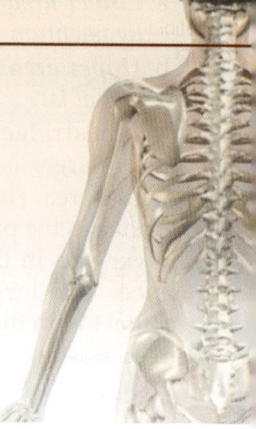

TERMINOLOGY

Tibia is also called *shin-bone*

PECULIARITIES

1. Tibia is the 2nd largest bone of body.
2. It is homologous with radius of forearm.
3. It is main weight bearing bone of leg in standing posture.

SIDE DETERMINATION

1. The broader end is the upper end of tibia.
2. A downward projection (*medial malleolus*) from the lower end is medial in position.
3. Keep the most prominent border of shaft anteriorly.

ANATOMICAL POSITION (Fig. 14.1)

1. Hold the bone in the hand of same side to which it belongs.
2. Keep the bone vertical.
3. *Tibial plateau* (superior surface of the upper end of tibia) lies in horizontal plane.

FEATURES AND ATTACHMENTS

Tibia consists of an upper end, a shaft and a lower end.

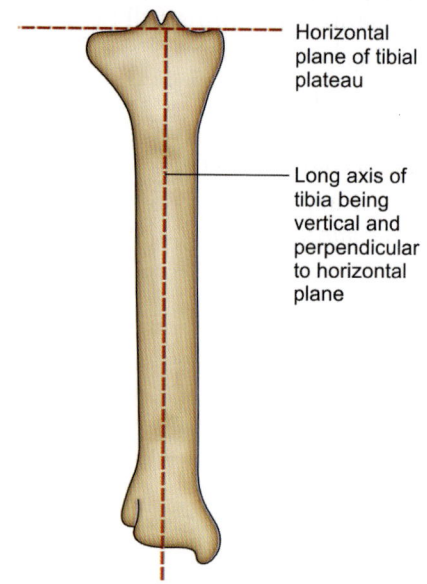

Horizontal plane of tibial plateau

Long axis of tibia being vertical and perpendicular to horizontal plane

Fig. 14.1: Normal anatomical position of tibia

I. UPPER END (Fig. 14.2)

It has two condyles (medial and lateral), an intercondylar area and tibial tuberosity.

A. Medial condyle

It is comprised 4 surfaces.

a. Superior surface

1. It is articular.
2. It is oval in shape with long axis directed anteroposteriorly.

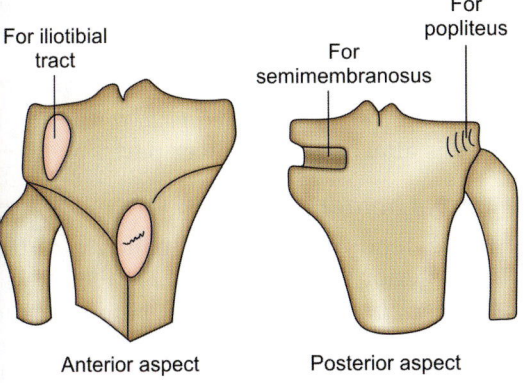

For iliotibial tract

For semimembranosus

For popliteus

Anterior aspect   Posterior aspect

Fig. 14.2: Upper end of right tibia

3. Its central part is concave to articulate with the convex medial femoral condyle.
4. Its peripheral part is flattened for the *medial meniscus*.
5. Its lateral border extends over the *medial intercondylar tubercle*.
6. Its margins receive attachment of *capsular ligament of knee*.

b. Posterior surface

It is deeply grooved for the attachment of *tendon of semimembranosus*.

c. Anterior surface

d. Medial surface

Anterior and medial surfaces receive the attachments of *medial patellar retinaculum*.

B. Lateral condyle

Like medial condyle, lateral condyle also has 4 surfaces.

a. Superior surface

1. It is articular.
2. It is circular in shape.
3. Its central part is concave to articulate with the convex lateral femoral condyle.
4. Its peripheral part is flattened for the *lateral meniscus*.
5. Its medial border extends over the *lateral intercondylar tubercle*.

6. Its margins provide attachment to the *capsular ligament*.

b. Posterior surface

1. Inferolaterally, this surface shows a circular smooth articular facet for head of fibula.
2. Between the articular facet for fibula and margin of superior surface there is a shallow groove for tendon of popliteus.

c. Anterior surface

It has *flat triangular facet for the attachment of iliotibial tract*.

d. Lateral surface

Anterior and lateral surfaces receive attachment of *lateral patellar retinaculum*.

C. Intercondylar area (Fig. 14.3)

1. It is the roughened area between the superior articular surfaces of two tibial condyles.
2. The middle of intercondylar area is marked by an elevation called *intercondylar eminence* which is formed by two small tubercles called *medial* and *lateral intercondylar tubercles*.

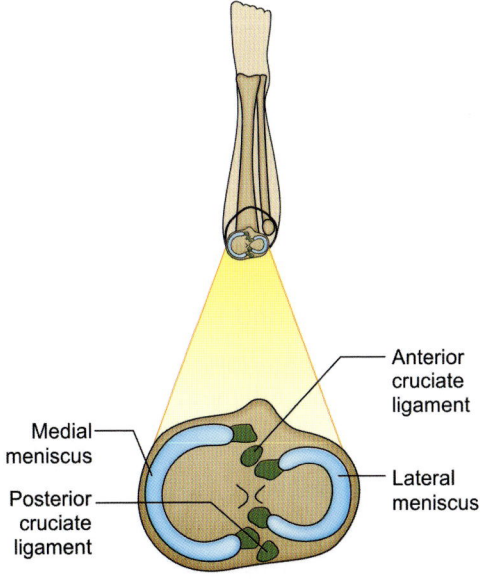

Anterior cruciate ligament

Medial meniscus

Posterior cruciate ligament

Lateral meniscus

Fig. 14.3: Proximal articular surface of right tibia

3. Intercondylar eminence divides the inter-condylar area into two parts.
   i. *Anterior intercondylar area.*
   ii. Posterior intercondylar area.
4. From before backwards, the intercondylar area provides attachments to following 6 structures, of which 3 are located in its anterior part and 3 in its posterior part:
   i. Anterior horn of medial meniscus.
   ii. Anterior cruciate ligament.
   iii. Anterior horn of lateral meniscus.
   iv. Posterior horn of lateral meniscus.
   v. Posterior horn of medial meniscus.
   vi. Posterior cruciate ligament.

Note: *To remember the sequence remember the rhyme "Medical College Lucknow, Lucknow Medical College. Also remember that both the Lucknow are together in the middle adjacent to intercondylar eminence.*

D. Tibial tuberosity

1. It is located on the anterior aspect and marks the upper end of anterior border of shaft.
2. It is divided into upper smooth and lower rough part.
3. *Ligamentum patellae* is attached to upper smooth part.
4. Lower rough part is related to subcuta-neous *infrapatellar bursa* which separates it from the skin.
5. Epiphyseal line at the upper end of tibia passes between the smooth and rough parts of the tibial tuberosity

II. SHAFT (Figs 14.4 and 14.6 to 14.10)

It has 3 borders (anterior, medial and lateral) and 3 surfaces (lateral, medial and posterior).

A. Borders

a. Anterior border

1. It is sharpest.
2. It extends from tibial tuberosity to anterior border of medial malleolus.

3. It is also called *shin*.
4. It is subcutaneous.
5. *Deep fascia* of leg is attached to it.
6. *Superior extensor retinaculum* of ankle is attached to its lower part.

b. Medial border

1. It extends from medial condyle to the posterior border of medial malleolus.
2. *Soleal line* (a roughened ridge on the posterior surface) joins the medial border at the junction of its upper 1/3rd with the lower 2/3rd.
3. Medial border above the soleal line receives attachment of *fascia covering the popliteus.*
4. Below the soleal line, the medial border provides attachments to (Fig. 14.5):
   i. *Deep fascia of leg.*
   ii. *Soleus in its upper part.*
   iii. *Deep transverse fascia.*

c. Lateral (interosseous) border

1. It extends from lateral condyle to the anterior border of fibular notch.
2. *Interosseous membrane* is attached to it
3. *Anterior tibiofibular ligament* is attached to the lower end of lateral border.

B. Surfaces

a. Lateral surface

1. It is between anterior and interosseous borders.
2. Its upper 2/3rd receives attachment of *tibialis anterior.*
3. Its lower 1/3rd is crossed by following structures from medial to lateral.
   i. *Tibialis anterior.*
   ii. *Extensor hallucis longus.*
   iii. *Anterior tibial artery.*
   iv. *Deep peroneal nerve.*
   v. *Extensor digitorum longus.*
   vi. *Peroneus tertius.*
4. *Superior extensor retinaculum* covers the lower part of the lateral surface.

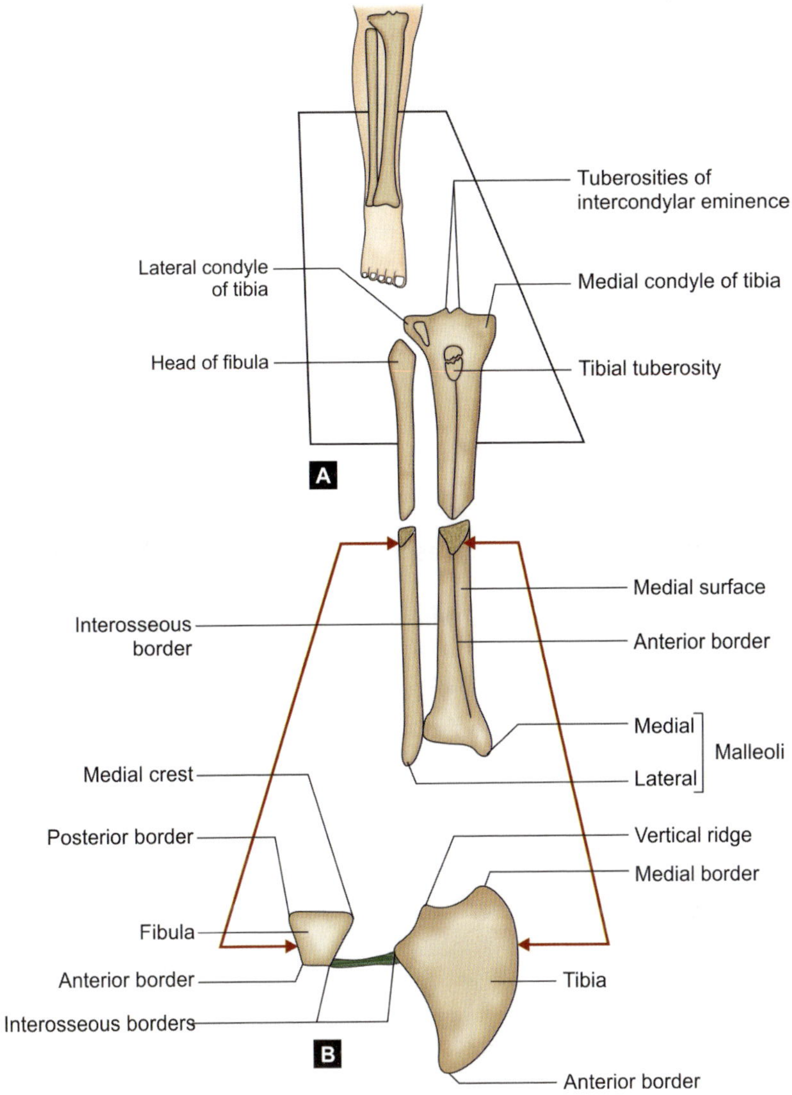

Tuberosities of
intercondylar eminence

Lateral condyle
of tibia

Medial condyle of tibia

Head of fibula

Tibial tuberosity

A

Medial surface

Interosseous
border

Anterior border

Medial ⎤
           ⎥ Malleoli
Lateral ⎦

Medial crest

Posterior border

Vertical ridge

Medial border

Fibula

Anterior border

Tibia

Interosseous borders

B

Anterior border

Fig. 14.4: Tibia and fibula. (A) Anterior aspect; (B) Cross-section

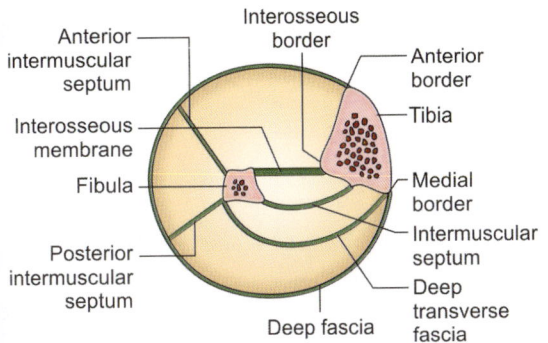

Anterior
intermuscular
septum

Interosseous
border

Anterior
border

Interosseous
membrane

Tibia

Fibula

Medial
border

Posterior
intermuscular
septum

Intermuscular
septum

Deep
transverse
fascia

Deep fascia

Fig. 14.5: Osseofascial compartments of leg

b. Medial surface

1. It is between anterior and medial borders.
2. It is mostly subcutaneous.
3. Its upper part receives attachments of following structures from before backwards:
   i. *Sartorius*
   iii. *Semitendinosus*
   ii. *Gracilis*
   iv. *Tibial collateral ligament*

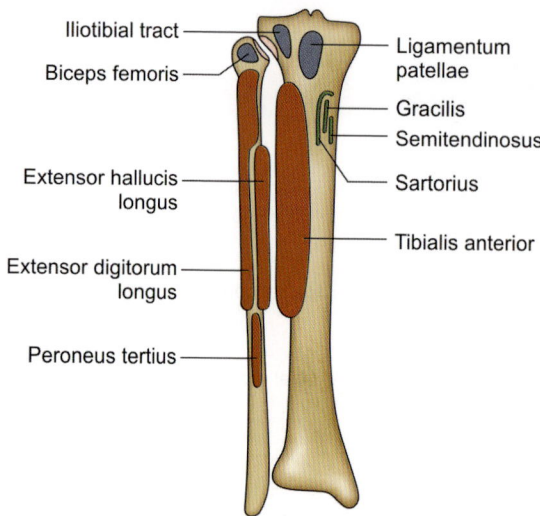

Fig. 14.6: Right tibia and fibula: Anterior aspect

Note: *To remember the names of three muscles attached to the upper part of medial surface of tibia, one can remember "General between two Sergeants".*

4. *Great saphenous vein* is related to lower 1/3rd of medial surface.

c. Posterior surface

1. It is between medial and lateral borders.
2. There is a roughened ridge extending from fibular facet to the junction of upper and middle 3rd of the medial border. This is named as *soleal line*. This line gives attachments to following structures from above downwards (Fig. 14.9):
   i. *Fascia covering popliteus.*
   ii. *Fascia covering soleus.*
   iii. *Soleus (origin).*
   iv. *Deep transverse fascia.*

   The *tendinous arch* for origin of soleus is attached to a tubercle at the upper end of soleal line.
3. A triangular area above the soleal line provides attachment to *popliteus*.

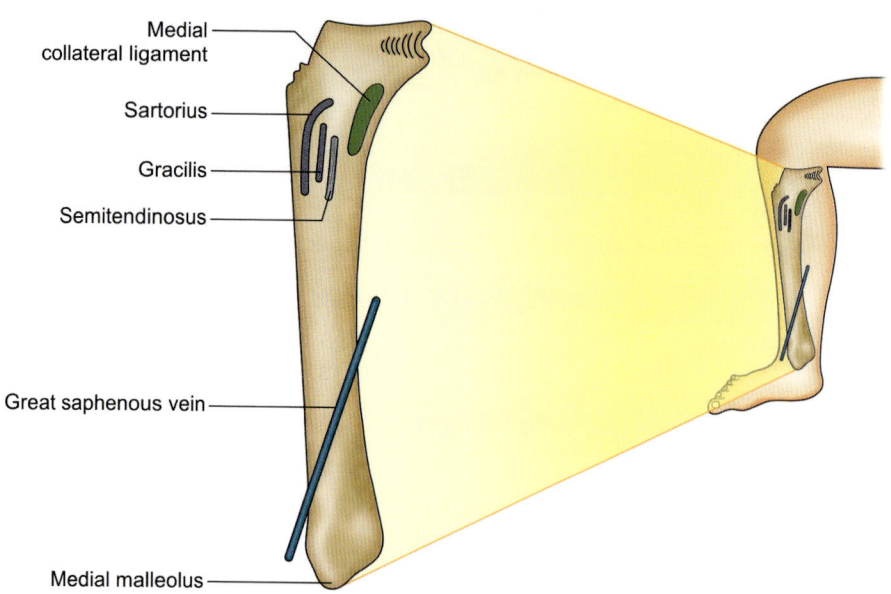

Fig. 14.7: Right tibia : Medial aspect

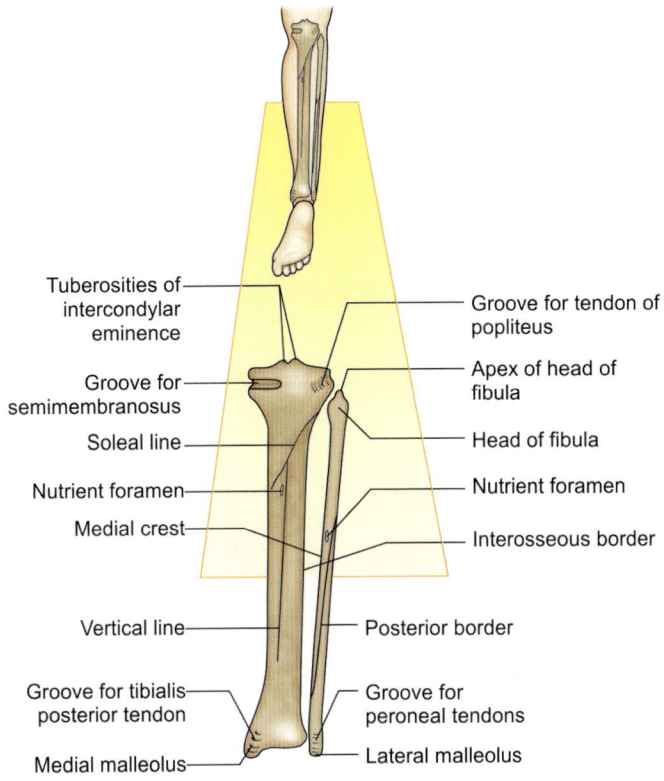

Tuberosities of intercondylar eminence

Groove for semimembranosus

Soleal line

Nutrient foramen

Medial crest

Vertical line

Groove for tibialis posterior tendon

Medial malleolus

Groove for tendon of popliteus

Apex of head of fibula

Head of fibula

Nutrient foramen

Interosseous border

Posterior border

Groove for peroneal tendons

Lateral malleolus

Fig. 14.8: Right tibia and fibula: Posterior aspect

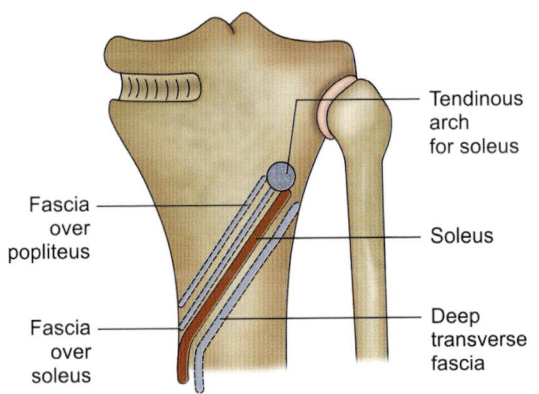

Fascia over popliteus

Fascia over soleus

Tendinous arch for soleus

Soleus

Deep transverse fascia

Fig. 14.9: Attachments to soleal line

4. The area below the soleal line is divided into a medial and a lateral parts by a vertical line which itself receives attachment of *fascia covering the tibialis posterior*.

5. *Nutrient foramen* is situated at the upper end of vertical line. Nutrient canal is directed downwards, i.e. away from the knee. Thus the upper end is the growing end of bone. *Nutrient artery*, a branch of posterior tibial artery, is the largest nutrient artery of the body.

6. *Flexor digitorum longus* is attached to the medial area below the soleal line.

7. *Tibialis posterior* is attached to the lateral area below the soleal line.

8. Lower 1/4th of the posterior surface is related to following structures from medial to lateral:
   i. Tibialis posterior.
   ii. Posterior tibial vessels.
   iii. Tibial nerve.
   iv. Flexor hallucis longus.

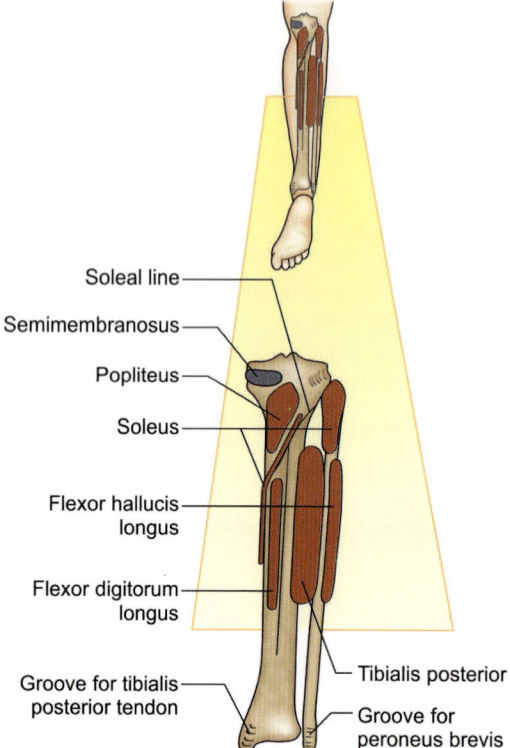

Soleal line

Semimembranosus

Popliteus

Soleus

Flexor hallucis longus

Flexor digitorum longus

Groove for tibialis posterior tendon

Tibialis posterior

Groove for peroneus brevis

Fig. 14.10: Right tibia and fibula: Posterior aspect

Note: *Flexor digitorum longus tendon is separated from the bone by tendon of tibialis posterior.*

III. LOWER END

It has 5 surfaces (anterior, posterior, medial, lateral and inferior) and a downward projection from the medial part called medial malleolus.

A. Surfaces

a. Anterior surface

1. It extends beyond inferior surface.
2. It is separated from the inferior surface by a groove.
3. This groove receives attachment of anterior part of *capsule of ankle joint*.
4. Anterior surface above the groove is related to following structures from medial to lateral:

    i. *Tibialis anterior.*
    ii. *Extensor hallucis longus.*
    iii. *Anterior tibial artery.*
    iv. *Deep peroneal nerve.*
    v. *Extensor digitorum longus.*
    vi. *Peroneus tertius.*

Note: *For remembering this sequence remember the rhyme "The Himalayas Are Not Dry Plateaus.*

b. Posterior surface

1. Its lower margin receives attachment of posterior part of *capsule of ankle joint*.
2. Area above the lower margin is related to following structures from medial to lateral:

    i. Tibialis posterior.
    ii. *Flexor digitorum longus.*
    iii. *Posterior tibial artery.*
    iv. *Tibial nerve.*
    v. *Flexor hallucis longus.*

Note: *For remembering this sequence remember the rhyme "The Doctors Are Not Hunters".*

c. Medial surface

1. It is subcutaneous.
2. It continues downwards as medial surface of medial malleolus.

d. Lateral surface

1. It forms the *fibular notch*.
2. Its anterior and posterior margins provide attachments to *anterior and posterior tibiofibular ligaments* respectively.
3. *Interosseous tibiofibular ligament* is attached to its upper rough part between anterior and posterior tibiofibular ligaments.
4. Its lower 4 mm is smooth and related to an upward prolongation of synovial membrane of talocrural (ankle) joint.

e. Inferior surface

1. It articulates with superior articular surface of talus to form *talocrural (ankle) joint.*

2. Medially it continues as the articular surface of medial malleolus.

3. Medial malleolus

It has 4 surfaces (anterior, posterior, medial and lateral) and an inferior border.

a. Anterior surface

Capsular ligament of ankle joint is attached to it.

b. Posterior surface

1. It is grooved by *tendon of tibialis posterior*.
2. Medial margin of groove gives attachment to the *flexor retinaculum*.

c. Medial surface

It is subcutaneous.

d. Lateral surface

It has a comma shaped facet for articulation with the malleolar facet on the medial surface of talus.

e. Inferior border

It provides attachment to capsular ligament and *deltoid ligament* of the ankle joint.

CAPSULAR ATTACHMENTS (Fig. 14.11)

At the upper end, capsule is attached to the margins of tibial plateau medially, laterally and posteriorly. Anteriorly the capsule blends with patellar retinacula and is indirectly attached to anterior surfaces of tibial condyles.

At the lower end the capsule is attached to the margins of articular surfaces except laterally where it shifts over the lower end of fibula.

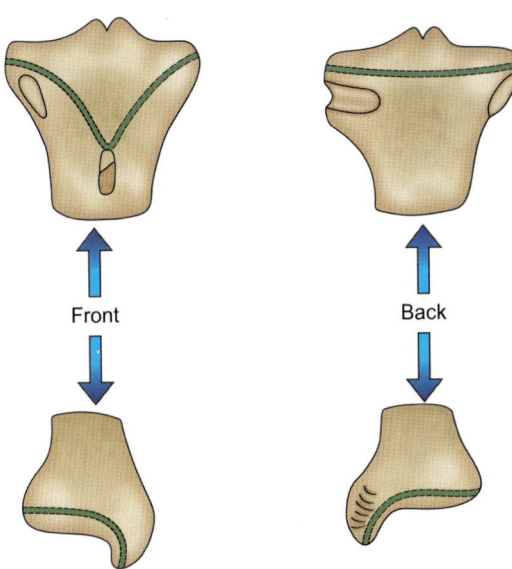

Front   Back

Fig. 14.11: Capsular attachments of right tibia

OSSIFICATION

A. Primary centre

One centre appears for the shaft at the age of 8th week of intrauterine life.

B. Secondary centres

Two in all, one for upper end and one for lower end.

a. Upper end

Appearance: At birth
Fusion: 20 years

b. Lower end

Appearance: 2 years
Fusion: 18 years

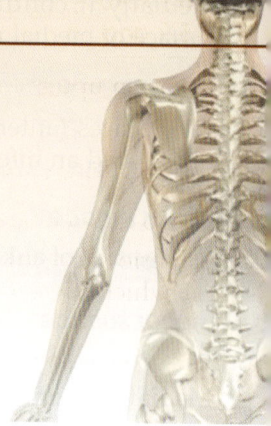

Fibula

TERMINOLOGY

Fibula is a Latin word which means pin. It is rightly named so because it is a long pin like bone.

PECULIARITIES

1. It is the lateral bone of leg.
2. It is homologous with ulna.
3. It is smaller of the two bones of leg.
4. Although fibula does not take part in transmission of body weight, it is very important for stability of ankle joint.

SIDE DETERMINATION (Fig. 15.1)

1. Rounded end of bone is called head which is always superior.
2. The lower end is relatively flattened. It is marked by a triangular articular facet which faces medially.
3. A depression (*malleolar fossa*) at the lower end is posterior to triangular articular facet.

Note: *Proper placement of malleolar fossa will help you in determining the side of fibula. Keep the fibula on the lateral side of leg in such a way that malleolar fossa faces downwards, backwards and medially.*

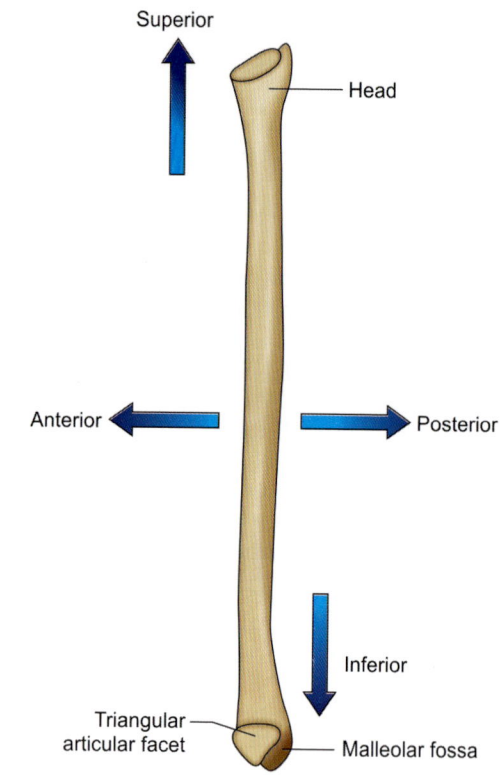

Fig. 15.1: Right fibula: Medial aspect

NORMAL ANATOMICAL POSITION

Hold the bone vertically with the hand of corresponding side keeping in the mind the direction of malleolar fossa.

FEATURES AND ATTACHMENTS
(Figs 15.2 and 15.4 to 15.8)

Fibula has an upper end, a shaft and a lower end.

I. UPPER END (Fig. 15.3)

1. It is also called *head* of fibula.

2. Its superior surface bears a circular articular facet which faces superiorly and antero-medially. It articulates with lateral condyle of tibia to form *superior tibiofibular* joint. Its margin provides attachment to capsule of this joint.

3. *Styloid process* is an upward projection from the posterolateral aspect of the head.

4. Front of styloid process provides attachment to the *fibular callateral ligament*.

5. Areas anterior, lateral and posterior to attachment of fibular callateral ligament

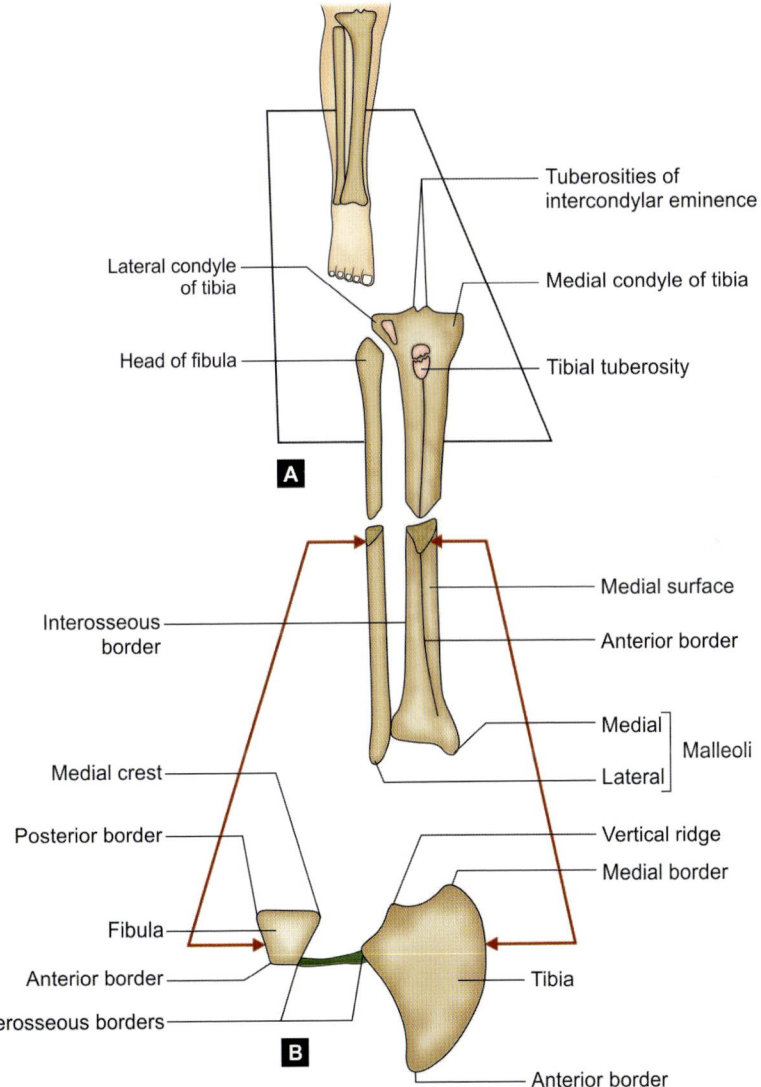

Fig. 15.2: Right tibia and fibula: (A) Anterior aspect; (B) Cross-section

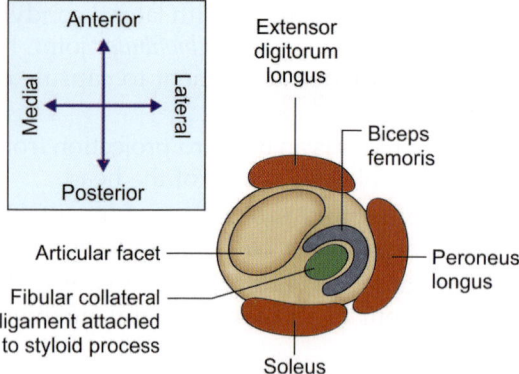

Fig. 15.3: Head of right fibula: Superior aspect

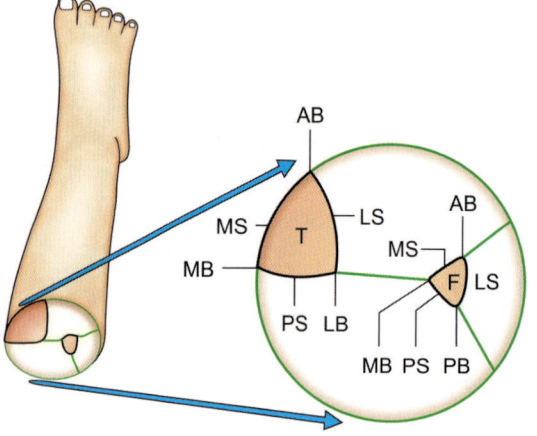

Fig. 15.4: Cross-sectional views of tibia and fibula. T: Tibia; F: Fibula; AB: Anterior border; MB: Medial border, PB: Posterior border; LB: Lateral border; MS: Medial surface; LS: Lateral surface; PS: Posterior surface

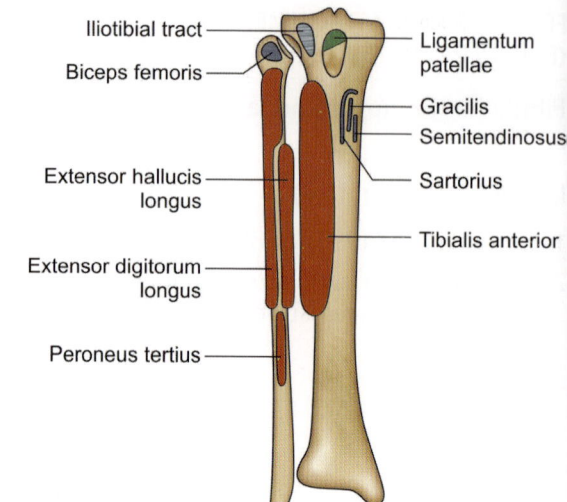

Fig. 15.5: Right tibia and fibula: Anterior aspect

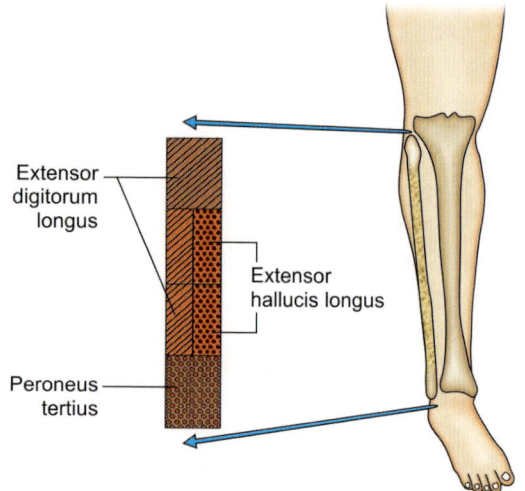

Fig. 15.6: Muscular attachments to the medial surface of right fibula

form a 'C' shaped attachment of *biceps femoris*.

6. *Extensor digitorum longus, peroneus longus and soleus* are attached to anterior, lateral and posterior surfaces of head respectively.

7. *Common peroneal nerve* is related to posterolateral aspect of neck (lower limit of head) of fibula.

II. SHAFT

It has 3 borders (anterior, posterior and medial) and 3 surfaces (medial, lateral and posterior).

A. Borders

a. Anterior border

1. Anterior intermuscular septum of leg is attached to the upper 3/4th of anterior border.

2. Inferiorly it splits to enclose a triangular area which continues with lateral surface of lateral malleolus.

3. *Superior extensor retinaculum* is attached to the anterior margin of the triangular area.

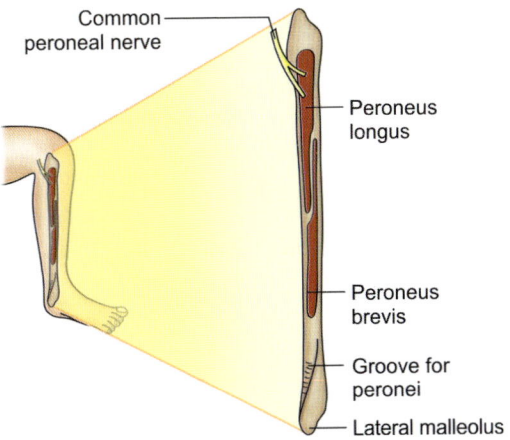

Fig. 15.7: Right fibula : Lateral aspect

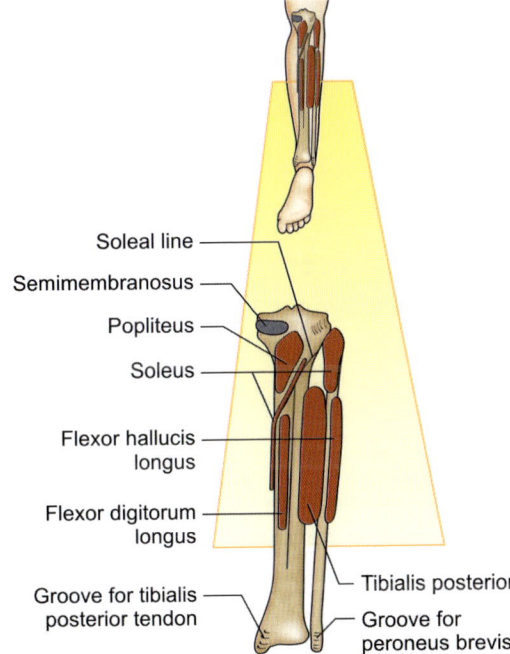

Fig. 15.8: Right tibia and fibula: Posterior aspect

4. *Superior peroneal retinaculum* is attached to the posterior margin of the triangular area.

b. Posterior border

1. It extends from the posterior aspect of head to the medial margin of groove on the back of lower end of fibula.

2. *Posterior intermuscular septum* of leg is attached to its upper 3/4th.

c. Medial (interosseous) border

1. It lies close and just medial to the anterior border.
2. Inferiorly it ends at the upper end of the roughened area for the interosseous ligament.
3. *Interosseous membrane* is attached to it except at the upper end where a gap between tibia and fibula transmits the *anterior tibial vessels.*

B. Surfaces

a. Medial surface

1. It is between anterior and medial borders.
2. It is very narrow.
3. *Extensor digitorum longus* is attached to the whole of its upper fourth and anterior half of its middle 2/4th.
4. *Extensor hallucis longus* is attached to the posterior half of the middle 2/4th.
5. Its lower 1/4th receives attachment of *peroneus tertius.*

b. Lateral surface

1. It is between anterior and posterior borders.
2. *Peroneus longus* is attached to its upper 1/3rd and posterior half of the middle 1/3rd.
3. *Peroneus brevis* is attached to its lower 1/3rd and the anterior half of its middle 1/3rd.

c. Posterior surface

1. It is between medial (interosseous) border and the posterior border.
2. Its upper 2/3rd is divided into medial and lateral areas by a sharp vertical ridge termed as *medial crest.*
3. Fascia covering the tibialis posterior is attached to the medial crest.
4. Lower part of the posterior surface presents a rough triangular area whose

anterior margin, intermediate area and posterior margin provide attachments to *anterior tibiofibular, interosseous tibiofibular* and *posterior tibiofibular* ligaments respectively.

5. Medial area (grooved surface between medial crest and medial border) gives origin to *tibialis posterior*.

6. Upper 1/4th of the lateral area gives origin to *soleus*.

7. Lower 3/4th of the lateral area gives origin to *flexor hallucis longus*.

8. *Peroneal artery* descends in relation to medial crest.

9. *Nutrient artery*, a branch of peroneal artery, enters the nutrient foramen present just above the middle of the posterior surface.

10. Nutrient canal is directed downwards and, therefore, the upper end of fibula is growing end.

III. LOWER END (LATERAL MALLEOLUS) (Fig. 15.9)

Lateral malleolus is 0.5 cm lower than the medial malleolus.

Note: *Remember that in case of bones of forearm, the styloid process of radius is lower than the styloid process of ulna. Therefore, it can be said that the lateral bones of both, forearm and leg project more downwards than the medial bones*

Lateral malleolus has four surfaces (medial, lateral, anterior and posterior) and an inferior border.

A. Surfaces

a. Medial surface

1. It bears a triangular articular surface anteriorly which articulates with talus.
2. More posteriorly there is *malleolar fossa*.
3. *Posterior tibiofibular ligament* is attached to the upper part of malleolar fossa.
4. Lower part of malleolar fossa receives attachment of *posterior talofibular ligament*.

b. Lateral surface

It is subcutaneous.

c. Anterior surface

It gives attachment to *anterior talofibular ligament*.

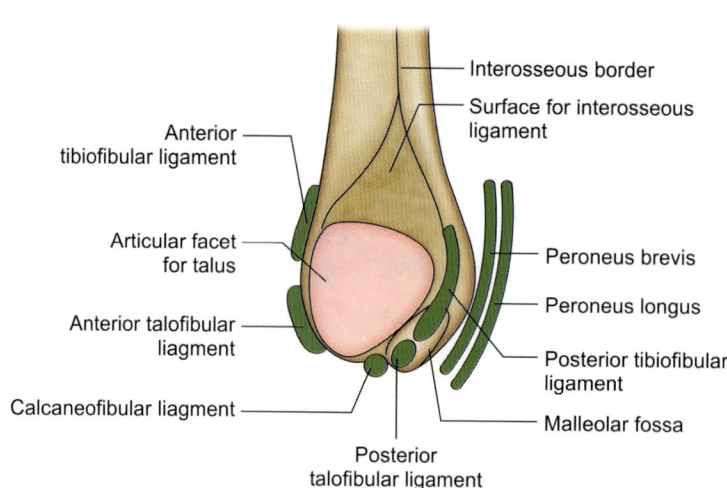

Fig. 15.9: Lower end of right fibula: Medial aspect

d. Posterior surface

1. It has a groove for *tendons of peroneus longus and peroneus brevis*. The former is more superficial.

Note: *Imagine brevis as a child and longus as an adult, because a child has to be protected that is why it is deep in the groove.*

2. Lateral border of the groove gives attachment to *superior peroneal retinaculum*.

B. Inferior border

It presents a notch to which is attached *calcaneofibular ligament*.

OSSIFICATION

A. Primary centre

One centre appears for the shaft of fibula at 8th week of intrauterine life.

B. Secondary centres

Two in all, one for upper end and one for lower end.

a. Upper end

Appearance: 4 years
Fusion with shaft: 20 years

b. Lower end

Appearance: 2 years
Fusion with shaft: 18 years

Note: *To remember the ossification of fibula, one can number the upper end as 420 and lower end as 218, i.e. times of appearance for upper end and lower end are 4 and 2 years respectively while fusion take place at 20 and 18 years respectively. Upper end is 420 in another sense also because it defies the law of ossification which states that the centre that appears first fuses last but in case of upper end of fibula, the centre appears late and fuses late as compared to lower end.*

Tarsal Bones

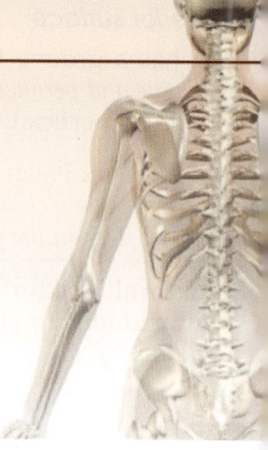

TARSUS

Seven tarsal bones together constitute the tarsus.

NAMES

Seven tarsal bones are named as follows:
1. Talus.
2. Calcaneus.
3. Navicular bone
4. Cuboid bone
5. Medial cuneiform.
6. Intermediate cuneiform.
7. Lateral cuneiform.

Talus and calcaneus form *proximal tarsal row*. Cuboid bone and three cuneiforms constitute the *distal tarsal row*. Navicular bone lies between the two rows.

IDENTIFICATION OF TARSAL BONES IN FOOT SKELETON (Figs 16.1 and 16.2)

1. *Calcaneus* is the largest tarsal bone. It forms heel and is located below the talus.
2. *Talus* is the second largest tarsal bone. It rests over the superior aspect of calcaneus. It has a head which is directed forwards and medially.
3. *Navicular* bone is identified on the basis of deep concavity on the proximal surface which meets with the talar head.

4. *Cuboid* bone is the next distal bone in the line of calcaneus.
5. *Cuneiforms* are the 3 small tarsal bones arranged from side to side along the distal surface of the navicular bone.

INDIVIDUAL TARSAL BONES

I. TALUS

Nomenclature

Talus is a Latin word meaning *ankle bone*.

Peculiarities

1. It is the second largest tarsal bone.
2. There is no muscular attachment to this bone.
3. It participates in the formation of three joints, i.e. talocrural (ankle), talocalcaneal (subtalar) and talocalcaneonavicular.

Side determination

1. Keep the rounded head forwards.
2. Keep the trochlear articular surface (which is convex anteroposteriorly and concave from side to side) upwards.
3. Each side has got an articular surface. The one which is triangular, faces laterally while the comma shaped articular facet is directed medially.

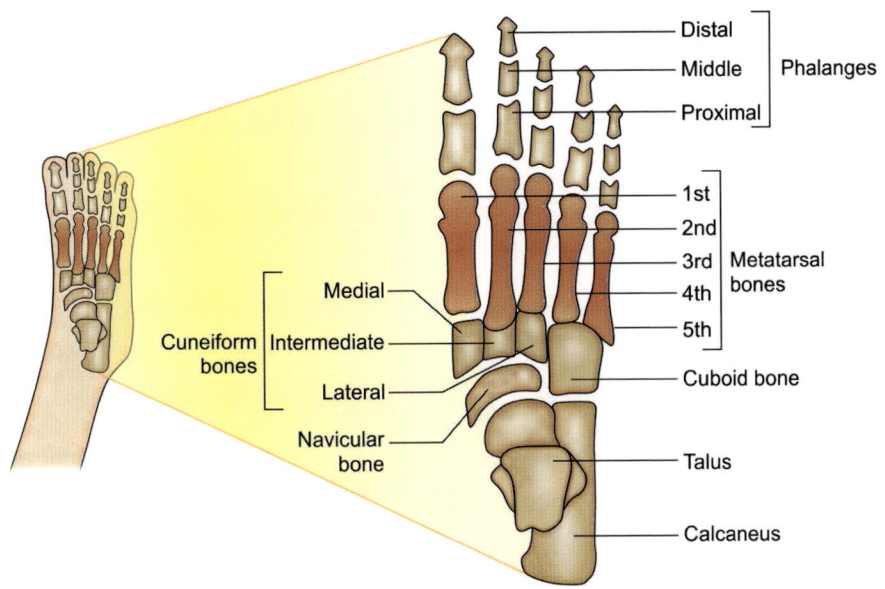

Fig. 16.1: Skeleton of the right foot: Dorsal aspect

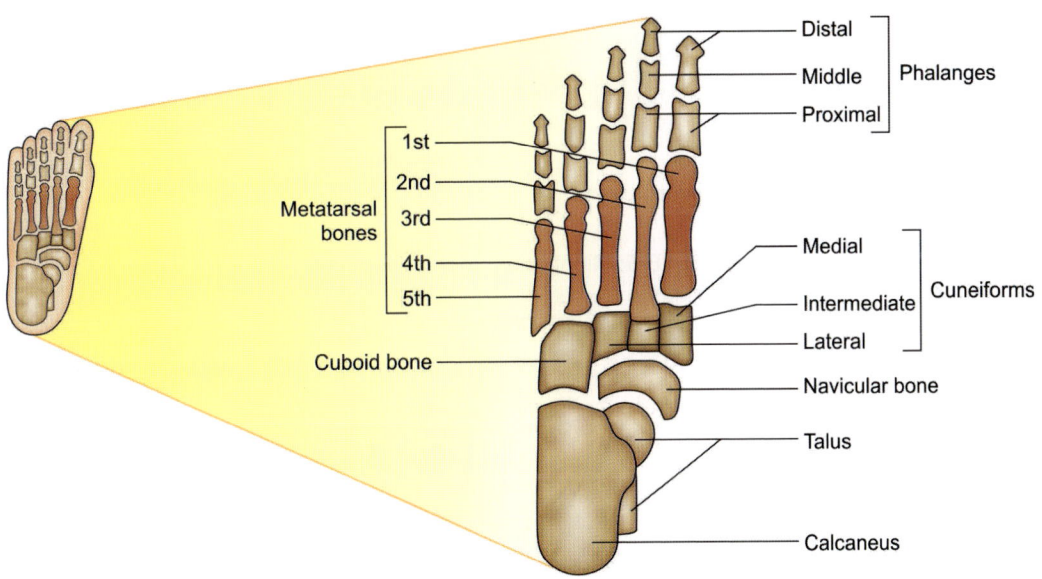

Fig. 16.2: Skeleton of right foot: Plantar aspect.

**Features and attachments
(Figs 16.3 to 16.6)**

Talus has got a head, a neck and a body.

A. Head

1. It is directed forwards, downwards and medially.

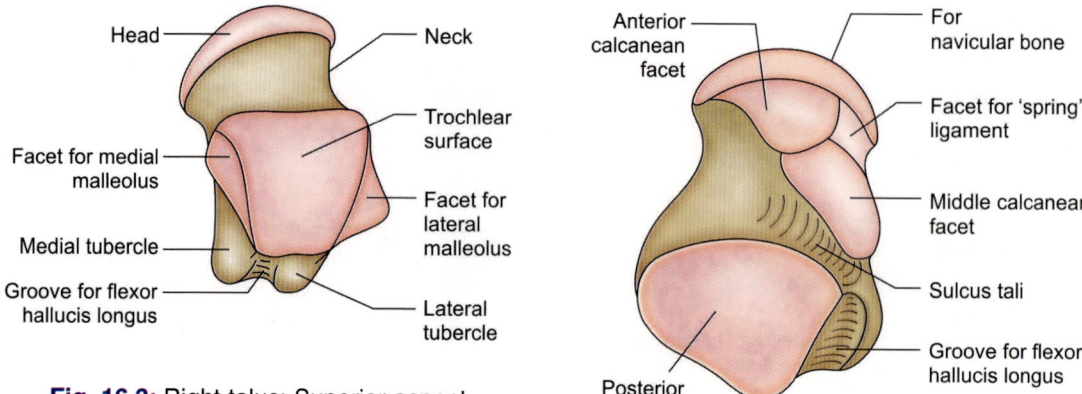

Fig. 16.3: Right talus: Superior aspect

Fig. 16.4: Right talus: Inferior aspect

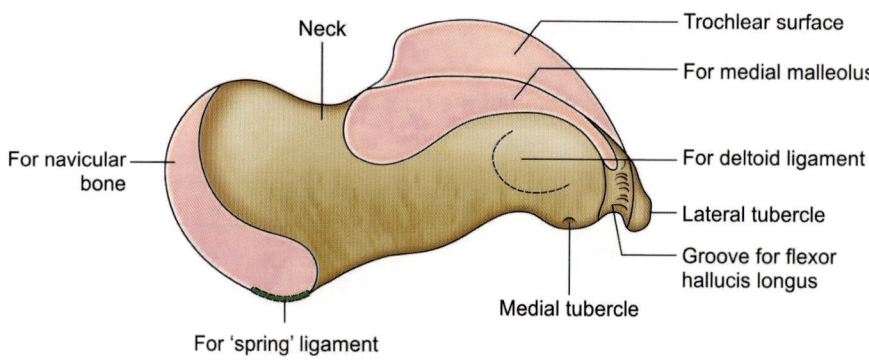

Fig. 16.5: Right talus: Medial aspect

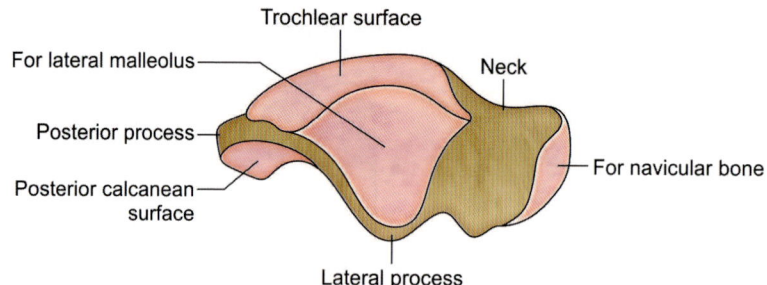

Fig. 16.6: Right talus: Lateral aspect

2. It has two surfaces, anterior and inferior.

3. Anterior surface is oval and convex to articulate with the concavity of navicular bone.

4. Inferior surface has 3 articular areas separated by ridges.

i. Posterior articular area is the largest and articulates with the middle facet of calcaneus.

ii. Medial facet articulates with the spring (*plantar calcaneonavicular*) ligament.

iii. Anterolateral facet articulates with the anterior facet of calcaneus.

B. Neck

1. It is the constriction between head and body.
2. Its long axis forms an angle of 150° with the long axis of body.
3. Distal part of its dorsal surface provides attachment to *dorsal talonavicular ligament and capsular ligament of ankle joint*.
4. Proximal part of dorsal surface is intra-capsular.
5. Laterally, there is attachment of *anterior talofibular ligament*.
6. Plantar surface medially, is narrow and called *sulcus tali*. It *opposes the sulcus calcanei* of calcaneus to form *sinus tarsi*.
7. Plantar surface of neck provides attachments to two ligaments, *interosseous talo-calcanean* (medially) and *cervical* (laterally).

C. Body

It has five surfaces (superior, inferior, medial, lateral and posterior).

i. Superior surface

1. It bears *trochlear articular surface*.
2. Trochlear articular surface is convex from anterior to posterior and concave from side to side.
3. The articular surface is broader anteriorly and narrower posteriorly.
4. It participates in the formation of *ankle joint*.

ii. Inferior surface

1. It is entirely articular.
2. This articular surface is oval and concave.
3. It articulates with the posterior facet of calcaneus to form *subtalar joint*.

iii. Medial surface

1. It is articular above and nonarticular below.
2. Its articular area is comma shaped to articulate with the medial malleolus.
3. *Deep part of the deltoid ligament* is attached to the nonarticular part.

iv. Lateral surface

1. It shows a triangular articular area.
2. It articulates with lateral malleolus.
3. Its anterior border gives attachment to *anterior talofibular ligament*.
4. Its lower end forms the apex of triangle also called the *lateral process of talus*.

v. Posterior surface

1. It is also called *posterior process of talus*.
2. *Tendon of flexor hallucis longus* grooves the posterior surface.
3. *Medial and lateral tubercles* bound the groove for flexor hallucis longus.
4. Deltoid ligament's superficial fibres (*posterior tibiotalar ligament*) are attached to the medial tubercle.
5. *Posterior talofibular ligament* is attached to the lateral tubercle.
6. *Os trigonum* is the name given to the lateral tubercle when it is a separate bone. Os trigonum is one of the examples of atavistic epiphysis.

Ossification

Talus ossifies from one centre which appears in its body during 6th month of intrauterine life.

II. CALCANEUS

Terminology

It is a Latin word which means heel. Clinicians often name it as *os calis*.

Peculiarities

1. It is the largest bone of foot.
2. It is the strongest bone of foot.
3. It is the first tarsal bone to ossify.
4. It contributes to subtalar as well as mid-tarsal joints.

Side determination

1. Keep the long axis of bone anteroposteriorly.
2. Look for the anterior and posterior surfaces.

Anterior surface is articular and concavoconvex. The posterior surface is larger and rough.

3. Keep the surface bearing large convex articular area dorsally.

4. Keep the concave surface medially. Medial surface is made concave by the shelf like projection called *sustentaculum tali*.

Features and attachments

It has six surfaces (anterior, posterior, superior, plantar, lateral and medial).

A. Anterior surface

1. It is the smallest of all.
2. It bears a concavoconvex articular facet.
3. It articulates with cuboid.

B. Posterior surface

1. It is divided into 3 areas.
2. Its upper part is smooth and is related to a bursa.
3. Its middle part receives insertion of *tendocalcaneus and plantaris*.
4. Its lowermost part is roughened. Dense fibrofatty tissue covers it. It is weight bearing during standing posture.

C. Superior surface (Fig. 16.7)

1. It is also called dorsal surface.
2. It is divided into 3 areas.
    i. Posterior 1/3rd is nonarticular.
    ii. Middle 1/3rd is articular.
    iii. Anterior 1/3rd is partly articular and partly nonarticular.
3. Posterior 1/3rd is rough and is related to fibrofatty tissue between tendocalcaneus and ankle.
4. Middle 1/3rd forms the *posterior facet for talus*.
5. Anteromedial area of anterior 1/3rd possesses two articular facets called *middle and anterior facets for talus*. Middle facet is situated over sustentaculum tali.
6. Nonarticular part of anterior 1/3rd can be divided into medial narrow and lateral wide parts.

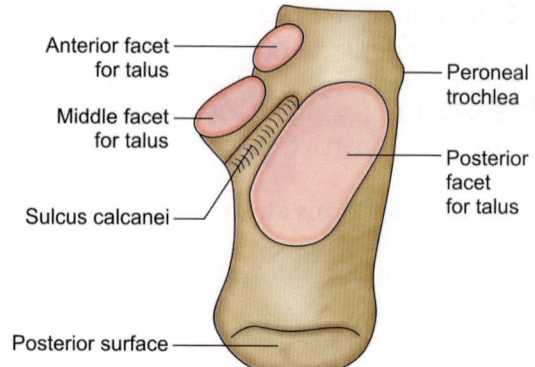

Fig. 16.7: Right calcaneus: Dorsal aspect

a. Medial narrow part is grooved and known as *sulcus calcanei*. It receives attachments of:
    i. *Interosseous talocalcanean ligament* medially.
    ii. *Cervical ligament laterally.*
b. Lateral part (area in front of the posterior facet for talus) provides attachments to:
    i. *Extensor digitorum brevis.*
    ii. *Stem of inferior extensor retinaculum.*
    iii. *Stem of bifurcated ligament.*

D. Plantar surface (Fig. 16.8)

1. It has a smaller tubercle at the anterior end called *anterior tubercle.*
2. The elevation at the posterior end is called *calcaneal teberosity.*

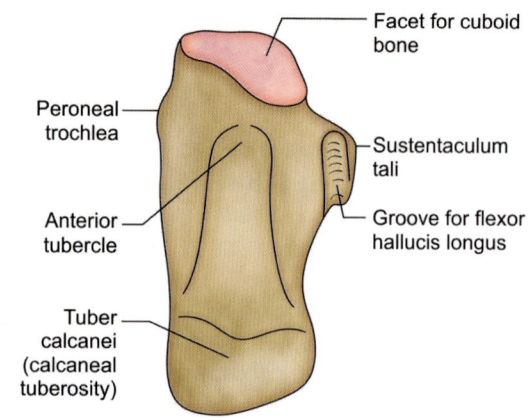

Fig. 16.8: Right calcaneus: Plantar aspect

3. Calcaneal tubersity is further divided into *larger medial* and *smaller lateral processes*.

4. *Flexor retinaculum* and *abductor hallucis* are attached to the medial margin of medial process.

5. *Plantar aponeurosis* and *flexor digitorum brevis* are attached to the distal margin of medial process.

6. *Abductor digiti minimi* is attached to the distal margins of both the processes.

7. To the anterior tubercle is attached *short plantar ligament*.

8. Triangular area between the anterior tubercle and calcaneal tuberosity gives attachment to *long plantar ligament*.

9. Lateral margin of triangular area in front of lateral process provides attachment to *lateral head of flexor digitorum accessorius*.

E. Lateral surface (Figs 16.9 and 16.11)

1. It is almost flat.

2. Most of it is subcutaneous.

3. A small elevation in its anterior part is called *peroneal trochlea (tubercle)*.

4. Peroneal trochlea lies between the tendons of peroneus brevis above and peroneus longus below.

5. Inferior peroneal retinaculum is attached to the peroneal trochlea and margins of the grooves for peronei muscles.

6. *Calcaneofibular ligament* is attached to this surface about a cm behind the peroneal trochlea.

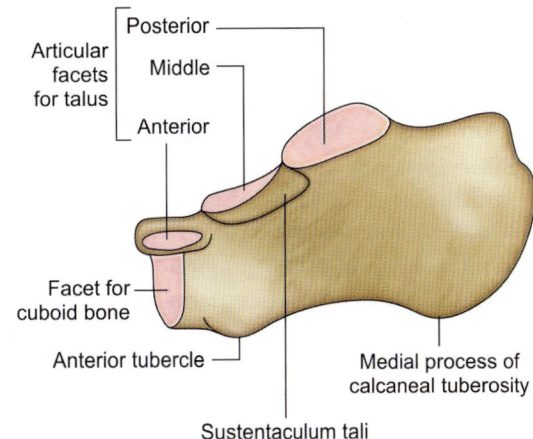

Fig. 16.10: Right calcaneus: Medial aspect

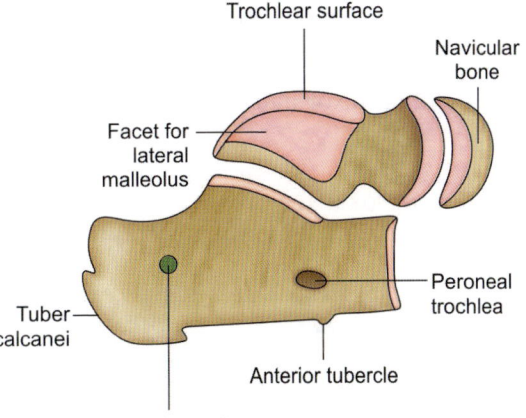

Fig. 16.11: Interrelationships between right talus, calcaneus and navicular bone: Lateral aspect

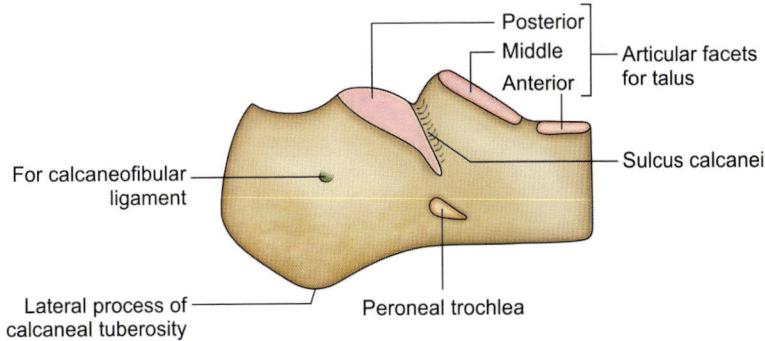

Fig. 16.9: Right calcaneus: Lateral aspect

F. Medial surface (Figs 16.10 and 16.12)

1. It is concave from above downwards.
2. *Sustentaculum tali* is a shelf like projection from its upper anterior part.
3. Superior surface of sustentaculum tali has middle facet for talus which contributes to *talocalcaneonavicular joint.*
4. *Tendon of flexor hallucis longus* grooves the inferior surface of sustentaculum tali.
5. *Tendon of flexor digitorum longus* is related to medial surface of sustentaculum tali.
6. Medial surface of sustentaculum tali provides attachments to:
    i. *Spring ligament.*
    ii. *Slip from tibialis posterior.*
    iii. *Some fibres of superficial part of deltoid ligament.*
7. Medial head of *flexor digitorum accessorius* arises from the medial surface below the groove of flexor hallucis longus.

Ossification

Calcaneus ossifies from a centre which appears during 3rd month of intrauterine life.

> **Note:** *Some times a secondary centre may appear for the posterior surface at the age of 6–8 years. If present, it fuses with the rest of bone at the age of 16 years.*

III. NAVICULAR BONE

Terminology

Navicular is a Latin word which means little ship.

Side determination

1. Deep concave surface faces posteriorly.
2. A prominent projection called *navicular tuberosity,* is directed medially.
3. A groove adjacent to tuberosity is the part of plantar surface and therefore faces inferiorly.

Features and attachments (Figs 16.13 to 16.15)

Navicular has 6 surfaces:

A. Anterior surface

It has 3 facets for corresponding 3 cuneiforms.

B. Posterior surface

It is deeply concave for articulation with head of talus.

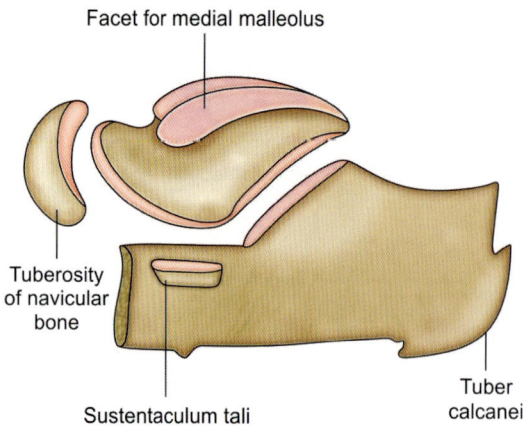

Fig. 16.12: Interrelationships between right talus, calcaneus and navicular bone: Medial aspect

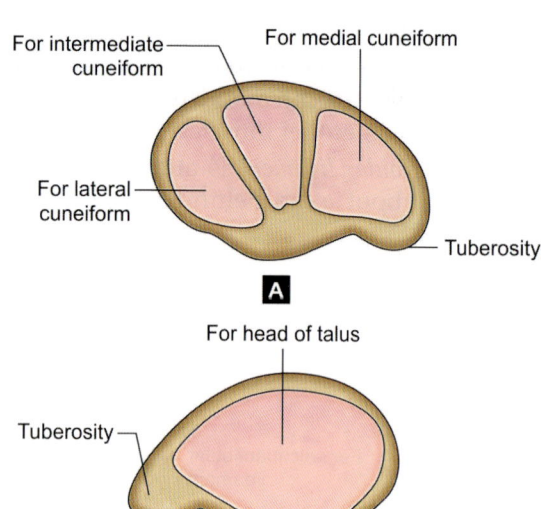

Fig. 16.13: The right navicular bone. (A) Distal aspect; (B) Proximal aspect

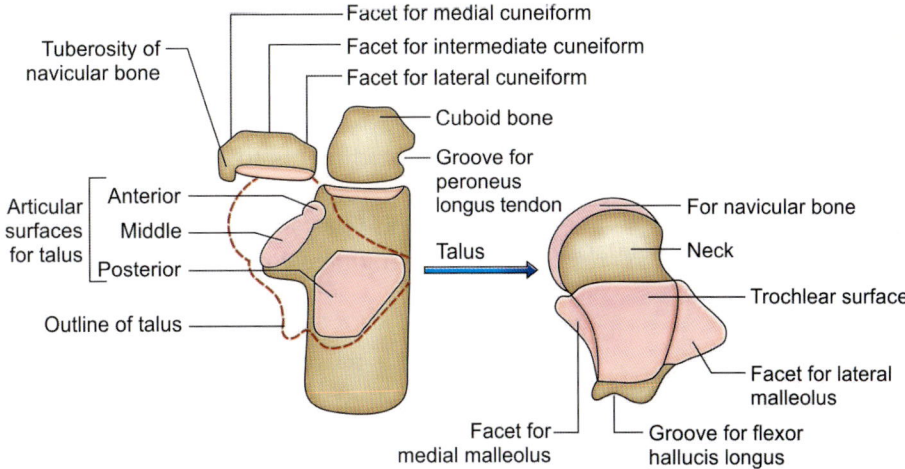

Fig. 16.14: Right talus, calcaneus and navicular and cuboid bones. Dorsal aspect

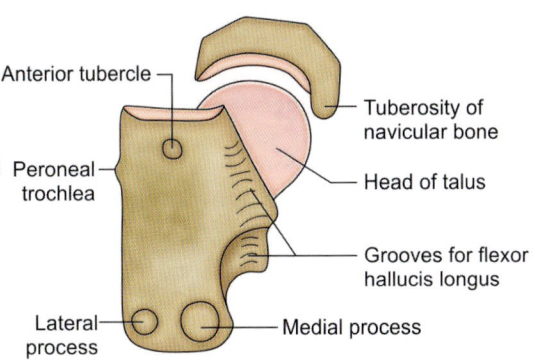

Fig. 16.15: Right talus, calcaneus and navicular bone: Plantar aspect

C. Dorsal surface

It receives attachments of:

1. Dorsal talonavicular ligament.
2. Dorsal cuneonavicular ligaments.
3. Dorsal cubonavicular ligament.

D. Plantar surface

1. Its medial part is marked by a groove through which passes *tendon of tibialis posterior.*
2. Its lateral part receives attachment of *plantar calcaneonavicular (spring) and plantar cuneonavicular ligaments.*

E. Medial surface

It presents the *navicular tuberosity* which receives the insertion of the main part of tendon of *tibialis posteriors.*

F. Lateral surface

It gives attachment to the *medial limb (calcaneonavicular part) of bifurcated ligament.*

Ossification

Navicular bone ossifies from single centre which appears during 4th year.

IV. CUBOID BONE

Terminology

The name of bone is derived from its shape which is approximately cubical.

Side determination

1. Articular surfaces of the cuboid bone are anterior (distal) and posterior (proximal). The proximal surface is one and concavoconvex while distal surface is divided into two by a vertical ridge.
2. Its inferior surface is marked by a groove.
3. Its lateral surface is less extensive and nonarticular while medial surface is more extensive and partly articular.

Features and attachments

Cuboid bone has got 6 surfaces:

A. Anterior surface

1. It is wholly articular.
2. It is divided by a vertical ridge into medial quadrangular and lateral triangular areas for the bases of 4th and 5th metatarsal bones respectively.

B. Posterior surface

It bears a concavoconvex surface for the anterior surface of calcaneus.

C. Plantar surface (Fig. 16.16)

1. A groove in this surface runs medially and forwards and is meant for *tendon of peroneus longus.*
2. There is a ridge behind the groove. This ridge and margins of groove provide attachments to *long plantar ligament.*
3. Surface behind the ridge gives attachment to *short plantar ligament.*

D. Dorsal surface (Fig. 16.17)

It receives attachments of following ligaments:

1. *Dorsal calcaneocuboid.*
2. *Dorsal cubometatarsal.*
3. *Dsorsal cubonavicular.*
4. *Dorsal cuneocuboid.*

E. Medial surface

1. Its anterior part is articular for lateral cuneiform bone.
2. Its posterior part is nonarticular and gives attachments to:
    i. *Calcaneocuboid part of bifurcated ligament.*
    ii. *Interosseous cubonavicular ligament.*
    iii. *Interosseous cuneocuboid ligament*

F. Lateral surface

1. It is narrow and nonarticular.
2. The groove for peroneus longus begins here.

Ossification

Cuboid bone ossifies from one centre which appears just before birth, i.e. at 9th month of intrauterine life.

V. CUNEIFORM BONES

Terminology

Cuneiform is a Latin word which means wedge shaped.

Names

There are three cuneiforms. These are named from medial to lateral as follows:

1. Medial or 1st cuneiform.
2. Intermediate or 2nd cuneiform.
3. Lateral or 3rd cuneiform.

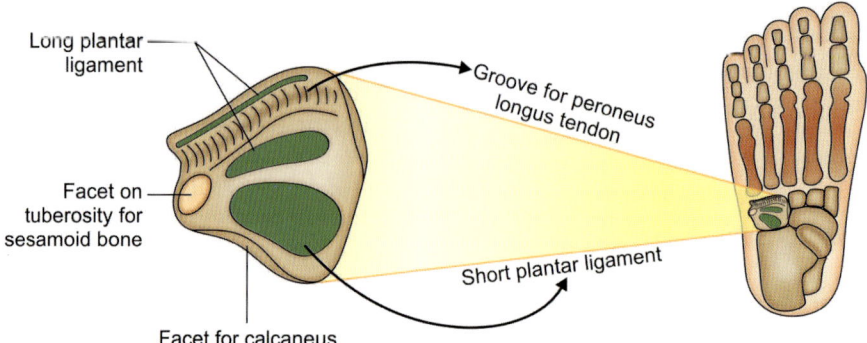

Fig. 16.16: Right cuboid bone: Plantar view

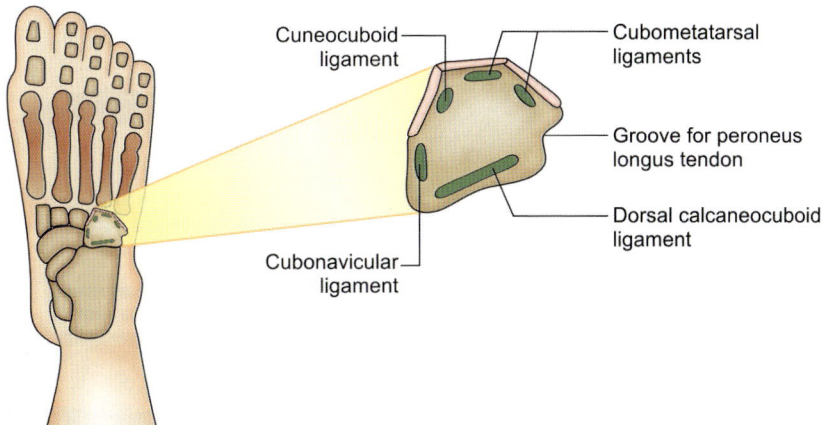

Fig. 16.17: Right cuboid bone: Dorsal view

Sizes

The medial cuneiform is largest while inter-mediate cuneiform is smallest.

Articulations (Fig. 16.18)

1. Proximal surfaces of cuneiforms articulate with navicular bone.
2. Distal surface of medial cuneiform arti-culates with the base of 1st metatarsal bone.
3. Distal surface of intermediate cuneiform articulates with the base of 2nd metatarsal bone.

4. Distal surface of lateral cuneiform arti-culates with the base of 3rd metatarsal bone.
5. Adjacent cuneiforms articulate with each other.
6. Medial and lateral cuneiform bones arti-culate with the corresponding sides of base of 2nd metatarsal.
7. Lateral surface of lateral cuneiform arti-culates with the base of 4th metatarsal and cuboid bones.

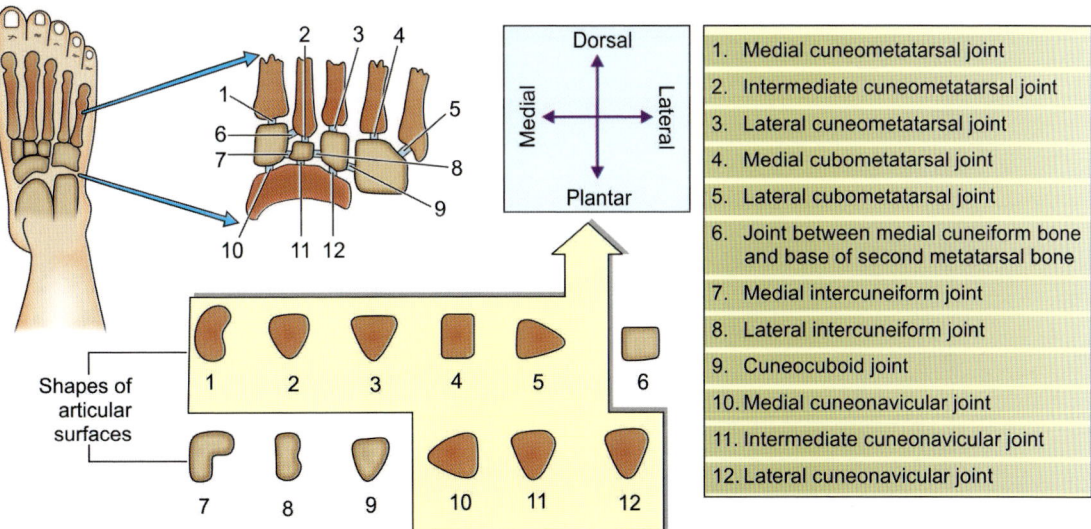

1.	Medial cuneometatarsal joint
2.	Intermediate cuneometatarsal joint
3.	Lateral cuneometatarsal joint
4.	Medial cubometatarsal joint
5.	Lateral cubometatarsal joint
6.	Joint between medial cuneiform bone and base of second metatarsal bone
7.	Medial intercuneiform joint
8.	Lateral intercuneiform joint
9.	Cuneocuboid joint
10.	Medial cuneonavicular joint
11.	Intermediate cuneonavicular joint
12.	Lateral cuneonavicular joint

Fig. 16.18: Right cuneiform bones: Dorsal aspect

Attachments

1. Medial cuneiform receives attachments of *tibialis anterior* and *peroneus longus*.
2. Slips of *tibialis posterior* extend to plantar surfaces of all cuneiforms.
3. In general three cuneiforms receive attachments of interosseous, dorsal and plantar ligaments (Fig. 16.19).

Ossification

Each cuneiform ossifies from one centre, the time of appearance for which is as follows:

Lateral cuneiform	: 1 year
Medial cuneiform	: 2 years
Intermediate cuneiform	: 3 years

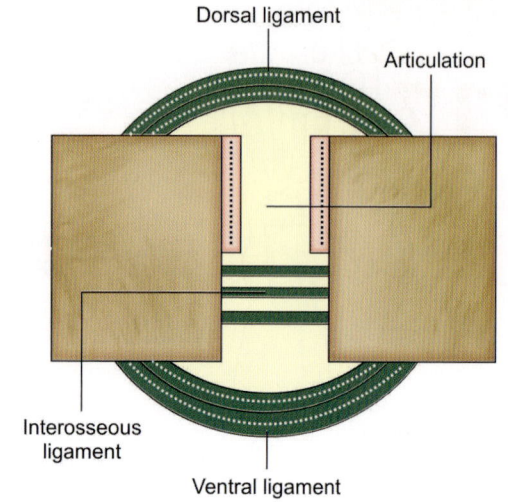

Fig. 16.19: Ligaments attached to cuneiform bones

Metatarsal Bones

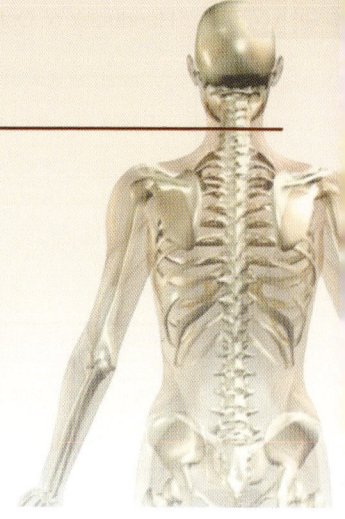

METATARSUS

Five metatarsal bones together constitute the metatarsus.

NAMING THE METATARSAL BONES (Fig. 17.1)

Metatarsal bones are named by numbering them. They are numbered from medial to lateral, i.e. the metatarsal bone along the great toe is called 1st metatarsal bone and the metatarsal bone along the little toe is known as 5th metatarsal bone.

IDENTIFICATION OF METATARSAL BONES (Fig. 17.2)

1st metatarsal bone

1. It is shortest and thickest.
2. Proximal surface of its base possesses a kidney shaped articular surface.

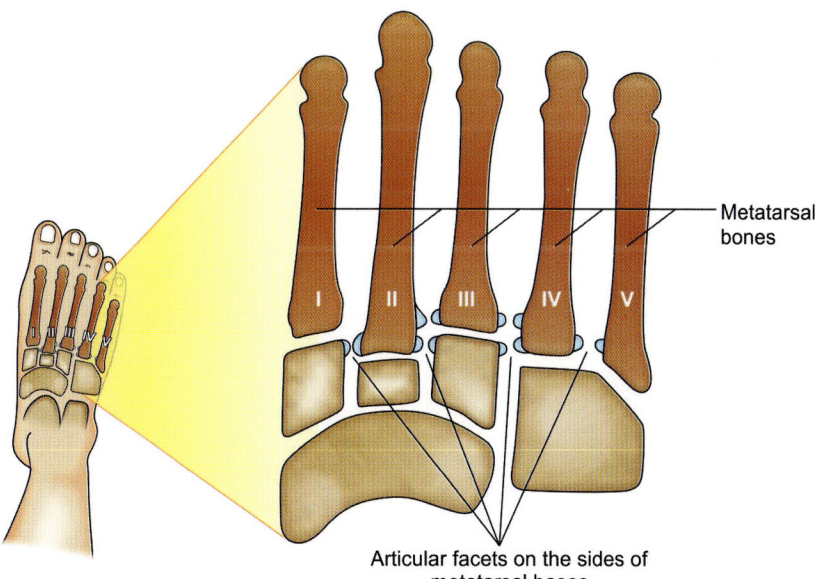

Articular facets on the sides of metatarsal bases

Fig. 17.1: Skeleton of right foot: Dorsal aspect

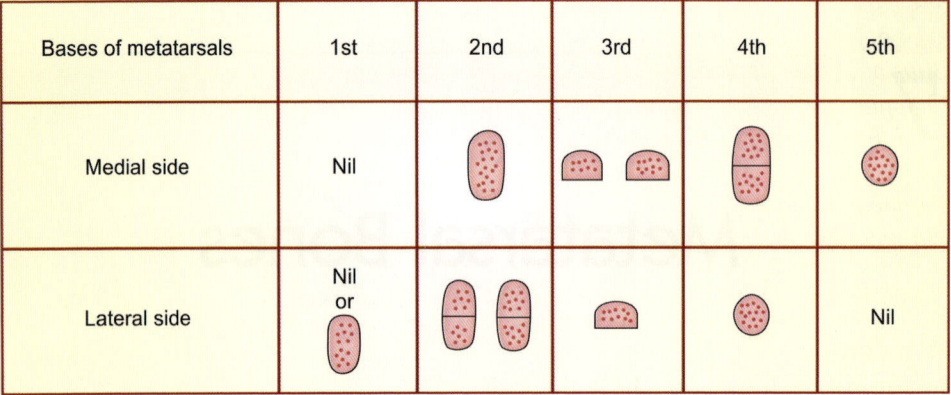

Bases of metatarsals	1st	2nd	3rd	4th	5th
Medial side	Nil				
Lateral side	Nil or				Nil

Fig. 17.2: Shapes of articular facets by the sides of bases of metatarsal bones

2nd metatarsal bone

1. Proximal surface of its base has triangular articular surface.
2. One side of the base has single facet while the other side possesses two facets divided into four.

3rd metatarsal bone

It has two facets on one side and one facet on the other side of the base.

4th metatarsal bone

It has a quadrilateral facet on the proximal surface of base and single facet on one side and one facet divided into two on the other side.

5th metatarsal bone

The lateral aspect of base projects proximally to form *styloid process*.

FEATURES AND ATTACHMENTS

Metatarsal bones are miniature long bones. Each metatarsal bone has got a distal end (head), a shaft or body and a proximal end (base).

I. HEAD

1. Its articular surface meets with the base of corresponding proximal phalanx.
2. Articular surface is more extensive on the plantar aspect.

3. Each side of the head shows a tubercle dorsally for callateral ligament of tarso-metatarsal joint.

II. SHAFT

1. It is concave on its plantar aspect.
2. Sides of the shaft provide attachments to interossei muscles.
3. Plantar aspect of 5th metatarsal bone gives origin to flexor digiti minimi.

III. BASE

1. Articulations of proximal surfaces and the shapes of articular surfaces are as follows:

Metatarsal-sal bone	Proximal bone	Shape of the articular surface
1st	Medial cuneiform bone	Kidney shaped
2nd	Intermediate cuneiform bone	Triangular
3rd	Lateral cunciform bone	Triangular
4th	Cuboid bone	Quadrangular
5th	Cuboid bone	Triangular

2. Both the sides of bases of middle 3 metatarsal bones and lateral side of 1st and medial side of 5th metatarsal bones possess articular facets the details of which are as follows:
3. Base of 1st metatarsal bone gives attach-ments to:
    i. Tibialis anterior.
    ii. Peroneus longus.

4. Plantar aspects of bases of middle 3 meta-tarsal bones provide attachments to:
    i. *Slips of tibialis posterior.*
    ii. *Oblique head of adductor hallucis.*
5. Base of 5th metatarsal bone receives insertions of:
    i. *Peroneus tertius.*
    ii. *Peroneus brevis.*

OSSIFICATION

A. Primary centre

One centre appears for the shaft of each metatarsal bone as follows:

1st metatarsal bone—10th week of intra-uterine life.

Rest of the metatarsal bone—9th week of intrauterine life.

B. Secondary centre

Only one secondary centre appears for each metatarsal bone.

Location

1st metatarsal bone	: Base
Rest of the metatarsal bones	: Head
Appearance	: 3 years
Fusion	: 18 years

Phalanges of the Foot

The total number of phalanges in each foot is 14. Great toe has got only two phalanges, i.e. proximal and distal. Rest of the toes have got three phalanges each, i.e. proximal, middle and distal (Fig. 18.1).

CHARACTERISTICS

1. Phalanges of the foot are very much similar to those of hand as far as features are concerned but in foot they are relatively smaller.
2. Each phalanx has *base* (proximal end), *shaft* and *head* (distal end).

3. Articular surfaces show similarities with those of phalanges of hand.
4. The distal phalanx of each toe bears a roughened tuberosity on the plantar aspect of its distal end. This gives attachment to the pulp of the tip of the toe and provides a wider area to take pressure.

OSSIFICATION

A. Primary centre

One centre appears for the shaft as follows:
Proximal phalanx : 12th week of IUL.

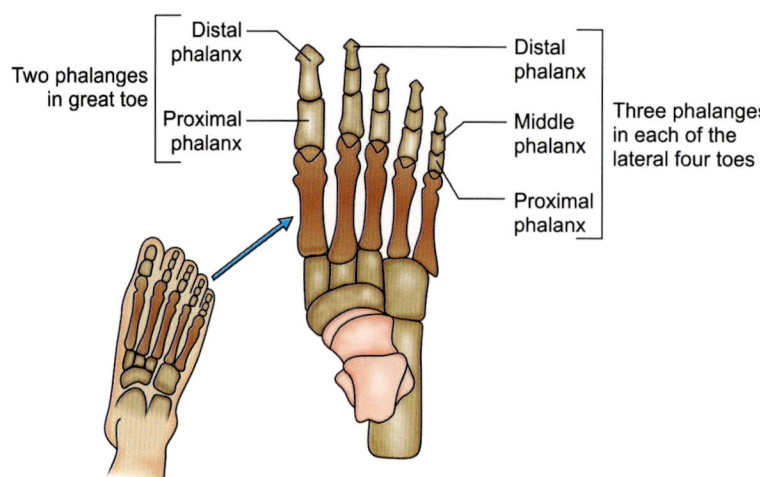

Fig. 18.1: Skeleton of right foot: Dorsal aspect

Middle phalanx : 15th week of intrauterine life

Distal phalanx : 9th week of intrauterine
life

B. Secondary centre

One centre appears for the base of each
phalanx.

Appearance

Proximal phalanx : 2 years

Middle phalanx : 4 years

Distal phalanx : 6 years

Fusion : 18 years

Vertebrae

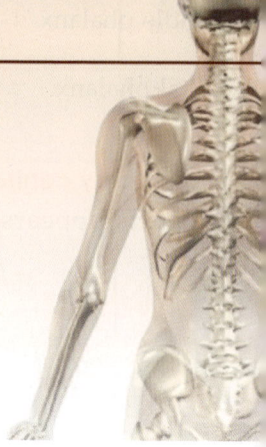

GENERAL CONSIDERATIONS

1. Vertebral column is made up of a number of irregular bones called vertebrae.
2. Vertebral column forms the central axis of the body.
3. There are 33 vertebrae.
4. Vertebrae are named according to regions they belong.
5. Following is the classification of vertebrae:

Cervical vertebrae	7
Thoracic vertebrae	12
Lumbar vertebrae	5
Sacral vertebrae	5 (these fuse to form single *sacrum*)
Coccygeal vertebrae	4 (these fuse to form single *coccyx*)

6. Vertebrae are mobile or fixed.
7. Mobile vertebrae are called *true vertebrae* while fixed vertebrae are called *false vertebrae*.
8. Movable vertebrae are cervical, thoracic and lumbar.
9. Sacral and coccygeal vertebrae are immobile.

CURVATURES OF VERTEBRAL COLUMN (Fig. 19.1)

a. Primary curvatures

1. During intrauterine life the whole vertebral column is concave ventrally and convex dorsally. This is *primary curvature*.
2. In adult primary curvatures are retained only in thoracic and sacral regions.
3. They are mainly due to the shape of vertebrae.

b. Secondary curvatures

1. Secondary curvatures are convex forwards.
2. They develop after birth.
3. They develop due to posture.
4. They are mainly due to the shape of intervertebral discs.
5. Secondary curvatures are observed in cervical and lumbar regions.
6. Cervical curvature appears around 6–9 months when the child starts holding his head by himself.
7. Lumbar curvature appears at about 12–18 months when the child starts walking.

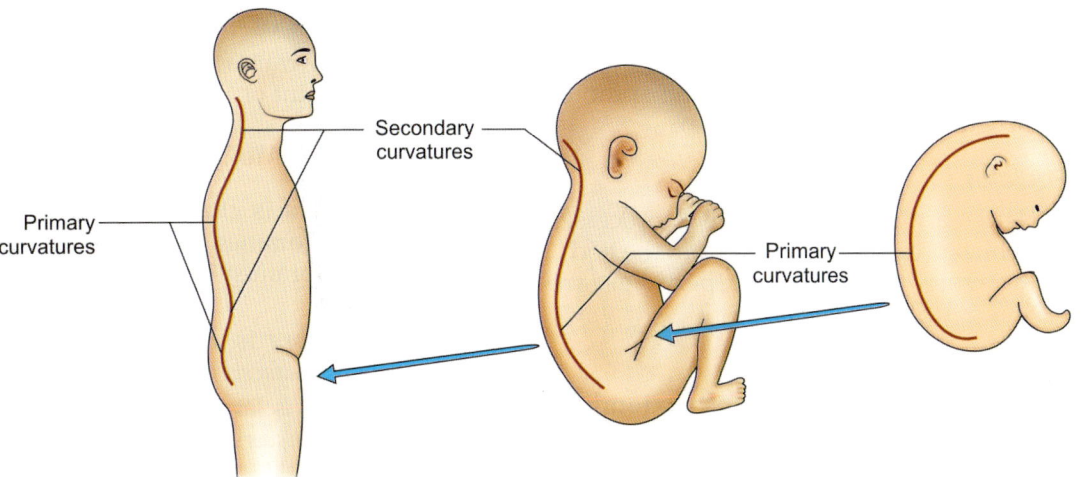

Fig. 19.1: Curvatures of vertebral column

MOVEMENTS OF VERTEBRAL COLUMN

Vertebral column shows following movements:

1. *Flexion*: Forward bending.
2. *Extension*: Backward bending.
3. *Lateral flexion*: Side bending.
4. *Rotation*: Twisting of trunk.
5. *Circumduction*: Combination of all the above movements.

FEATURES OF A TYPICAL VERTEBRA (Fig. 19.2)

A typical vertebra is made up of 2 parts, body and vertebral arch.

a. Body

1. It is ventral part of a vertebra.
2. It is cylindrical in shape.
3. It has 4 surfaces, anterior, posterior, superior and inferior.
4. Anterior surface is convex from side to side and concave from above downwards.
5. Posterior surface is slightly concave from side to side but flat from above downwards. It has number of foramina for exit of *basivertebral veins*. It forms anterior boundary of vertebral foramen.
6. Upper and lower surfaces are rough for the intervertebral discs.

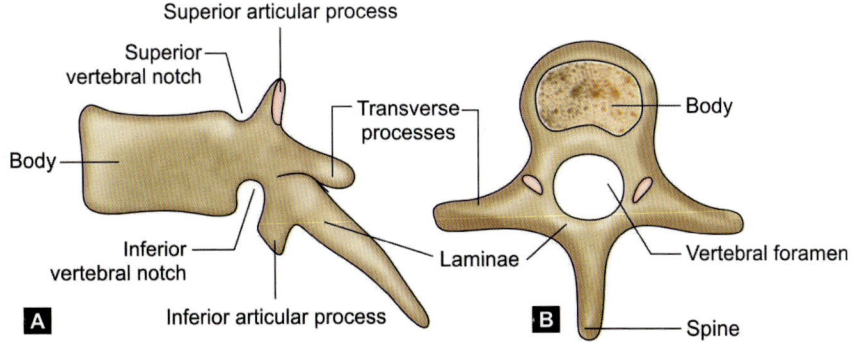

Fig. 19.2: A typical vertebra. (A) Left lateral view; (B) Superior view

b. Vertebral arch

It consists of a pair of pedicles, a pair of laminae and seven processes (one spinous, four articular and two transverse).

i. Pedicles

1. These are pair of short thick processes which project backwards from the body.
2. Between the adjacent pedicles are *intervertebral foramina*.

ii. Laminae

1. These are bony plates extending backwards and medially from posterior end of the pedicles.
2. Posteriorly they fuse to form spine in the midline.
3. Body, pedicles and laminae together enclose the foramen of vertebra called *vertebral foramen*.

iii. Transverse process

It projects laterally on each side from the junction of pedicle and lamina.

iv. Articular processes

1. They are two on each side and four in total.
2. They are *superior and inferior articular processes* projecting upwards and downwards respectively from the junction of pedicle and lamina.

v. Spinous process (spine)

It projects backwards in the midline from the meeting point of laminae.

DISTINGUISHING FEATURES (Fig. 19.3)

1. *Cervical vertebra* is characterized by the presence of a foramen in each transverse process. This foramen is named as *foramen transversarium*.
2. *Thoracic vertebra* is recognized by the presence of *costal facets* on the sides of body.
3. *Lumbar vertebra* is larger in size and lacks both *foramen transversarium* as well as *costal facets*.
4. There is no isolated sacral vertebra. Five *sacral vertebrae* fuse to form single piece of triangular and curved **sacrum**.
5. Similarly there is no isolated coccygeal vertebra. Four *coccygeal vertebrae* fuse to form single piece of **coccyx**. Coccyx is relatively very small in size than sacrum.

REGIONAL VERTEBRAE

I. CERVICAL VERTEBRAE

These are classified as *typical* and *atypical*. 3rd to 6th cervical vertebrae are typical. 1st, 2nd and 7th cervical vertebrae are atypical.

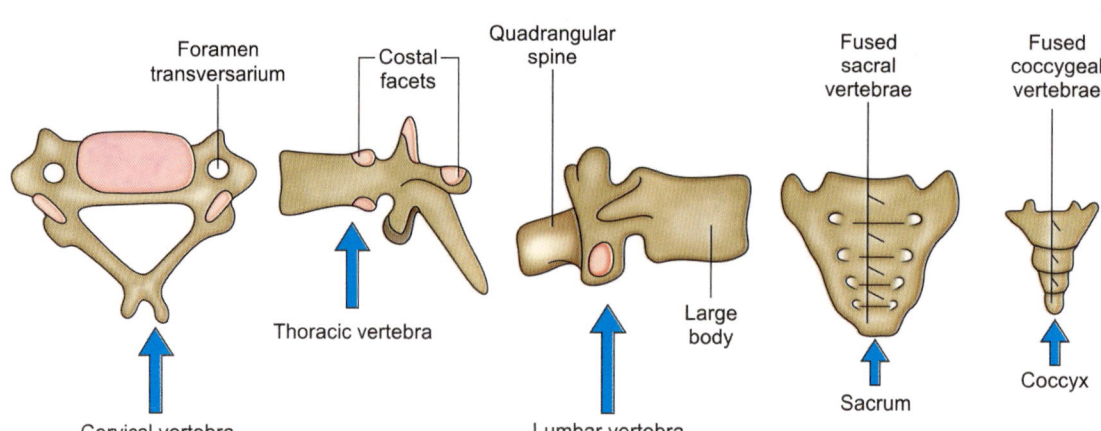

Fig. 19.3: Distinguishing features of vertebrae

A. Typical cervical vertebra (Fig. 19.4)

It has a *body* and a *vertebral arch*. These enclose *vertebral foramen*.

a. Body

1. It is smallest among all vertebrae.
2. It is narrower anteroposteriorly.
3. It has 4 surfaces; *superior, inferior, anterior* and *posterior*.
4. Its superior surface is concave from side to side with an upward projecting lip on either side. This surface is mainly related to *intervertebral disc*.
5. The inferior surface is convex from side to side. The anterior border of inferior surface projects downwards to hide the intervertebral disc. Inferior surface, like superior surface is also related to *intervertebral disc*.

6. Anterior surface provides attachments to *anterior longitudinal ligament* in the middle and *longus colli muscle* on either side of it.
7. Posterior surface has number of foramina for *basivertebral veins*. Its superior and inferior margins provide attachments to *posterior longitudinal ligament*.

b. Vertebral foramen

1. It is triangular in shape.
2. It is bigger than the body.

c. Vertebral arch

It is comprised of *pedicles, laminae*, the *superior* and *inferior articular processes*, the *transverse processes* and *spine*.

i. Pedicles (Fig. 19.5)

1. They are directed backwards and laterally. It is this direction which is

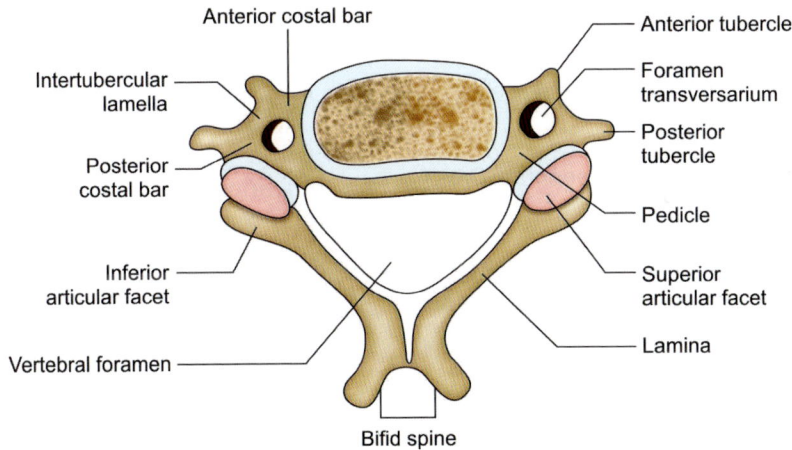

Fig. 19.4: Typical cervical vertebra: Superior aspect

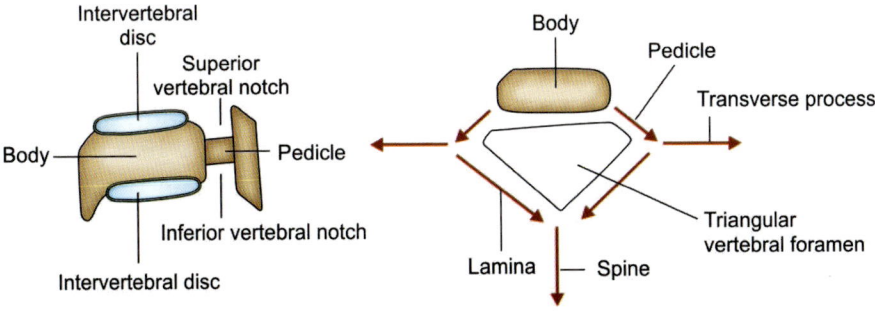

Fig. 19.5: The pedicle of cervical vertebra

responsible for triangular shape of vertebral foramen.

2. Above and below the pedicles are *superior* and *inferior vertebral notches* respectively. These notches are equal in size.

ii. Laminae (Fig. 19.6)

1. These are long and narrow.
2. The superior border is thinner than the inferior border.
3. *Ligamentum flavum* is attached to its superior border and lower part of its anterior surface.

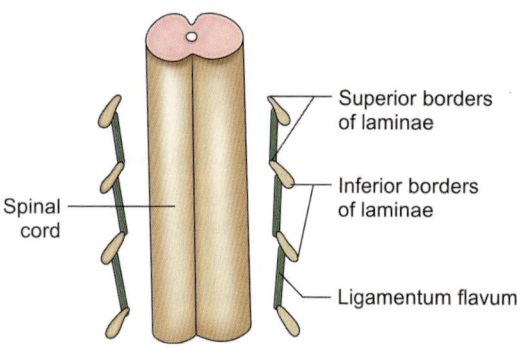

Fig. 19.6: The laminae of cervical vertebrae: Cross-sectional view

iii. Articular processes

1. *Superior* and *inferior articular processes* are located on each side, above and below the junction of pedicle and lamina.
2. *Superior articular process* faces upwards and backwards.
3. *Inferior articular process* is directed downwards and forwards.
4. Superior articular process of a vertebra articulates with inferior articular process of the vertebra above.
5. Articular processes lie in one line forming an *articular pillar*.

iv. Transverse process

1. It has got a foramen called *foramen transversarium*, which forms a characteristic feature of *cervical vertebra*.

2. *Vertebral artery, vertebral vein* and *sympathetic nerves* pass through foramen transversarium (vertebral artery passes through upper 6 foramina only).

3. The foramen transversarium is bounded anteriorly and posteriorly by *anterior and posterior roots* respectively.

4. The lateral ends of the anterior and posterior roots are connected by *costotransverse bar* or *intertubercular lamella* (Fig. 19.7).

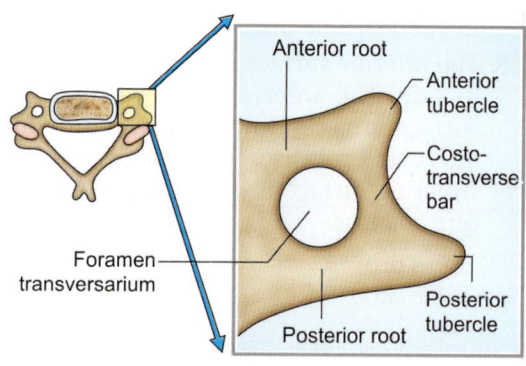

Fig. 19.7: Foramen transversarium

5. Junctions of anterior and posterior roots with costotransverse bar are marked by *anterior and posterior tubercles* respectively.

6. The enlarged anterior tubercle of the sixth cervical vertebra is called *carotid tubercle*. This is related to *common carotid artery*.

7. Anterior tubercles give origins to *scalenus anterior, longus capitis* and *longus colli muscles*.

8. Posterior tubercles provide attachments to *levator scapulae, scalenus medius, scalenus posterior* and some *deep muscles of the back*

9. The anterior root, anterior tubercle, costotransverse bar, posterior tubercle and adjoining (lateral part of) posterior root represent the *costal element* while the medial part of posterior root represents the *transverse element* of the developing vertebra (Fig. 19.8).

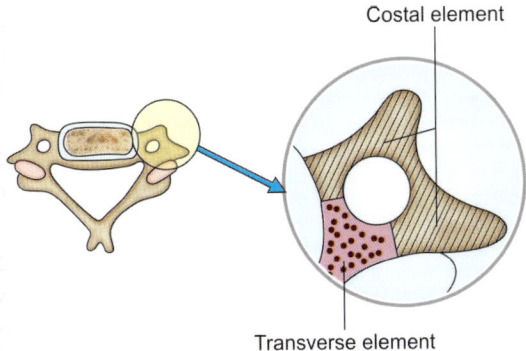

Costal element

Transverse element

Fig. 19.8: Costal and transverse elements of transverse process

v. Spine

1. It is small and bifid.
2. *Ligamentum nuchae* is attached to the *spinous notch*.
3. *Interspinous ligaments* are attached to its superior and inferior borders.
4. Sides provide attachments to *deep muscles of the back* (Fig. 19.9).

B. Atypical cervical vertebrae

First cervical vertebra

Terminology

It is also named as *atlas* because it supports the skull. According to Greek mythology, Atlas is the God who supported the earth on his shoulders.

Distinguishing features

1. It is ring shaped with narrow anterior and posterior arches.
2. It has no body.
3. It has no spine.
4. It has a large *lateral mass* on either side.
5. The two *transverse processes* are widest apart relative to other cervical vertebrae.

Normal anatomical position

1. Two arches lie in same horizontal plane.
2. *Anterior arch* is smaller than the *posterior arch*.
3. *Superior articular facets* on lateral masses are elongated.

Features and attachments
(Figs 19.10 and 19.11)

Atlas has got an *anterior arch*, a *posterior arch* and two *lateral masses*.

a. Anterior arch

1. It is smaller than the posterior arch.
2. It connects the two lateral masses.

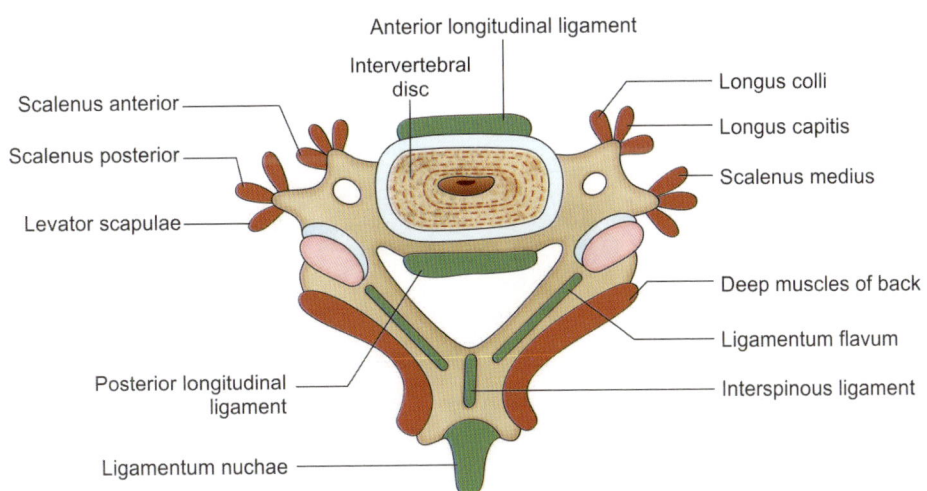

Anterior longitudinal ligament

Intervertebral disc

Scalenus anterior

Scalenus posterior

Levator scapulae

Posterior longitudinal ligament

Ligamentum nuchae

Longus colli

Longus capitis

Scalenus medius

Deep muscles of back

Ligamentum flavum

Interspinous ligament

Fig. 19.9: Main attachments and relations of typical cervical vertebra

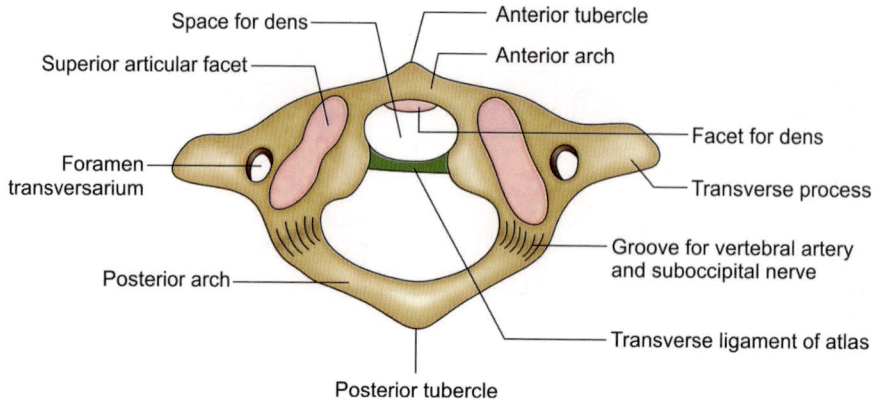

Fig. 19.10: Atlas: Superior aspect

3. *Anterior tubercle* is present on its anterior aspect in the midline. Midline part of upper end of *anterior longitudinal ligament* is attached to it.
4. Its anterior surface on each side of anterior tubercle provides attachment to *longus colli muscle.*
5. An *oval facet* is present on its posterior surface in the midline for articulation with dens of 2nd cervical vertebra to form the *atlantoaxial joint.*
6. *Anterior atlanto-occipital membrane* is attached to the upper border of anterior arch.

7. Lateral part of upper end of *anterior longitudinal ligament* is attached to the lower border of anterior arch.

b. Posterior arch

1. It is longer than the anterior arch.
2. Midline *posterior tubercle* on its posterior surface represents the spine.
3. *Ligamentum nuchae* is attached to the posterior tubercle.
4. On each side of posterior tubercle is attached the *rectus capitis posterior minor.*
5. *Vertebral artery (3rd part)* and *first cervical nerve* lie in the shallow groove on the

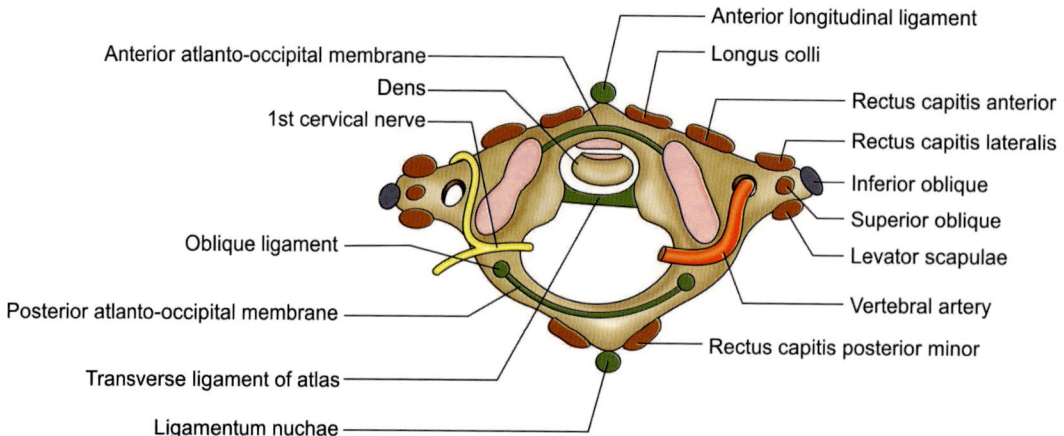

Fig. 19.11: Attachments and relations of atlas: Superior view

superior surface of posterior arch just behind the lateral mass.

6. *Posterior atlanto-occipital membrane* is attached to the superior border behind the grooves.

7. *Ligamentum flavum* is attached to its lower border on each side of midline.

c. *Lateral masses*

Each lateral mass has got two articular facets (superior and inferior), two surfaces (anterior and medial) and a transverse process.

1. *Superior articular facet* is concave and elongated. It articulates with occipital condyle to from *atlanto-occipital joint.*

Note: *Remember, we say 'No' at atlanto-axial joint, i.e. move the head from side to side while we say 'Yes' at atlanto-occipital joint, i.e. perform nodding movement of the head.*

2. *Inferior articular facet* is flat and circular. It articulates with axis.

3. *Medial surface* has got a *tubercle for transverse ligament of atlas.*

4. *Anterior surface* gives origin to *rectus capitis anterior.*

5. *Transverse process* is long and strong. It has *foramen transversarium* which transmits *vertebral artery, vertebral vein* and *sympathetic nerve. Rectus capitis lateralis, levator scapulae* and *superior oblique muscles* are attached to its superior aspect around the foramen transversarium. *Inferior oblique muscle* is attached to its inferior surface. Anterior aspect of transverse process is related to *ventral ramus of 1st cervical nerve* and *accessory nerve.*

Second cervical vertebra (Figs 19.12 and 19.13)

Terminology

It is also called *axis* because atlas carrying the skull rotates on it.

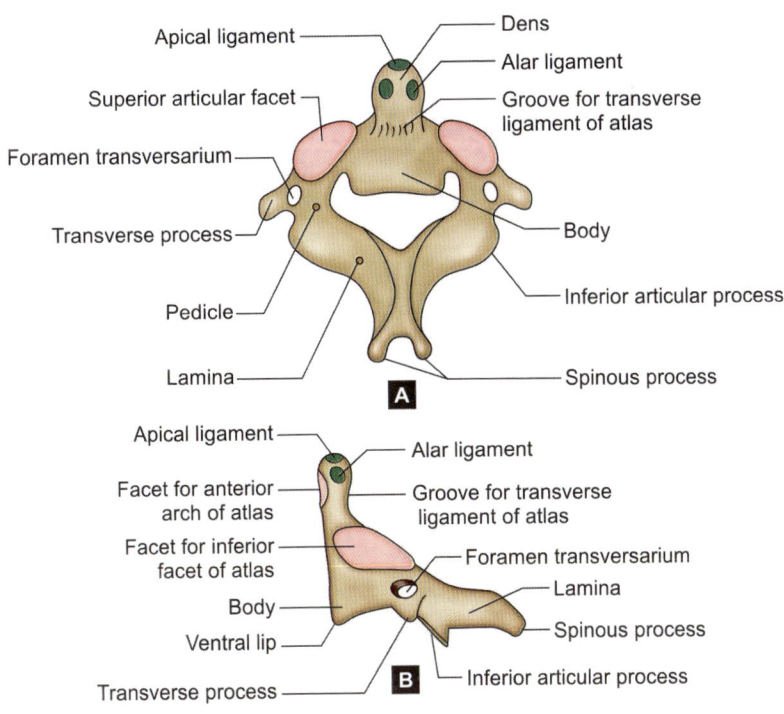

Fig. 19.12: Axis: (A) Posterosuperior aspect; (B) Lateral aspect

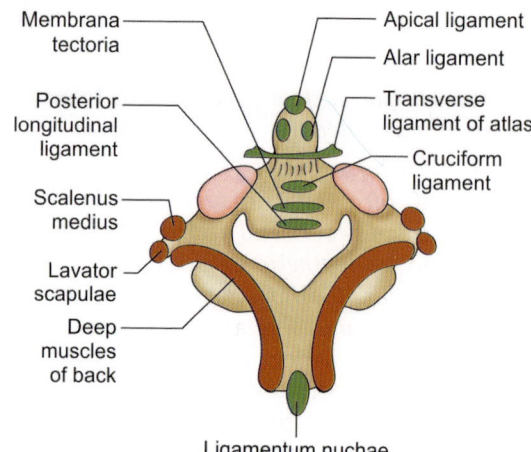

Membrana tectoria — Apical ligament — Alar ligament

Posterior longitudinal ligament — Transverse ligament of atlas

Scalenus medius — Cruciform ligament

Lavator scapulae

Deep muscles of back

Ligamentum nuchae

Fig. 19.13: Attachments and relations of axis: Posterosuperior view

Peculiarities

1. It is strongest of the cervical vertebrae.
2. It is easily identified by the presence of an *odontoid process (dens)* which is a strong tooth like projection from the superior surface of body.

Features and attachments

a. Body and odontoid process

1. Apex of odontoid process gives attachment to *apical ligament*.
2. On each side of the apex, the sloping gives attachment to *alar ligament*.
3. Anterior surface of odontoid process possesses an oval facet for articulation with anterior arch of atlas.
4. Posterior surface of odontoid process is grooved to lodge *transverse ligament of atlas*.
5. Inferior surface of body is related to *intervertebral disc*.
6. The anterior surface of body gives attachments to *anterior longitudinal ligament* in the midline and *longus colli muscle* on each side.
7. The posterior surface of the body provides attachments to following 3 structures from above downwards:

   i. *Lower vertical limb of cruciform ligament.*
   ii. *Membrana tectoria.*
   iii. *Posterior longitudinal ligament.*
8. *Superior articular facet* (for articulation with the inferior facet of atlas) is situated lateral to odontoid process, partly over the body and partly on the pedicle.

b. Vertebral arch

1. The pedicle passes backwards from the upper part of body.
2. *Superior articular facet* is large, flat and circular. It is directed upwards and laterally.
3. *Inferior articular facet* is situated posterior to transverse process and is directed downwards and forwards.
4. *Spine* is short, thick and strong. Its tip is bifid and receives attachment of *ligamentum nuchae*.
5. *Ligamentum flavum* is attached to superior border and lower part of anterior surface of *lamina on each side*.
6. Side of spine provides attachment to *rectus capitis posterior major*.
7. External surface of lamina is meant for the attachment of *inferior oblique* in its upper part and *deep muscles of back* in its lower part.
8. *Transverse processes* are very small. They represent the true posterior tubercles only.
9. The tip of transverse process receives attachments of following 3 muscles from anterior to posterior:

   i. *Scalenus medius*
   ii. *Levator scapulae*
   iii. *Deep muscles of back*

Seventh cervical vertebra

Terminology

It is also called *vertebra prominens* because it has a very long spine which may be palpated under the skin of lower part of the back of neck.

Peculiarities (Fig. 19.14)

1. *Spine* is long, horizontal and nonbifid.
2. *Transverse process* is large with prominent posterior tubercle.
3. *Foramen transversarium* is smaller and some times may be absent.

Important attachments and relations

1. *Spine* provides attachments to *ligamentum nuchae, trapezius, rhomhoideus minor* and *deep muscles of back.*
2. *Posterior tubercle* of transverse process receives attachments of *suprapleural membrane* and *scalenus minimus.*
3. *Foramen transversarium* transmits *accessory vertebral vein.*

Note: *Vertebral artery occupies the foramina transversaria of the upper 6 cervical vertebrae only*

II. THORACIC VERTEBRAE

There are 12 thoracic vertebrae. They can be classified as *typical* and *atypical*. 2nd to 8th thoracic vertebrae are typical while 1st and 9th to 12th thoracic vertebrae are atypical.

A. Typical thoracic vertebra
Peculiarities

1. *Articular facets* are present by the side of body and front of transverse processes.
2. *Body* is heart shaped.
3. *Vertebral foramen* is circular.
4. *Spinous process* is long, pointed and directed downwards.
5. *Pedicle* is attached to the upper part of the body making the *inferior vertebral notch* deeper.

Features and attachments (Figs 19.15 to 19.17)

Typical thoracic vertebra has got a *body* and a *vertebral arch*. These enclose a relatively smaller and circular vertebral foramen.

a. Body

1. It is heart shaped.
2. Its anteroposterior and transverse dimensions are almost equal.
3. On each side, the body is characterized by the presence of 2 *costal facets, superior* and *inferior.*

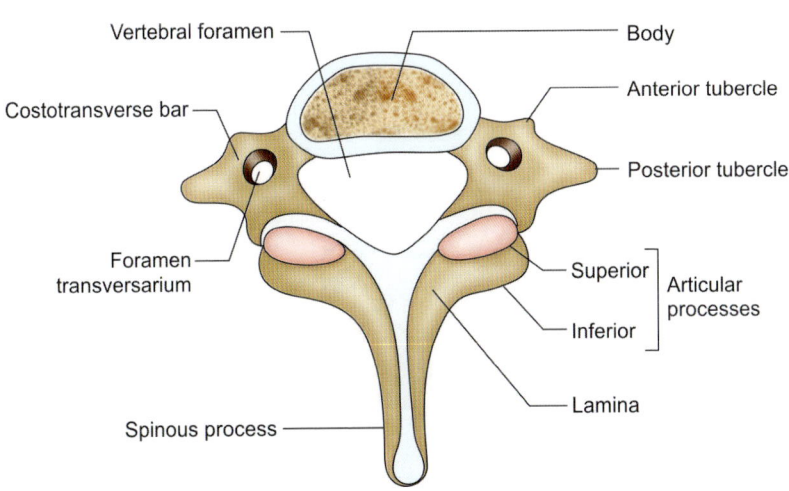

Fig. 19.14: Vertebra prominens: Superior aspect

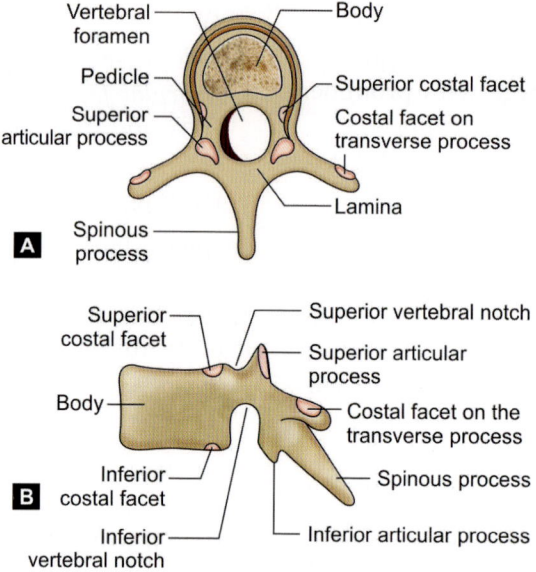

Fig. 19.15: Typical thoracic vertebra. (A) Superior aspect; (B) Left lateral aspect

4. *Superior costal facet* is larger and situated on the upper border of body near the pedicle.
5. *Inferior costal facet* is smaller and placed near the lower border just in front of inferior vertebral notch.
6. Anterior surface of body provides attachment to anterior *longitudinal ligament.*
7. Posterior surface is marked by *vascular foramina for basivertebral veins* which are covered by *posterior longitudinal ligament.*

The latter is attached to the upper and lower borders of the posterior surface of body.

b. *Vertebral arch*

Vertebral arch consists of a pair of *pedicles, laminae,* the *superior* and *inferior articular processes,* the *transverse processes* and a *spine.*

i. **Pedicles**

1. These are directed backwards, i.e. do not diverge and therefore making the vertebral foramen circular.

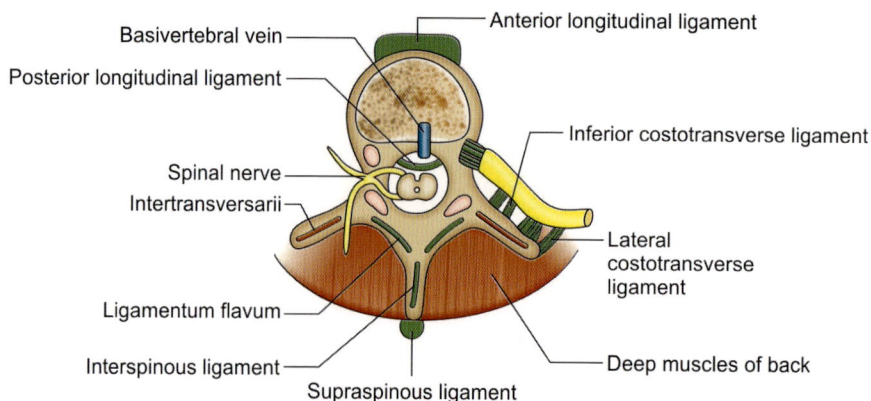

Fig. 19.16: Attachments and relations of thoracic vertebra: Superior view

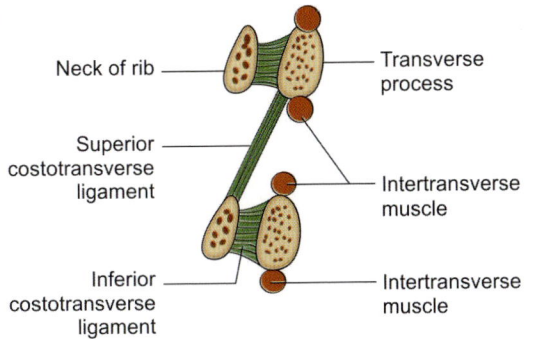

Fig. 19.17: Attachments of transverse process of a thoracic vertebra

2. Pedicles are attached nearer the superior border of body and thus the *superior vertebral notch* is shallow where as the *inferior vertebral notch* is deep.

ii. *Laminae*
1. They overlap each other from above downwards.
2. *Ligamenta flava* are attached to their upper borders and lower parts of anterior surfaces.
3. *Deep muscles of back* are attached to the posterior surfaces of laminae.

iii. *Superior articular processes*
1. These are flat surfaces located on the superior aspects of junctions of pedicles and laminae.
2. These facets are directed *backwards* and slightly laterally.

iv. *Inferior articular processes*
1. They are fused with the lateral ends of laminae.
2. Each articular facet is flat and faces forwards and little downwards and medially.

v. *Transverse processes*
1. They project backwards and laterally from the junction of pedicles and laminae between the superior and inferior articular processes.
2. A *facet* is observed on its anterior surface near the tip for articulation with the tubercle of numerically corresponding rib.

3. Tip provides attachment to *lateral costotransverse ligament.*
4. Its anterior surface medial to facet receives attachment of *(inferior) costotransverse ligament.*
5. *Superior costotransverse ligament* is attached to lower border of transverse process.

Note: *Superior costotransverse ligament is superior in relation to the neck of rib below.*

6. *Intertransverse mucles* are attached to superior and inferior borders of transverse processes.
7. Posterior surfaces of transverse processes near their lateral ends provide attachments to *levatores costarum.*

vi. *Spine*
It is long, pointed and in general directed downwards.

Note: *In the middle four vertebrae the spinous processes are almost vertical.*

Thoracic spines provide attachments to the following structures:
1. *Trapezius* (all the thoracic spines) and *latissimus dorsi* (lower six thoracic spines) *muscles.*
2. *Interspinous and supraspinous ligaments.*
3. *Rhomboideus major* (2nd to 5th thoracic spines) and rhomboideus minor (1st thoracic spine) muscles.
4. *Serratus posterior superior* (upper three thoracic spines) and *serratus posterior inferior* (lower two thoracic spines) muscles.
5. *Deep muscles of the back.*

B. Atypical thoracic vertebrae (Fig. 19.18)

First thoracic vertebra

1. Its *body* is more like a cervical vertebra with the upper surface of body showing lateral lipping and is bevelled anteriorly.
2. *Superior costal facet* on the lateral aspect of body is complete for articulation with the head of 1st rib.

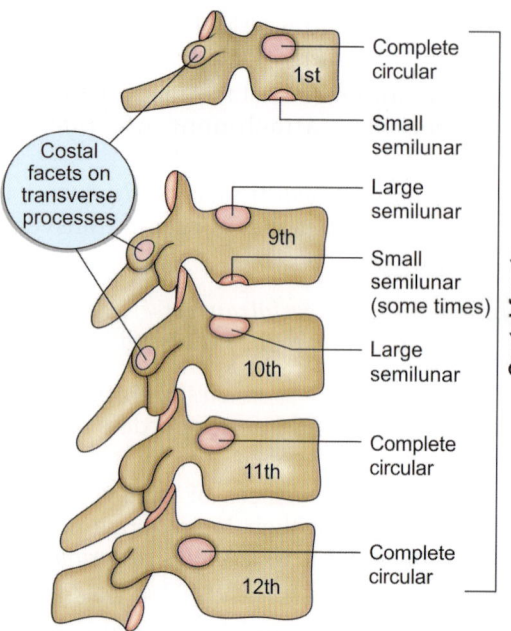

Fig. 19.18: Atypical thoracic vertebrae: Right lateral aspect

3. *Inferior costal facet* is half (demifacet) for 2nd rib.
4. *Spine* is nearly horizontal.
5. *Superior vertebral notches* are well marked.

Ninth thoracic vertebra

1. *Body* has got only *superior costal facets* (demifacets).
2. Inferior costal facets are absent.

Tenth thoracic vertebra

1. *Body* has single complete *costal facet* on each side superiorly.
2. *Costal facets* extend on the roots of pedicles.

Eleventh thoracic vertebra

1. *Body* has single *costal facet* on each side.
2. *Costal facet* extends on the upper part of pedicle.
3. *Transverse process* has no articular facet.

Twelfth thoracic vertebra

1. Shape is similar to lumbar vertebra.

2. Single *costal facet* is seen on each side of vertebra.
3. *Costal facet* is more on lower part of pedicle than on the body.
4. Transverse process has no articular facet but has *superior, inferior* and *lateral tubercles*.
5. The *superior articular facets* are thoracic in type whereas the *inferior articular facets* are lumbar in type.

III. LUMBAR VERTEBRAE

Peculiarities (Fig. 19.19)

1. A lumbar vertebra has *massive body*.
2. *Vertebral foramen* is triangular.
3. *Spine* is quadrangular.
4. *Superior articular facet* is concave.
5. *Inferior articular facet* is convex.
6. Posteroinferior part of root of transverse process has a rough elevation called *accessory process*.

Classification

There are 5 lumbar vertebrae. They are classified as *typical* and *atypical*. First to fourth lumbar vertebrae are typical. Last (5th) lumbar vertebra is atypical.

A. Typical lumbar vertebra (Figs 19.20 and 19.21)

a. Body

1. It is large.
2. Its transverse diameter is more than the anteroposterior diameter.
3. Its upper and lower surfaces are covered by *hyaline cartilages* which in turn are related to *intervertebral discs*.
4. Anterior surface in the midline provides attachment to the *anterior longitudinal ligament*.
5. *Crura of diaphragm* are attached to anterior surface on either side of anterior longitudinal ligament. Right crus is attached to upper three while left crus to upper two lumbar vertebrae.

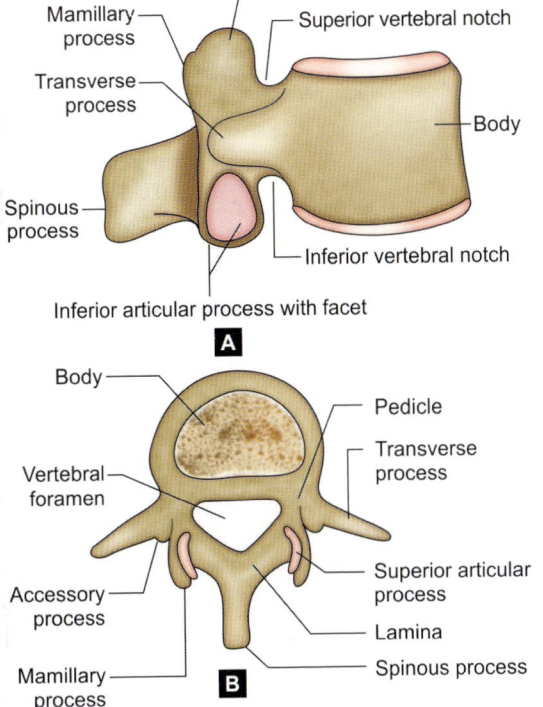

Superior articular process
Superior vertebral notch
Mamillary process
Transverse process
Body
Spinous process
Inferior vertebral notch
Inferior articular process with facet

A

Body
Pedicle
Transverse process
Vertebral foramen
Accessory process
Superior articular process
Lamina
Spinous process
Mamillary process

B

Fig. 19.19: Typical lumbar vertebrae. (A) Right lateral aspect; (B) Superior aspect

6. *Psoas major and its tendinous arches* are attached to upper and lower margins of sides of body.

7. *Posterior longitudinal ligament* is attached to margins of its posterior surface.

Note: *Remember, when lumbar vertebral body is seen from the side, attachments of following structures are appreciated from anterior to posterior; (i) anterior longitudinal ligament, (ii) crus of diaphragm, (iii) psoas major and (iv) posterior longitudinal ligament.*

b. Vertebral foramen

1. It is triangular in cross-section.
2. Outer two spinal meninges, i.e. *dura mater* and *arachnoid mater*, are found in the vertebral foramina of all the lumbar vertebrae.
3. *Conus medullaris with pia mater* occupies the vertebral foramen of 1st lumbar vertebra.
4. *Cauda equina* is contained in the foramina of lower four lumbar vertebrae.

c. Vertebral arch

i. Pedicles

1. They are short and strong.
2. *Inferior vertebral notches* are deeper than the superior vertebral notches.
3. Vertebral notches of adjacent vertebrae complete the formation of *intervertebral foramen.*
4. *Intervertebral foramina* are traversed by *spinal nerves* and *radicular vessels.*

ii. Laminae

1. These are short and thick.
2. They are directed posteromedially.

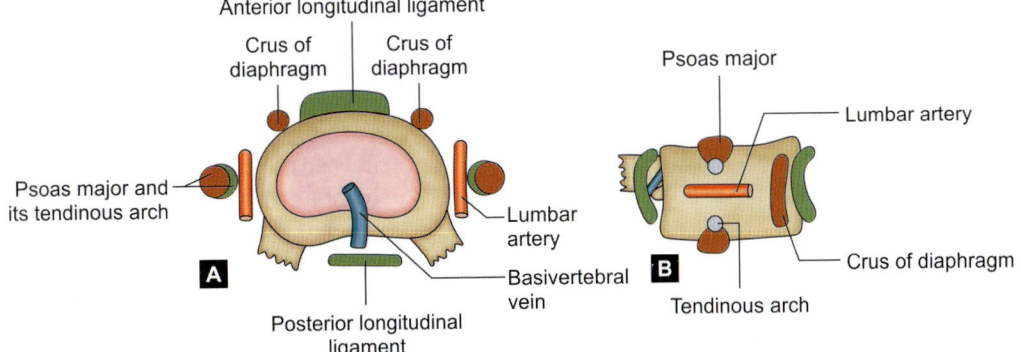

Anterior longitudinal ligament
Crus of diaphragm
Crus of diaphragm
Psoas major
Lumbar artery
Psoas major and its tendinous arch
Lumbar artery
Basivertebral vein
Crus of diaphragm
Tendinous arch
Posterior longitudinal ligament

A

B

Fig. 19.20: Attachments and relations of body of lumbar vertebra. (A) Superior view; (B) Right lateral view

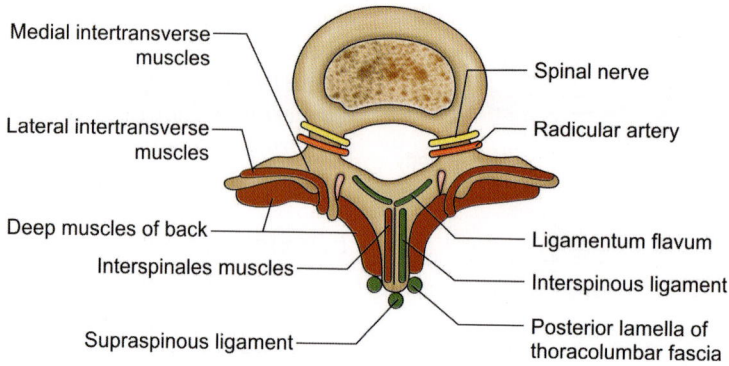

Medial intertransverse muscles

Lateral intertransverse muscles

Deep muscles of back

Interspinales muscles

Supraspinous ligament

Spinal nerve

Radicular artery

Ligamentum flavum

Interspinous ligament

Posterior lamella of thoracolumbar fascia

Fig. 19.21: Relations and attachments of vertebral arch of lumbar vertebra

3. *Ligamentum flavum* is attached to its upper border and lower half of its anterior surface.

4. Posterior surface of lamina gives attachments to *deep muscles of back.*

iii. Spine

1. It is quadrilateral in shape.

2. Its posterior border provides attachments to *supraspinous ligament* in the midline and *posterior lamella of thoracolumbar fascia* on each side.

3. Its superior and inferior borders receive attachments of *interspinous ligaments* in the midline and *interspinales muscles* on each side.

4. Sides of spine give attachments to *deep muscles of back.*

iv. Transverse processes

1. These are tapering and thin.

2. These are homologous with the ribs in the thoracic region.

3. *Medial and lateral arcuate ligaments* are attached to the tip of transverse process of 1st lumbar vertebra.

4. *Iliolumbar ligament* is attached to the tip of 5th lumbar vertebra.

5. *Middle lamella of thoracolumbar fascia* is attached to the tips of transverse processes of all vertebrae.

6. The anterior surface is marked by a faint ridge to which is attached the *anterior lamella of thoracolumbar fascia.*

7. Its anterior surface medial to ridge gives attachment to *psoas major* while the area lateral to ridge receives attachment of *quadratus lumborum muscle.*

8. Posterior surfaces of transverse processes are meant for attachments of *deep muscles of back.*

9. The upper and lower borders of transverse processes give attachments to *intertransversarii muscles.*

10. *Accessory process* gives attachment to medial intertransverse (medial part of intertransversarii) muscle.

v. Articular processes

1. *Superior articular facet* is concave and faces mainly medially while *inferior articular facet* is convex and faces mainly laterally.

2. The distance between the superior articular processes is relatively more than that between inferior articular processes in upper three lumbar vertebrae. This relation is reversed in case of 5th lumbar vertebra. In 4th lumbar vertebra both superior and inferior articular processes are at equal distances (Fig. 19.22).

3. Posterior border of superior articular process is marked by a roughened elevation called *mamillary process.*

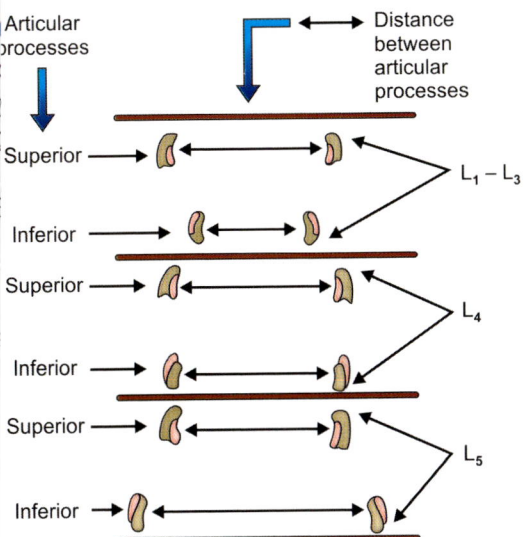

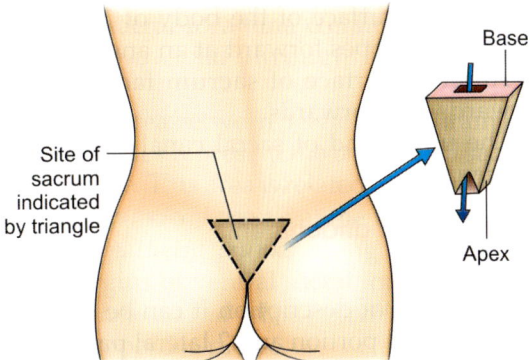

Fig. 19.23: Wedge shaped sacrum (arrow is passing through the sacral canal)

inferior apex. It has 4 surfaces, *pelvic (anterior)*, *dorsal (posterior)* and *2 lateral*. The canal of sacrum is called *sacral canal*.

Fig. 19.22: Interrelationships of distances between lumbar articular processes

4. Mamillary process provides attach-ments to *medial intertransverse muscles* and *deep muscles of back*.

B. Atypical (5th) lumbar vertebra

1. Thick and short *transverse processes* are connected to whole of the pedicles and part of body.
2. The distance between *inferior articular processes* is more than that between *superior articular processes*.
3. The *body* is very much deeper anteriorly than posteriorly.

IV. SACRUM

Terminology

The word sacrum is derived from the Latin word *sacred*. It is considered to be a 'sacred bone' because it occupies the lowest part of the back which is invariably covered as mark of respect.

General form (Fig. 19.23)

Sacrum is a wedge shaped triangular bone. The base of wedge is superior and forms the base of sacrum. Edge of the wedge forms the

Anatomical position (Fig. 19.24)

1. Sacrum is a midline bone placed between hip bones (on each side), 5th lumbar vertebra (superiorly) and coccyx (inferi-orly).

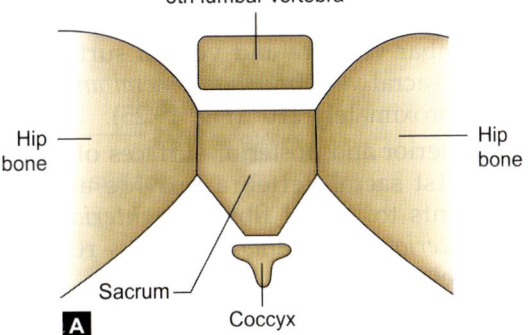

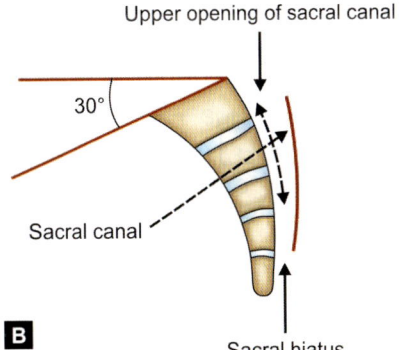

Fig. 19.24: Position of sacrum. (A) Posterior view; (B) Side view

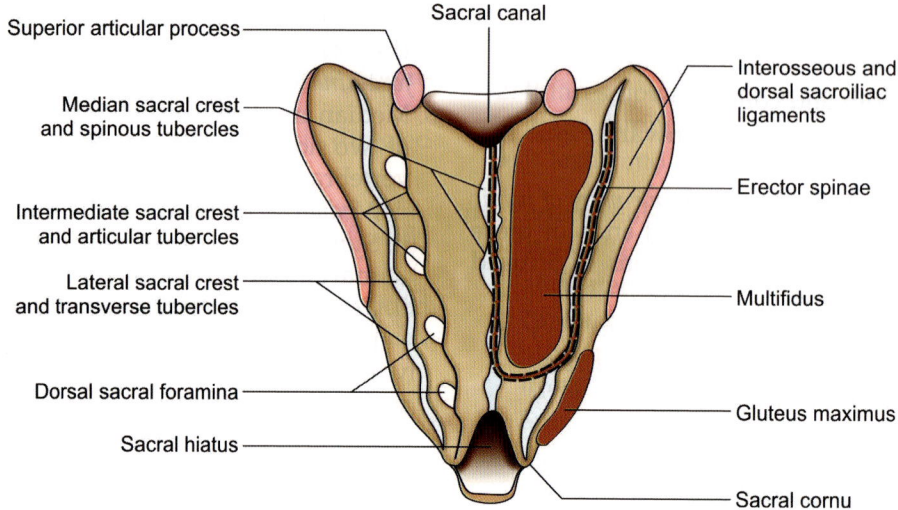

Superior articular process

Sacral canal

Interosseous and dorsal sacroiliac ligaments

Median sacral crest and spinous tubercles

Erector spinae

Intermediate sacral crest and articular tubercles

Lateral sacral crest and transverse tubercles

Multifidus

Dorsal sacral foramina

Sacral hiatus

Gluteus maximus

Sacral cornu

Fig. 19.28: Sacrum: Dorsal surface

7. The *lateral mass* (bony mass lateral to pelvic sacral foramina) is formed by the fusion of costal elements with each other and with the transverse processes of sacral vertebrae.

8. *Piriformis* orginates from the middle 3 pieces of sacral vertebrae.

b. *Dorsal surface* (Fig. 19.28)

1. This surface is relatively rough.

2. It is convex and faces backwards and upwards.

3. Five vertical uneven ridges are the most prominent features on the dorsal surface.

4. A median ridge called *median sacral crest* is formed by the fusion of sacral spines. Elevations along this crest are therefore known as *spinous tubercles*.

5. On either side of median sacral crest is *intermediate sacral crest*. Tubercles along the crest are called *articular tubercles* because this crest is formed by the fusion of articular processes of sacral vertebrae.

6. The lower end of the intermediate sacral crest projects as *sacral cornu*. This represents the inferior articular process of 5th sacral vertebra.

7. Most lateral crest, on each side, is called *lateral sacral crest*. Its tubercles are called *transverse tubercles* because this crest is formed by the fusion of transverse processes of sacral vertebrae.

8. There are four pairs of *dorsal sacral foramina*. These are located just lateral to intermediate sacral crest (Fig. 19.29).

9. Dorsal sacral foramina communicate with the sacral canal through intervertebral foramina.

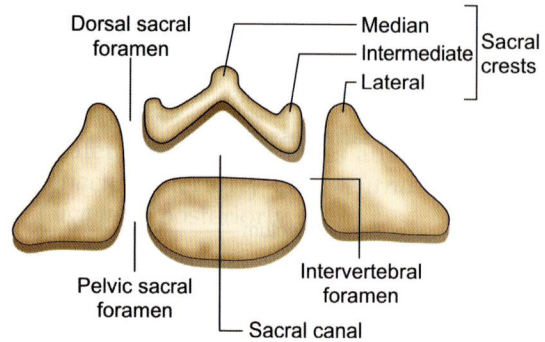

Dorsal sacral foramen

Median
Intermediate } Sacral crests
Lateral

Pelvic sacral foramen

Intervertebral foramen

Sacral canal

Fig. 19.29: Sacral canal and its communications

10. The *erector spinae* muscle takes origin in a 'U' shaped manner from lateral and median sacral crests on each side.

11. The area enclosed by 'U' gives origin to *multifidus muscles*.

c. Lateral surface (Fig. 19.30)

It is tapering, being wider above and narrower below.

i. Upper wider part

1. Anteriorly it has an 'L' shaped articular surface called *auricular surface*. Angle between the two limbs of 'L' faces backwards.

> **Note:** *It is named as auricular surface because it is shaped like the auricle or pinna. Remember that 'auricular' is 'articular'.*

2. Auricular surface articulates with ilium to form *sacroiliac joint*.
3. Anterior and inferior margins of auricular surface provide attachment to *ventral sacroiliac ligament*.
4. *Interosseous sacroiliac ligament* is attached to the area just behind the auricular surface.
5. More posteriorly is attached the *dorsal sacroiliac ligament*.

ii. Lower narrower part

It gives attachments to following structures from anterior to posterior:

  i. *Coccygeus muscle.*

  ii. *Sacrospinous ligament.*

  iii. *Sacrotuberous ligament.*

  iv. *Gluteus maximus muscle.*

> **Note:** *Remember on the lower narrow part of the lateral area there are 2 muscles and 2 ligaments. We can also say that 2 ligaments are sandwiched between two muscles.*

D. Sacral canal

1. It is formed by sacral vertebral foramina.
2. It is triangular in cross-section.
3. The laminae of 5th sacral vertebra do not fuse giving rise to *sacral hiatus* which marks the lower end of sacral canal.
4. Sacral canal communicates with the pelvic and dorsal sacral foramina through four *intervertebral foramina* present in its lateral wall on each side.
5. The contents of sacral canal are as follows:

   i. Lower part of *cauda equina* (sacral and coccygeal nerve roots).

   ii. *Filum terminale.*

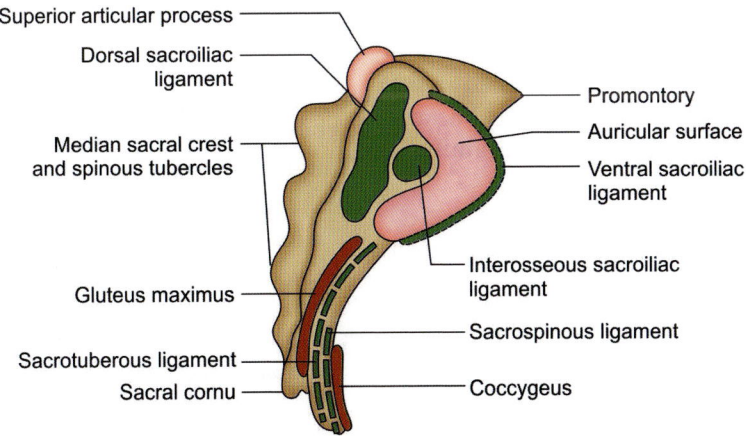

Fig. 19.30: Sacrum: Right lateral aspect

iii. *Spinal meninges.*

iv. *Lateral sacral vessels.*

6. Following structures emerge through sacral hiatus:

   i. *5th sacral nerves.*

   ii. *Coccygeal nerves.*

   iii. *Filum terminale.*

Note: *Remember that the 2nd sacral vertebra marks the lower limit of dura mater, arachnoid mater and subarachnoid space.*

7. Lower part of sacral hiatus is bounded on each side by *sacral cornu* which represents the inferior articular process of 5th sacral vertebra. Sacral cornu gives attachment to *intercornual ligament.*

Sex differences (Table 19.1)

Table 19.1: Sexual dimorphism in sacrum

Features	Male sacrum	Female sacrum
1. Length	More	Less
2. Ratio between the transverse width of body of 1st sacral vertebra and the entire width of sacral base.	More than 1/3rd	Less than 1/3rd
3. Auricular surface	Relatively longer, encroaches on the 3rd segment also in addition to upper two segments.	Smaller, occupies only upper two segments of sacrum
4. Anterior surface of sacrum	Shallower	Deeper
5. Sacral index $\dfrac{\text{Breath of the base}}{\text{Lenght}} \times 100$	Lesser	Greater
6. Width	Relatively narrower	Wider
7. Curvature	Uniformly curved	Flattened in the upper part but sharply curved in the lower part

V. COCCYX

Terminology

The word coccyx is derived from Greek word 'cuckoo', the name of a bird. This is due to the fact that the bone resembles the beak of a bird. Another name of coccyx is 'tail bone' because it is highly developed in animal with tail.

Normal anatomical position

Coccyx is directed downwards and forwards.

Features and attachments (Fig. 19.31)

Coccyx is formed by the fusion of four coccygeal vertebrae. It is triangular in shape with the base upwards and apex downwards. It has two surfaces (pelvic and dorsal) and two lateral borders (right and left).

A. Base

1. It is formed by the superior surface of the body of 1st coccygeal vertebra.

2. It articulates with the apex of sacrum.

3. *Coccygeal cornua* project from the postero-lateral part of the base.

4. Coccygeal and sacral cornua are connected by *intercornual ligaments.*

5. *Transverse process* projects laterally from the base.

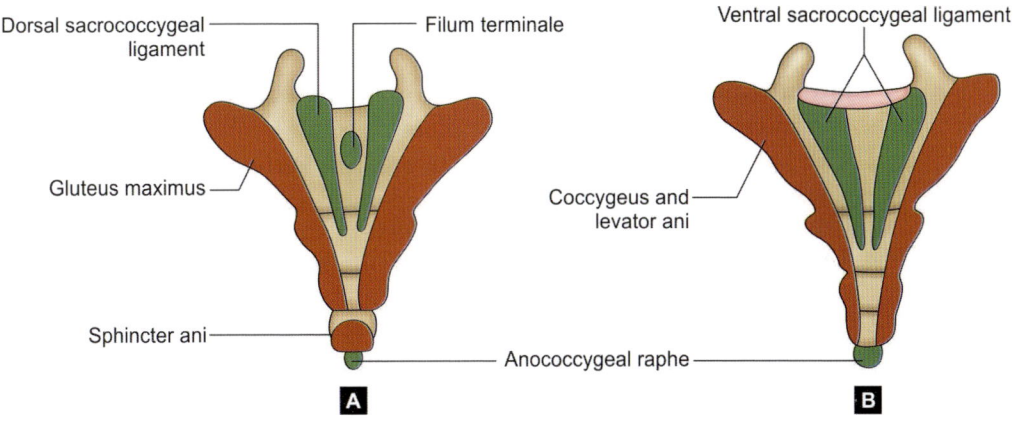

Fig. 19.31: Coccyx. (A) Dorsal aspect; (B) Ventral aspect

B. Apex

It is formed by the last coccygeal segment. It provides attachment to *anococcygeal raphe*.

C. Surfaces

a. Pelvic surface

1. *Ganglion impar* is related to it.

2. It provides attachment to *ventral sacrococcygeal ligament*.

3. *Coccygeus* and *levator ani* are attached to either side of it.

b. Dorsal surface

It provides attachments to following structures:

   i. Gluteus maximus.

   ii. Sphincter ani externus.

   iii. Dorsal sacrococcygeal ligament.

   iv. Filum terminale.

Note: *Remember filum terminale is a fibrous cord which connects the tip of spinal cord with the dorsum of coccyx.*

D. Lateral borders

Following ligaments are attached to either side (lateral border) of coccyx:

   i. Sacrotuberous ligament.

   ii. Sacrospinous ligament.

OSSIFICATION OF VERTEBRAE

1. GENERAL MODE OF OSSIFICATION

A. Primary centres: Three in all, one for body (centrum) and one for each half of the vertebral (neural) arch.

Appearance : 9–16 weeks of intrauterine life

Fusion : Each half of the neural arch with each other 1 year

: Neural arch with centrum, 3–6 years.

Note: *Before fusion, neural arch is united with centrum by synchondrosis called neurocentral joint.*

B. Secondary centres: 5 in total, one each for circumferential parts (*annular epiphyseal ring*) of upper and lower surfaces of the body, one each for tips of transverse processes and one for the tip of spine.

Appearance : Puberty

Fusion : 25 years.

II. EXCEPTIONS TO GENERAL MODE OF OSSIFICATION

a. Atlas : 3 centres in all.

1 each for lateral mass and half of posterior arch.

1 for anterior arch.

Appearance : For lateral mass—7 weeks of intrauterine life.

For anterior arch—1 year

Fusion : Two halves of posterior arch (derived from lateral mass) fuse with each other— 4 years

Anterior arch with each lateral mass—7 years.

b. Axis: 5 Primary and 2 secondary centres appear for axis.

Appearance

Primary centres:

1 for centrum : 2 months of intrauterine life.

2 for vertebral arch : 4 months of intrauterine life

2 for dens : 6 months of intrauterine life

These two centres for dens fuse to form one centre just before birth

Secondary centres

1 for tip of dens : 2 years

1 for lower surface of body : Puberty

Fusion

Two halves of the neural arches, with each other : 3 years

Body with neural arch and dens : 4 years

Apex of dens with

rest of the dens : 12 years

Body with the inferior epiphyseal plate : 25 years

c. 7th cervical vertebra

A separate centre appears for each costal element of transverse process at 6 months of intrauterine life. This fuses with the body and transverse element of transverse process at 6 years. Sometimes this part of the vertebra remains independent and then forms cervical rib.

d. Lumbar vertebrae

Two additional centres appear, one each for mamillary process.

e. Sacrum

Sacrum ossifies from 21 primary and 14 secondary centres. Primary centres appear in the bodies (5), arches (10) and costal elements (6). Secondary centres appear in the epiphyses of bodies (10), auricular surfaces (2) and margins below auricular surfaces (2).

i. Primary centres

Appearance : 2–8 months of intrauterine life

Fusion : 2–8 years

ii. Secondary centres

Appearance : Puberty

Fusion : 25 years

f. Coccyx

Coccyx ossifies from 4 primary centres, one each for individual coccygeal vertebra.

Appearance : 1–10 years

Fusion : 20–30 years

Sternum

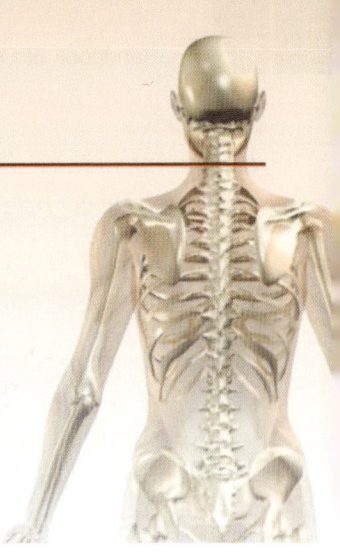

TERMINOLOGY

'Sternum' is derived from Greek word *sternon* which means chest. Sternum is also called 'breast bone'. It has three parts, *manubrium, body* and *xiphoid process*. Manubrium is a Latin word which means 'handle'. Term 'xiphoid' is borrowed from Greek word *xiphos* which means 'sword'.

LOCATION (Fig. 20.1)

It is a flat bone whose long axis is vertical. It lies in the median part of anterior thoracic wall. Its surfaces are anterior and posterior. Its anterior surface also faces a little upwards.

LENGTH

It is about 7 inches (17 cm) long.

STRUCTURE

It is made up of mainly spongy bone and thus it is rich in red bone marrow.

FEATURES AND ATTACHMENTS

Sternum is made up of three pieces from above downwards:

    I. Manubrium.
   II. Body.
  III. Xiphoid process.

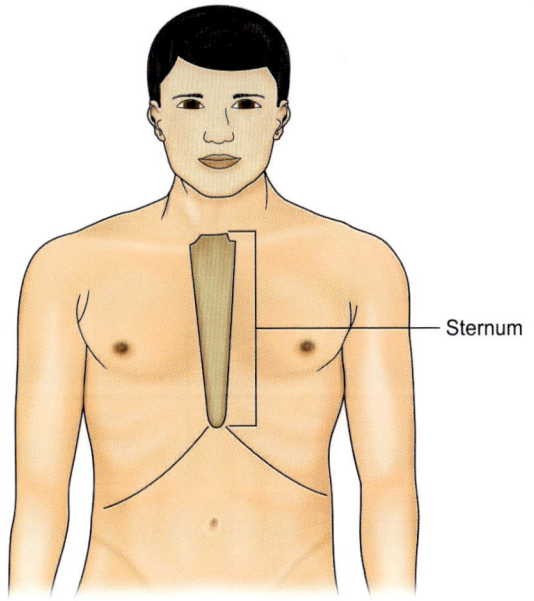

Fig. 20.1: Location of sternum

I. MANUBRIUM (PRESTERNUM OR EPISTERNUM)

It is somewhat triangular in shape and is wider above than below. It has two surfaces (anterior and posterior) and four borders (superior, inferior and 2 lateral).

A. Surfaces

a. Anterior surface (Fig. 20.2)

1. *Pectoralis major* originates from this surface on each side.
2. *Sternal head of sternocleidomastoid* takes origin from each side of its upper part.

b. Posterior surface (Figs 20.4 and 20.5)

1. It forms anterior boundary of the superior mediastinum (Fig. 20.3).
2. Two muscles originate from this surface:
   i. *Sternohyoid* at the level of the clavicular notch.
   ii. *Sternothyroid* at the level of facet for 1st costal cartilage.
3. Each half is related to corresponding parietal pleura.
4. Following vessels are related to this surface:
   i. *Arch of aorta* in its lower half.

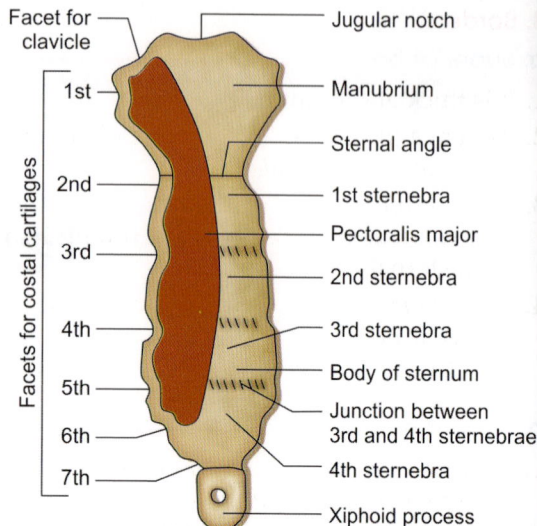

Fig. 20.2: Sternum: Anterior aspect

   ii. *Left brachiocephalic vein, brachiocephalic artery, left common carotid artery* and *left subclavian artery* in its upper half.

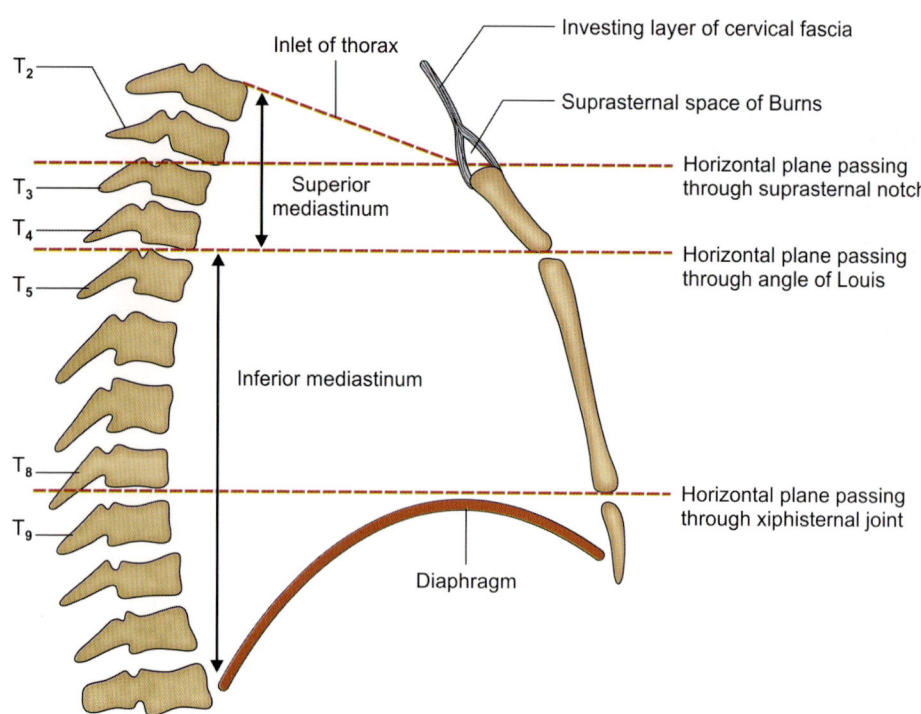

Fig. 20.3: Side views of sternum and thoracic vertebrae

B. Borders

a. Superior border

1. It is thick and rounded.
2. Its concavity in the middle is called suprasternal notch (*jugular notch*).
3. *Deep cervical fascia (investing layer)* and *interclavicular ligament* are attached to suprasternal notch.
4. *Clavicular notch* on either side of suprasternal notch forms *sternoclavicular joint* with the medial end of clavicle.

b. Inferior border

1. It articulates with the upper end of body of sternum to form *manubriosternal joint* which is a secondary cartilaginous joint.
2. Manubrium forms a little angulation at its junction with body. This is called *angle of Louis* or *sternal angle*.
3. Sternal angle articulates on either side with the 2nd costal cartilage, thus forms an important landmark for counting the ribs.

c. Lateral borders (Fig. 20.6)

1. There are two lateral borders, right and left.
2. Its upper part forms primary cartilaginous joint with the first costal cartilage.
3. A demifacet is seen on the lower part of the lateral border which along with similar one on the upper angle of the body, forms two synovial joints with the 2nd costal cartilage.

II. THE BODY (MESOSTERNUM OR GLADIOLUS)

It has two surfaces (anterior and posterior), two borders (right lateral and left lateral) and two ends (upper and lower).

A. Surfaces

a. Anterior surface (Fig. 20.2)

1. Body of the sternum is formed by the fusion of 4 small segments called *sternebrae*.
2. The sites of fusion of sternebrae are represented on the anterior surface of body in the form of 3 ill-defined horizontal ridges.

3. *Pectoralis major* originates from its corresponding half.

b. Posterior surface (Figs 20.4 and 20.5)

1. The transverse lines are less prominent than those on anterior surface.
2. *Transversus thoracis* originates from both the lower halves.

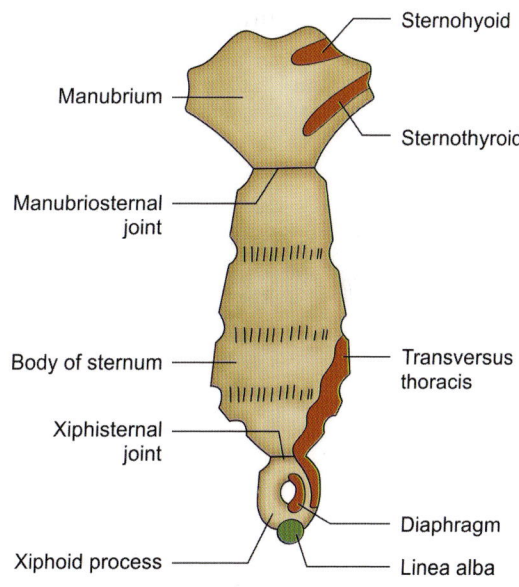

Fig. 20.4: Sternum: Posterior aspect

3. *Right lung and pleura* are related to the posterior surface on the right side of median plane.
4. *Left lung and pleura* are related to the upper two pieces on the left of midline.
5. *Pericardium* is related to lower two pieces on the left of the median plane.

B. Lateral borders (Fig. 20.6)

1. At their upper and lower ends, they articulate on either side with the lower part of 2nd and upper part of 7th costal cartilages by demifacets respectively.
2. It has 4 complete facets for 3rd to 6th costal cartilages.
3. Facets for the 3rd, 4th and 5th costal cartilages lie at the junction of sternebrae

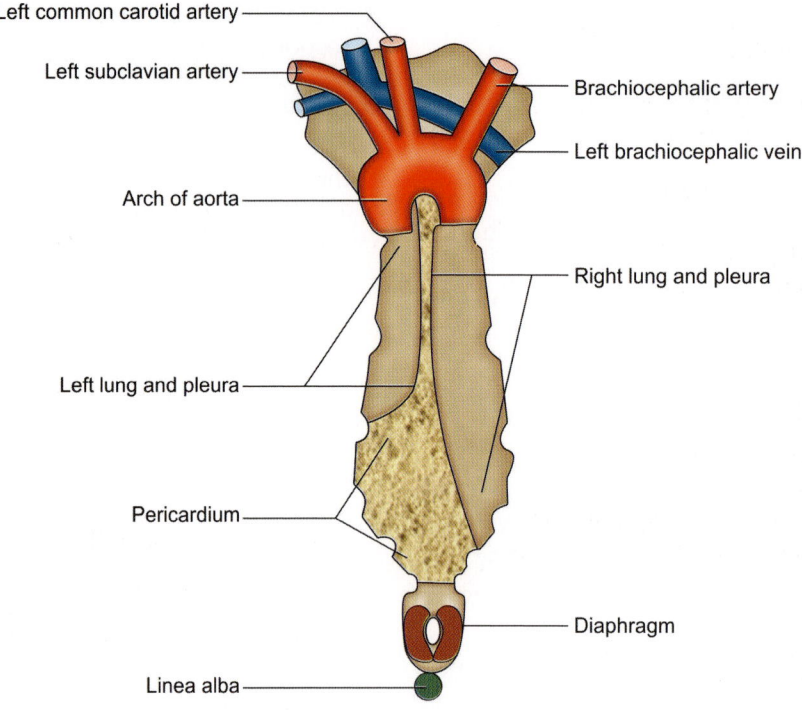

Fig. 20.5: Sternum: Posterior aspect

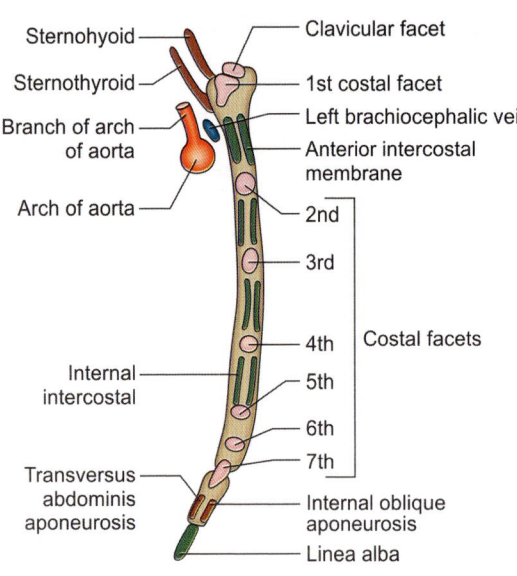

Fig. 20.6: Right lateral view of sternum

while that for 6th one lies at the side of 4th sternebra.

4. To the margins between the facets, follo wing structures are attached:
    i. *Internal intercostal muscles.*
    ii. *External intercostal membranes.* Attach ment of (ii) is anterior to (i).

C. Ends

a. Upper end

1. It is oval in shape.
2. It articulates with the lower end of the manubrium sterni to form *manubriosternal joint* which is secondary cartilaginous joint.

b. Lower end

1. It is quite narrow.
2. It articulates with xiphoid process to form *xiphisternal joint* which is a secondary cartilaginous joint.

3. Xiphisternal joint usually becomes a syn-ostosis by 40th year.

II. XIPHOID PROCESS (XIPHISTERNUM OR METASTERNUM OR ENSIFORM CARTILAGE)

It is lowest and smallest part of sternum and is of variable shapes. It has two surfaces (anterior and posterior), two borders (right lateral and left lateral) and two ends (upper and lower).

A. Surfaces

a. Anterior surface

It gives insertions to following:

   i. *Rectus abdominis muscle.*
   ii. *Aponeuroses of external and internal oblique muscles* (anterior lamina of rectus sheath).

b. Posterior surface

1. It gives origin to following:
   i. *Diaphragm.*
   ii. *Transversus thoracis*
2. It is related to *liver.*

B. Lateral borders

1. Each gives attachments to *aponeuroses of internal oblique and transversus abdominis muscles* (posterior lamina of rectus sheath).
2. The superior angle possesses a demifacet for 7th costal cartilage.

C. Ends

a. Upper end

It articulates with lower end of body to form xiphisternal joint.

b. Lower end

It gives attachment to *linea alba.*

SEX DIFFERENCES

Body of sternum in males is more than twice the length of manubrium. In females, the body is shorter and less than twice the length of manubrium.

OSSIFICATION

Sternum ossifies from 6 centres, one for manubrium, 4 for sternebrae (one for each sternebra) and one for xiphoid process.

A. *Appearance*

Centres appear as follows:

Manubrium	: 5th month	
1st sternebra	: 6th month	
2nd sternebra	: 7th month	Intrauterine life
3rd sternebra	: 8th month	
4th sternebra	: 9th month	

Xiphisternum : 3rd year

B. *Fusion:*

Between manubrium and 1st sternebra	: Ununited
Upper 3 sternebrae	: Between puberty and 25 years
Between 3rd and 4th sternebrae	: Puberty
Between 4th sternebra and xiphoid process	: 40 years

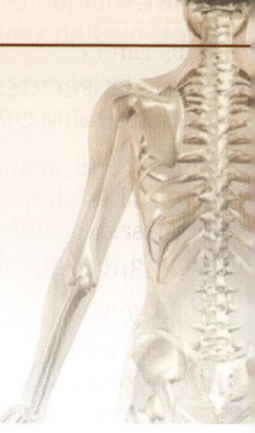

Ribs

GENERAL CONSIDERATIONS (Fig. 21.1)

1. Ribs are bilateral bony arches forming greater part of the thoracic wall.

2. Normally there are 12 pairs of ribs which are numbered from above downwards.

3. The length of the ribs increases from 1st to 7th rib and then decreases from 7th to 12th rib. Therefore the 7th rib is the longest rib.

4. The ribs are arranged obliquely, i.e. the anterior end is at a lower level than the posterior end. The obliquity is maximum in the 9th rib.

5. The 8th rib is the most laterally projected rib

6. Width of the rib gradually reduces from above downwards.

7. Intercostal spaces (gaps between adjacent ribs) are deeper in front than behind and deeper in the upper part than the lower part

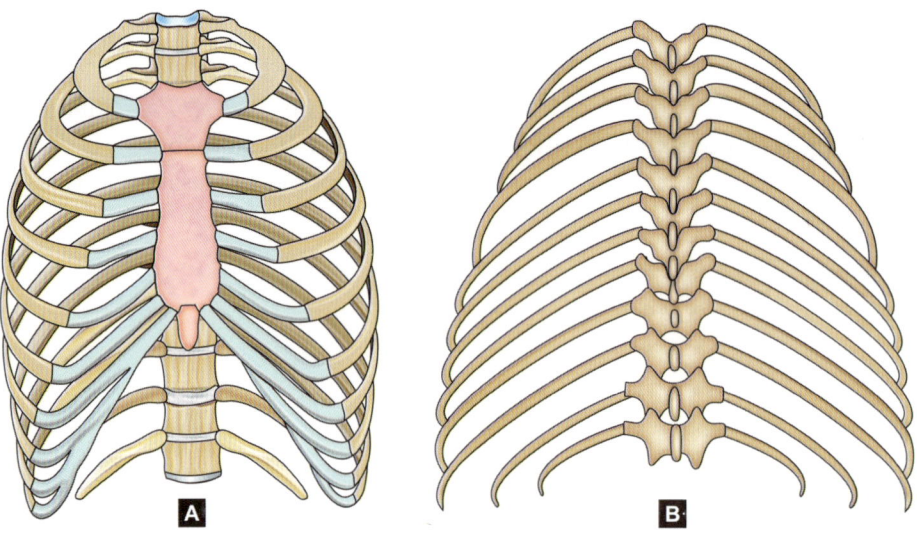

Fig. 21.1: The thoracic cage. (A) Anterior view; (B) Posterior view

CLASSIFICATION OF RIBS

The ribs can be classified differently.

A. According to the similarities and dissimilarities of features

a. Typical ribs
1. These are the ribs which are having same features.
2. 3rd to 9th ribs are typical ribs.

b. Atypical ribs
1. They have some special features and therefore can be differentiated from rest of the ribs.
2. 1st, 2nd, 10th, 11th and 12th ribs are the examples of atypical ribs.

B. According to the relations of ribs with the sternum

a. True ribs
1. These are the ribs which articulate with sternum anteriorly.
2. Upper seven ribs are true ribs.

b. False ribs
1. These are not connected to sternum anteriorly.
2. 8th to 12th ribs are false ribs.

C. According to articulation of ribs

a. Vertebrosternal ribs
1. Ribs which are connected posteriorly with vertebrae and anteriorly (directly or indirectly through its cartilage) with sternum, are called vertebrosternal ribs.
2. Upper seven ribs are examples of vertebrosternal ribs.

b. Vertebrochondral ribs
1. These ribs are connected posteriorly with the vertebrae but anteriorly they do not reach the sternum, instead their cartilages are joined together.
2. 8th, 9th and 10th ribs are examples of vertebrochondral ribs.

c. Vertebral ribs
1. Posteriorly they are attached to vertebrae but anteriorly they are free.
2. Last two ribs (11th and 12th) are vertebral ribs.

D. According to state of anterior end

a. Floating ribs
1. If the anterior end is free and does not articulate with sternum or adjacent cartilage then the rib is said to be floating rib.
2. 11th and 12th ribs are floating ribs.

b. Nonfloating ribs
1. If anterior end of bone is fixed due to its attachment to sternum or the adjacent cartilage then it is called as nonfloating rib.
2. All the ribs are nonfloating except last two.

Note: *Remember 'nonfloating rib' is usually not considered as terminology but has been used to differentiate it from 'floating rib'. Some of the terms used in classification reflect similar meaning, e.g. true ribs—vertebrosternal ribs and floating ribs—vertebral ribs. The 10th rib is also floating in Japanese.*

DESCRIPTION OF RIBS

I. TYPICAL RIB (Figs 21.2 to 21.4)

Side determination

The side of a typical rib can be determined by considering the following points:
1. The end of the rib having head, neck and tubercle is directed posteriorly.
2. Concavity of the rib faces medially.
3. The sharp border of the rib is inferior.

Normal anatomical position

Keep the bone on the corresponding side in such a way that the posterior end is higher and nearer the median plane than the anterior end.

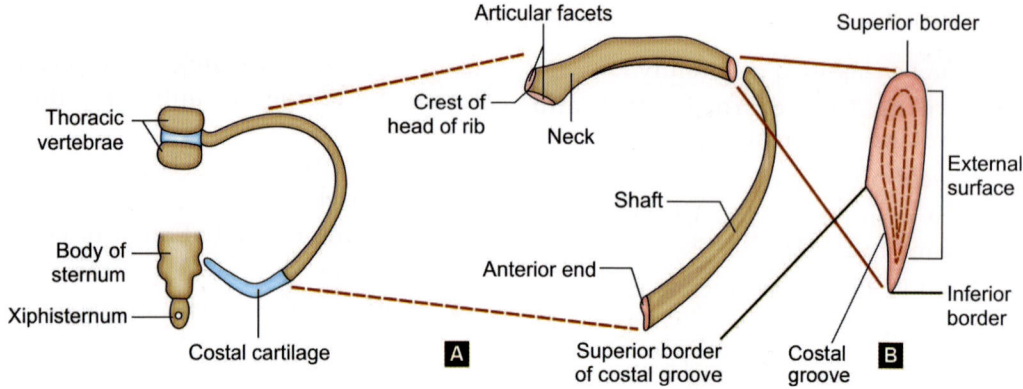

Fig. 21.2: Left typical rib. (A) Anterior aspect; (B) Cross section

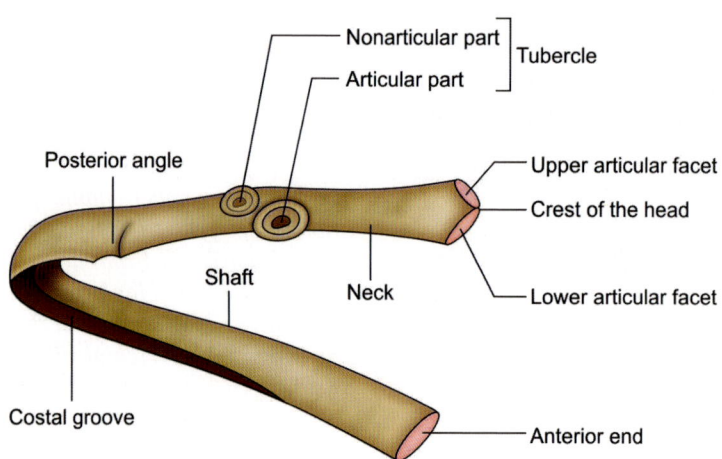

Fig. 21.3: Left typical rib: Posterior aspect

Features and attachments

Each rib has an anterior end, a posterior end and a shaft.

A. Anterior end

1. It is oval in shape.
2. It has a cup-shaped depression.
3. Anterior end forms *costochondral joint* (a primary cartilaginous joint) with the lateral end of corresponding costal cartilage.

B. Posterior end

It consists of head, neck and tubercle.

a. Head

1. The head lies at the junction of two vertebrae and therefore comprises two *articular facets* (Fig. 21.5).
2. The lower articular facet is larger and meets with the corresponding vertebra.

Note: *Remember 'L' for lower and 'L' for larger*

3. The upper smaller facet articulates with vertebra above.

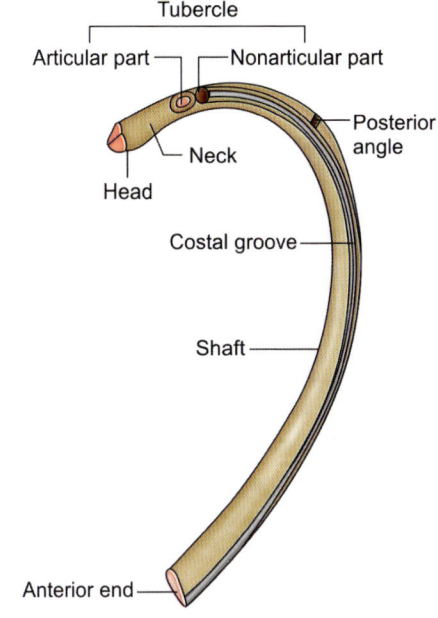

Fig. 21.4: Right typical rib: Inferior aspect

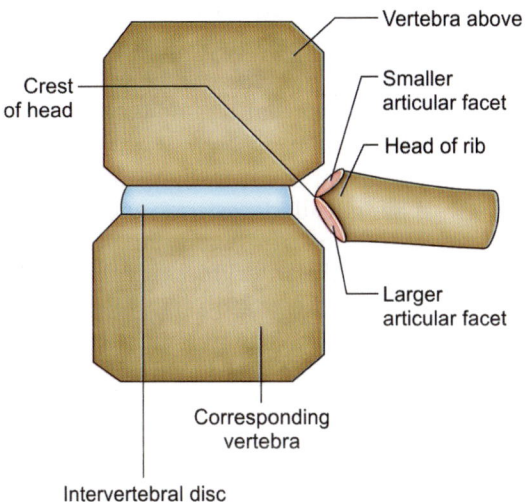

Fig. 21.5: Relations between the head of a typical rib and vertebrae

Note: *Remember 'S' for superior and 'S' for Smaller*

4. The articular facets are separated from each other by a transverse ridge called as the *crest of head* which lies opposite the intervertebral disc.

5. *Capsular ligament* is attached to margins of articular facets while *intra-articular ligament* is attached to the crest of head.
6. *Radiate ligament* is attached to the front of head (Fig. 21.6).
7. Anterior aspect of head is also related to *costal pleura and sympathetic chain.*

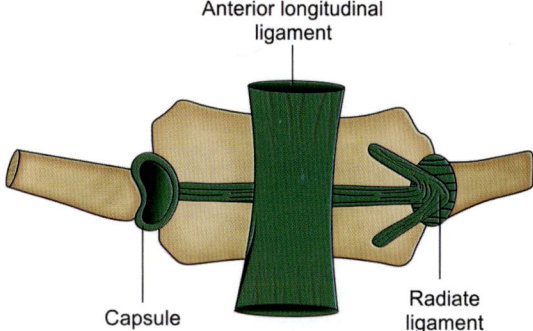

Fig. 21.6: Attachments on the head of 1st rib: Anterior view

b. *Neck* (Fig. 21.7)
1. It lies in front of the transverse process of corresponding vertebra.
2. It is flat part of rib adjacent to head.
3. It is 1 cm in length.
4. It has 2 borders (superior and inferior) and 2 surfaces (anterior and posterior).
   i. *Superior border*
      1. It is also called *crest of neck.*
      2. It is thin and sharp.
      3. *Superior costotransverse ligament* is attached to it.

Note: *Remember there are two crests at the posterior end of rib. Crest of head is between two articular facets while crest of neck is its sharp superior border.*

   ii. *Inferior border*
      1. It is smooth and round.
      2. It receives attachment of *internal (posterior) intercostal membrane.*
   iii. *Anterior surface*
      1. It is divided by an *oblique ridge* into an upper medial area and a lower lateral area.

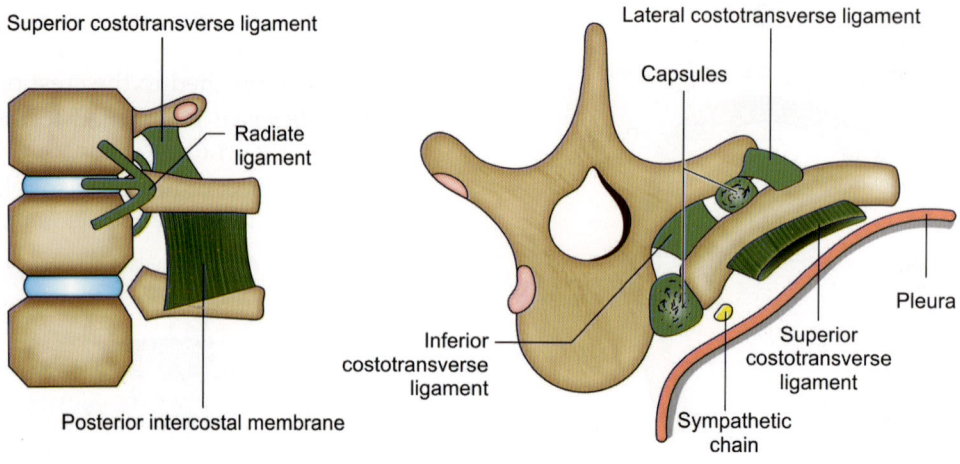

Superior costotransverse ligament

Radiate ligament

Posterior intercostal membrane

Lateral costotransverse ligament

Capsules

Pleura

Inferior costotransverse ligament

Superior costotransverse ligament

Sympathetic chain

Fig. 21.7: Attachments on the posterior end of a typical rib

2. The ridge gives attachment to *posterior intercostal membrane.*

3. Upper area is related to *posterior intercostal membrane* but separated from it by *fatty tissue.* Lower area is related to *costal pleura.*

iv. Posterior surface

1. It is rough.

2. It receives attachment of *inferior costotransverse ligament.*

c. Tubercle

1. It is situated on the outer surface of rib at the junction of neck with the shaft.

2. It is divided into medial articular and lateral nonarticular parts.

3. Medial part articulates with the transverse process of corresponding vertebra to form *costotransverse joint.*

4. Lateral part gives attachment to *lateral costotransverse ligament.*

Note: *Remember there are three costotransverse ligaments, lateral, superior and inferior, which are attached to the regions as follows:*

Lateral: Lateral part of tubercle

Superior: Crest of neck

Inferior: Back of neck.

C. Shaft

1. It is the major part of rib which intervenes between the anterior and posterior ends of rib.

2. It is thin and flat.

3. A typical rib has three qualities:

    i. It is *curved.* This can be appreciated by the fact that it is never straight.

    ii. It is *angulated.* There is a bend in the rib about 5 cm in front of tubercle. This is called *posterior angle* or only 'angle' of rib. A similar bend 2 cm behind the anterior end of rib is called *anterior angle* of rib (Fig. 21.8).

    iii. It is *twisted.* The twisting of the shaft can be appreciated by the fact that the inner surface faces slightly upwards behind the angle but it faces slightly downwards in the front of angle. Moreover due to twisting, the two ends of the rib cannot touch a horizontal plane simultaneously.

4. The shaft has two borders (superior and inferior) and two surfaces (outer and inner).

a. Borders

    i. *Superior border*

    1. It is thick and rounded.

    2. It has outer and inner lips.

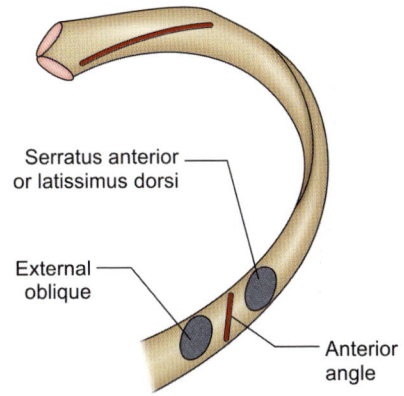

Fig. 21.8: Left typical rib: Anterior aspect

3. Outer lip receives insertion of *external intercostal muscle*.
4. Inner lip receives insertion of *internal intercostal* and *intercostalis intimus muscles*.

ii. *Inferior border*

1. It is sharp and forms the lower border of the costal groove.
2. *External intercostal muscle* originates from the lower border.

Note: *Remember that the upper border is for insertion whereas the lower border is for origin. Also that the external intercostal originates from the lower border of upper rib and gets inserted on the upper border of lower rib.*

b. Surfaces

i. *Outer surface*

1. It is smooth and convex.
2. *Angle (posterior angle)* of rib is marked by a ridge which provides attachment to *posterior layer of thoracolumbar fascia*.
3. *Levator costarum* and *sacrospinalis (erector spinae) muscles* are attached to outer surface, medial to the angle.
4. Anterior angle is marked by an indistinct oblique line which separates the origin of external oblique (anterior to angle) from serratus anterior (in cases of middle 4 ribs) or latissimus dorsi (in cases of 9th and 10th ribs) (Fig. 21.9).

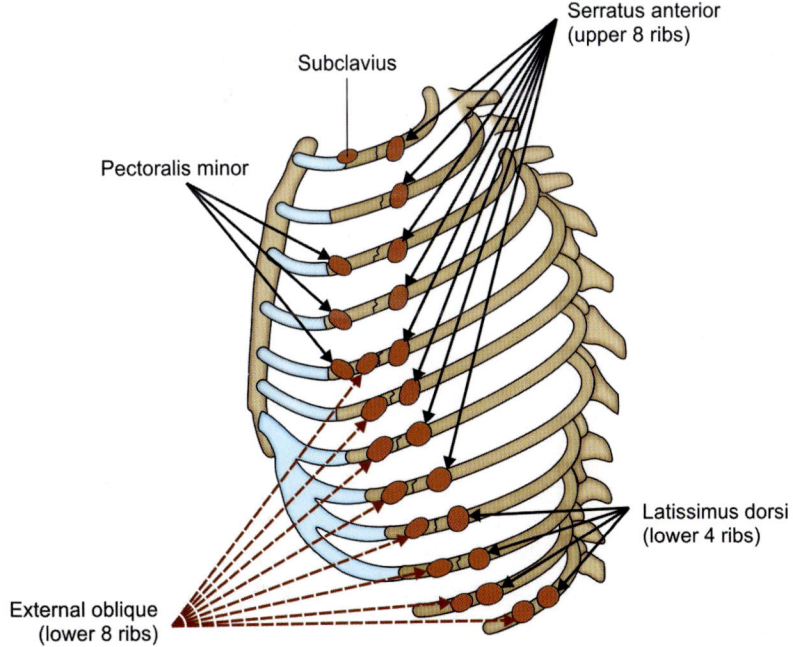

Fig. 21.9: The thoracic cage: Left lateral view

5. *Serratus anterior* (in cases of upper 8 ribs) or *latissimus dorsi* (in cases of 9th and 10th ribs) arises from the outer surface of rib just behind the anterior angle (Fig. 21.9).

ii. *Inner surface*

1. It is concave and smooth.
2. It has a *costal groove* in its lower part.
3. Costal groove lodges the following structures from above downwards:
   - *Intercostal vein.*
   - *Intercostal artery.*
   - *Intercostal nerve.*

Note: *Remember VAN to consider the sequence of Vein, Artery and Nerve.*

4. *Internal intercostal muscle* originates from the floor of costal groove.
5. *Intercostalis intimus* originates from middle 2/4th of the upper lip of costal groove.

Note: *Remember that internal intercostal is internal in the costal groove, i.e. it is in the floor of the groove whereas intercostalis intimus is intimately attached to the upper lip of costal groove.*

II. ATYPICAL RIBS

A. First Rib

Distinguishing features

1. It is shortest.
2. It is broadest.
3. It is most curved.
4. It has no twisting.
5. Angle coincides with tubercle.
6. Head has got only single facet.
7. Costal groove is absent.
8. Neck is rounded and elongated.
9. It is flattened from above downwards and therefore has inner and outer borders and superior and inferior surfaces.

Side determination

1. Keep the larger end anteriorly and th smaller end posteriorly.
2. Keep the surface of the shaft having two grooves separated by a ridge, superiorly.
3. Keep the concave border towards inner side and convex border towards outer side.

Note: *Keep the rib on a flat surface considering its position in your own body. The rib belongs to the side on which both the ends touch the surface simultaneously. If the rib is placed on the wrong side then only the anterior end will be touching the table top.*

Anatomical position

1. Posterior end is nearer the midline than the anterior end.
2. Posterior end is 3.5 cm higher than the anterior end.
3. Upper surface faces upwards as well as forwards.

Features and attachments

Just like typical rib, the first rib is comprised of two ends (anterior and posterior) and a shaft.

a. Anterior end

1. It is larger end.
2. It meets with 1st costal cartilage.

b. Posterior end

It consists of head, neck and tubercle.

i. *Head*

1. It is small and rounded.
2. It has a single rounded facet for articulation with the body of 1st thoracic vertebra to form *costovertebral joint.*
3. *Capsular ligament* of 1st costovertebral joint is attached to the margins of facet.
4. *Radiate ligament* is attached to the anterior margin of head.

ii. *Neck*

1. It is rounded.

2. It is directed upwards, backwards and laterally.
3. *Inferior costotransverse ligament* is attached to its posterior surface.
4. Following structures form the anterior relations of the neck from medial to lateral (Fig. 21.11):
   - *Sympathetic chain.*
   - *First posterior intercostal vein.*
   - *Superior intercostal artery.*
   - *First thoracic root (T_1) of brachial plexus.*

Note: *Remember SVAN for the relations of anterior aspect of neck from medial to lateral in which S—Sympathetic chain, V—Vein, A—Artery and N—Nerve.*

iii. Tubercle

1. It is large and prominent.
2. It articulates with the transverse process of 1st thoracic vertebra.
3. *Lateral costotransverse ligament* is attached laterally to the tubercle.

c. Shaft

It consists of two borders (outer and inner) and two surfaces (upper and lower).

i. Outer border

1. It is convex.
2. It is thick posteriorly and thin anteriorly.
3. *1st digitation of serratus anterior* arises from its middle.
4. It is related to scalenus posterior muscle in its posterior part while clavipectoral fascia and pectoralis major muscle in its anterior part.

ii. Inner border

1. It is concave.
2. *Scalene tubercle* is situated near its middle.
3. *Sibson's fascia* (suprapleural membrane) is attached to it.

iii. Upper surface (Figs 21.10 and 21.11)

1. It is rough and irregular.
2. It presents two shallow grooves separated by a ridge.
3. The ridge continues medially with the scalene tubercle along the inner border.
4. *Scalenus anterior* is inserted on the ridge and scalene tubercle.

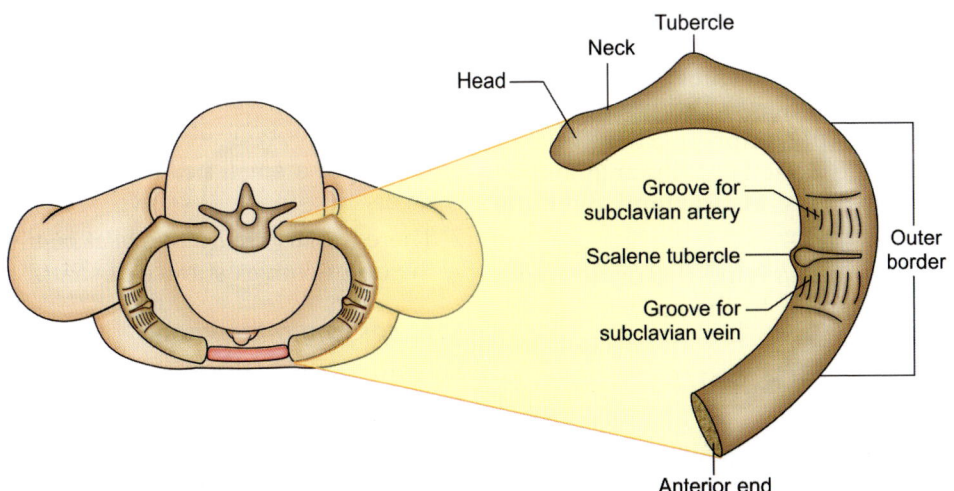

Fig. 21.10: First rib of left side. Superior aspect

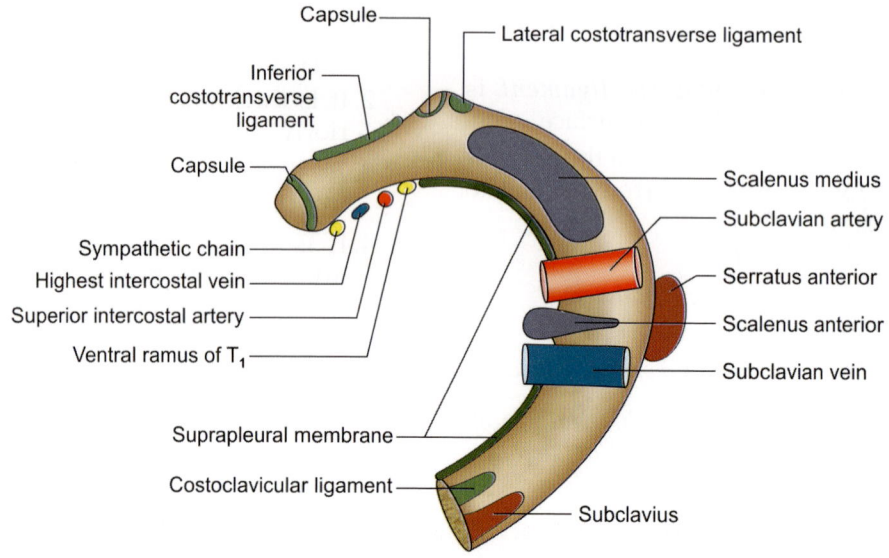

Fig. 21.11: First rib of left side: Superior view

5. *Subclavian vein* lies in the groove anterior to ridge.

6. *Subclavian artery* along with *lower trunk of brachial plexus* occupies the posterior groove.

Note: *Remember VAN is the sequence of structures occupying the grooves on the superior surface from anterior to posterior, i.e. Vein, Artery and Nerve.*

7. Area anterior to groove for subclavian vein provides attachments to *subclavius muscle* (anteriorly) and *costoclavicular ligament* (posteriorly). These attachments are located near the anterior end because they also extend over the costal cartilage.

8. *Scalenus medius* is inserted on the rough area posterior to the groove for subclavian artery.

iv. Lower surface **(Fig. 21.12)**

1. It is smooth.

2. It is related to *costal pleura*.

3. *Intercostal muscles* are attached to this surface near its outer border.

4. *1st intercostal nerve and vessels* are related to this surface mainly in its posterior part.

B. Second Rib (Fig. 21.13)

Distinguishing features

1. It is highly curved like first rib.

2. It is twice the length of 1st rib.

3. It has no twisting and therefore both the ends are in contact with the horizontal surface of table top.

4. Slight angle is present close to tubercle.

5. Like the 1st rib there is slight upward convexity of bone at the tubercle.

6. It has got a small head with two articular facets.

7. There is a *large rough muscular impression* on the outer convex surface of shaft.

Features and attachments

Second rib has the following additional features as compared to the typical ribs.

1. 2nd rib is a transitional rib therefore outer surface faces more upwards than outwards and inner surface faces more downwards than inwards.

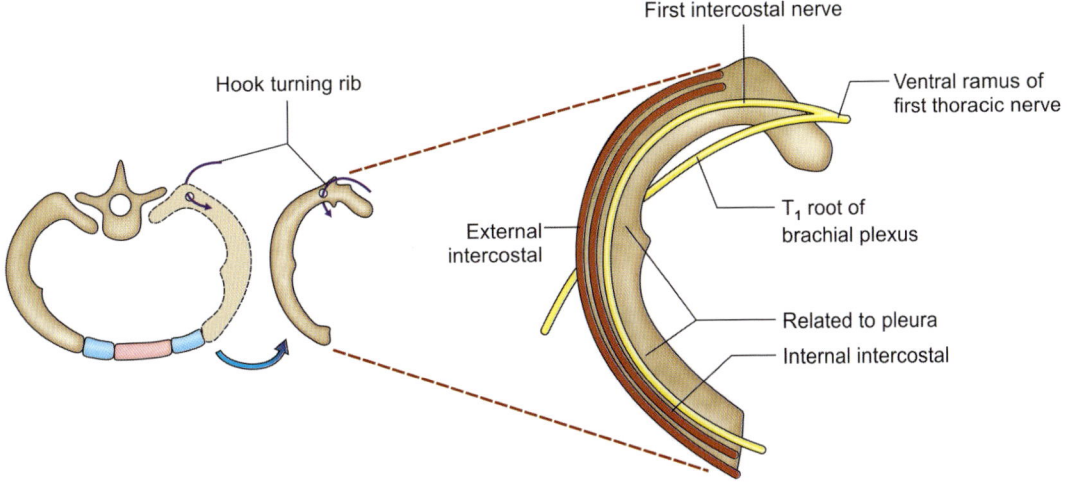

Fig. 21.12: First rib of left side: Inferior aspect

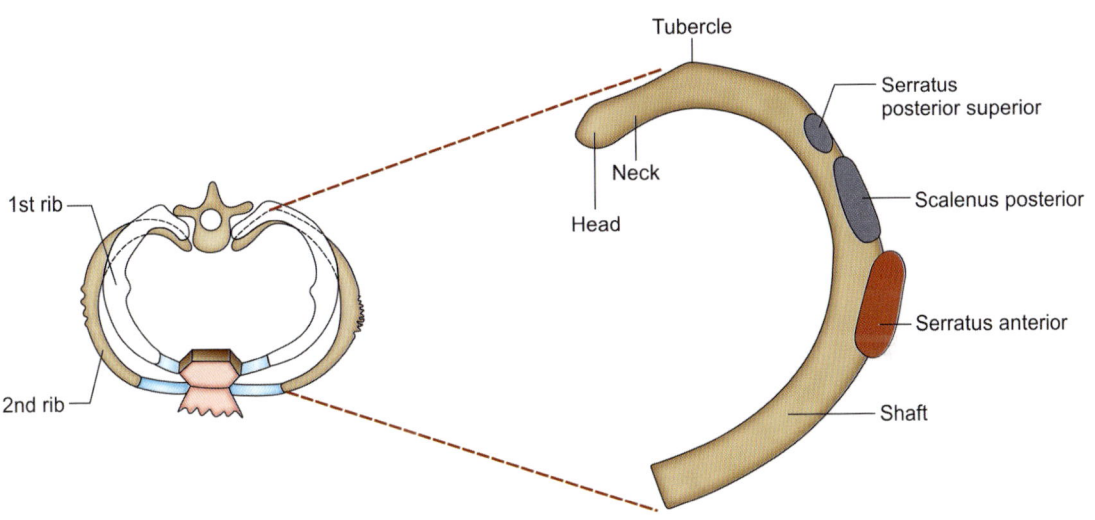

Fig. 21.13: Second rib of left side: Superior aspect

2. There is a *prominent rough impression* on the outer surface just behind its middle which gives origin to *serratus anterior muscle* (lower part of the 1st and whole of the 2nd digitations).
3. *Scalenus posterior* is attached to upper border and adjoining outer surface behind the rough impression.
4. 1st slip of *serratus posterior superior* is attached to the superior border further behind.

5. A short costal groove is visible in the posterior part of inner smooth concave surface.

C. Tenth Rib

It shows all the features of a typical rib except that it is shorter than the typical rib and head bears single facet to articulate with the body of corresponding (tenth) thoracic vertebra.

D. Eleventh Rib

The common features of eleventh and twelfth ribs differentiating them from typical ribs are as follows:

1. There is only one facet on the head.
2. There is no neck.
3. There is no tubercle.
4. Anterior ends are pointed.
5. They are quite shorter than typical ribs.

The features of eleventh rib which differentiate it from twelfth rib are as follows:

1. It is much longer than the twelfth rib.
2. A faint costal groove is observed on the inner surface.
3. Slight angle is present in the eleventh rib.

E. Twelfth Rib

Identifying features

1. There is only one facet on the head.
2. There is no neck.
3. There is no tubercle.
4. Anterior end is pointed.
5. It is smaller than the eleventh rib.
6. There is no costal groove.
7. There is no angle.

Side determination

1. Keep the pointed end anterolaterally and broader end posteromedially.
2. Keep the slightly concave surface inwards and upwards (Fig. 21.14).
3. Keep the sharper border inferiorly.

Features and attachments

It has two ends (posterior and anterior), two surfaces (outer and inner) and two borders (upper and lower).

a. Ends

i. Anterior end

It meets with a small costal cartilage.

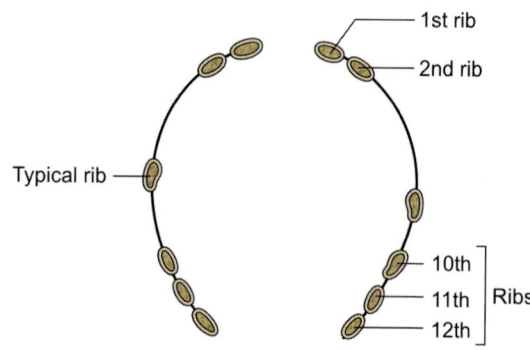

Barrel shaped chest

Fig. 21.14: Directions of surfaces of shafts of ribs

ii. Posterior end (head)

Capsular and radiate ligaments are attached to the head.

b. Surfaces

i. Outer surface (Fig. 21.15)

Following structures are attached to the outer surface:

1. Close to head: *Costotransverse ligament* above and *lumbocostal ligament* below.
2. Near the tip: *Latissimus dorsi muscle* above and *external oblique muscle* below.
3. Rest of the surface: *Posterior lamella of thoracolumbar fascia* and *levator costae, erector spinae* and *serratus posterior inferior muscles*.

ii. Inner surface (Fig. 21.16)

1. An oblique line crossing the middle of this surface marks the *line of pleural reflection.*
2. *Quadratus lumborum with anterior lamella of thoracolumbar fascia* is attached to the lower part of the medial half.
3. *Internal intercostal muscle* is inserted near the upper border of its middle two fourth.
4. *Diaphragm* arises from the upper part of its anterior one fourth.

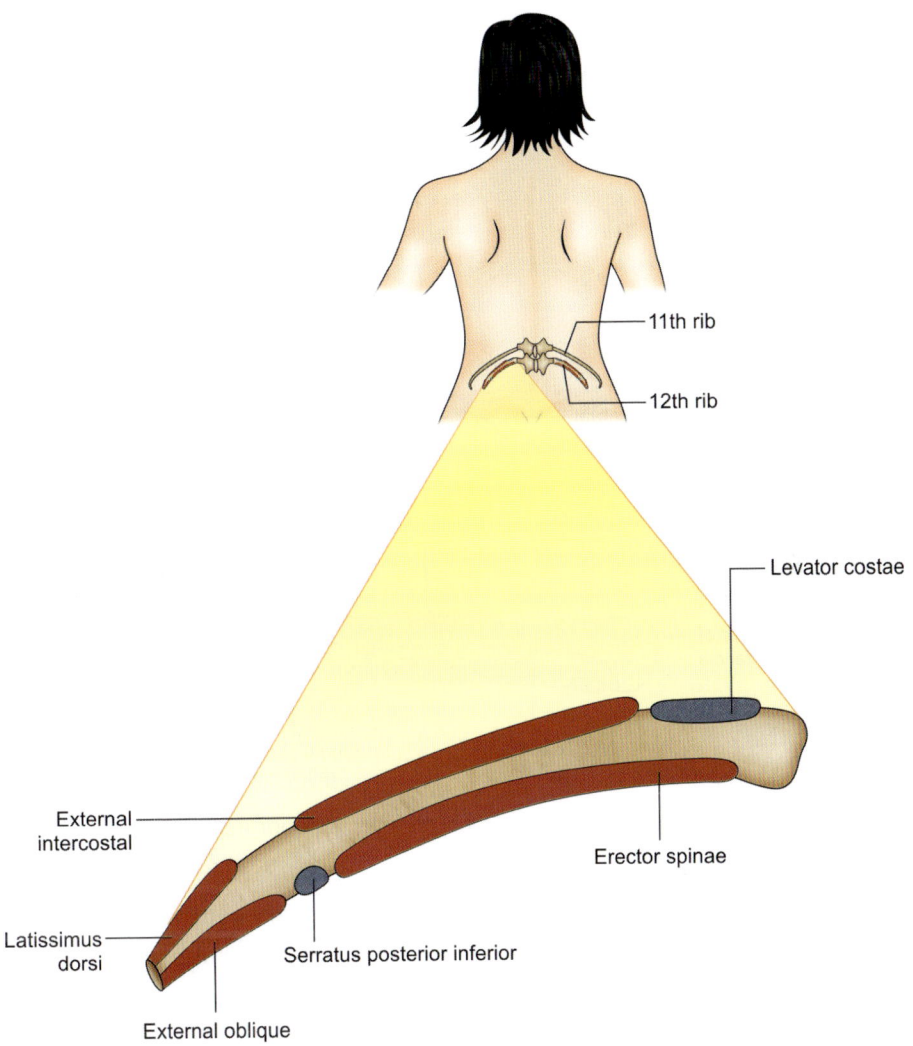

Fig. 21.15: Twelfth rib of left side: Posterior aspect

C. Borders

i. Upper border

External and internal intercostal muscles are inserted on this border.

ii. Lower border

1. Its medial half provides attachment to the *middle lamella of thoracolumbar fascia* which corresponds with the extent of quadratus lumborum.
2. Just beyond the lateral border of quadratus lumborum there is attachment of *lateral arcuate ligament*.

3. Lateral part of inferior border receives attachment of *posterior lamella of thoracolumbar fascia*.

OSSIFICATION OF RIBS

I. Second to tenth ribs

Four ossification centres appear in total, one primary and three secondary.

A. Appearance

Primary centre
• 1 for shaft: 8th week of intrauterine life.

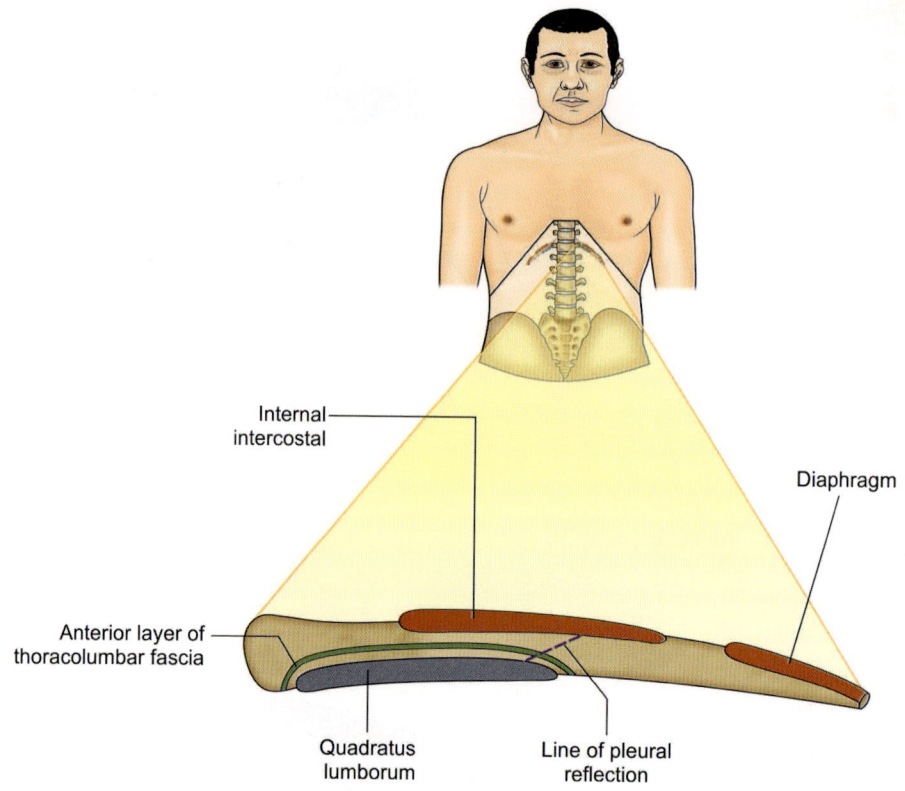

Internal intercostal

Diaphragm

Anterior layer of thoracolumbar fascia

Quadratus lumborum

Line of pleural reflection

Fig. 21.16: Twelfth rib of left side: Anterior aspect

Secondary centres
- 1 for head
- 1 for articular part of tubercle
- 1 for nonarticular part of tubercle
- All appear at puberty.

B. *Fusion:* 20 years

II. First rib

Three centres of ossification appear in total. One primary centre appears for shaft and two secondary centres appear one each for head and tubercle.

A. *Appearance*

Primary centre: 8th week of intrauterine life.

Secondary centres: Puberty

B. *Fusion:* 20 years.

III. Eleventh and twelfth ribs

Only two primary centres of ossification appear in total, i.e. one primary centre for shaft and one secondary centre for head.

A. *Appearance*

Primary centre: 8th week of intrauterine life.

Secondary centres: Puberty

B. *Fusion:* 20 years.

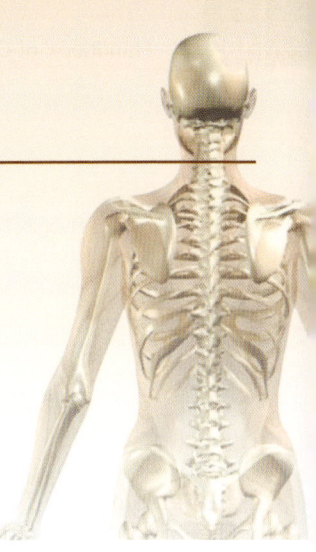

Hyoid

'Hyoid' is a Greek word which means U-shaped.

LEVEL

Hyoid lies at the level of 3rd cervical vertebra.

LOCATION (Fig. 22.1)

1. Hyoid is situated in the anterior midline of neck above the thyroid cartilage.
2. Its body (the bend of 'U') is the first resistant structure felt in the midline of neck, inferior to chin.
3. The tip of the greater cornu (the limb of 'U') of the hyoid can be palpated in the relaxed neck near the anterior border of sterno-cleidomastoid muscle midway between laryngeal prominence and mastoid process.

FEATURES AND ATTACHMENTS

Hyoid bone consists of a central body, a pair of greater cornua and a pair of lesser cornua.

I. BODY

It has two surfaces (anterior and posterior), two borders (upper and lower) and two lateral ends.

A. Surfaces

a. Anterior surface (Figs 22.2 and 22.3)

1. It is convex.
2. A median ridge divides it into two lateral halves.

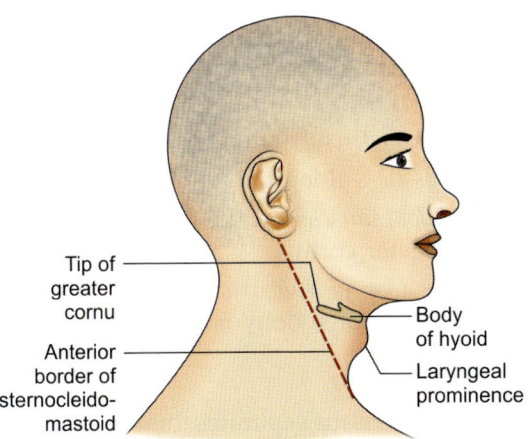

Fig. 22.1: Location of hyoid bone

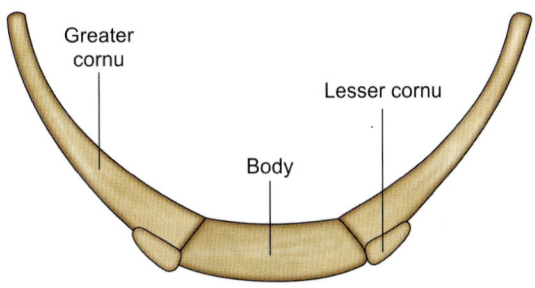

Fig. 22.2: The hyoid bone: Anterior aspect

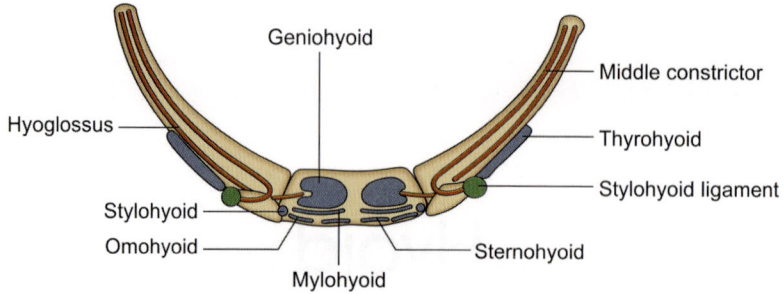

Fig. 22.3: The hyoid bone: Anterior aspect

3. *Geniohyoid* and *mylohyoid muscles* are inserted on this surface in its upper and lower parts respectively.
4. *Hyoglossus* partly originates from anterior surface.
5. *Investing layer of cervical fascia* is attached below the insertion of mylohyoid.

b. Posterior surface

1. It is concave.
2. It is related to following structures (Fig. 22.4).
   i. *Bursa*
   ii. *Thyrohyoid membrane*
   iii. *Epiglottis*

B. Borders

a. Upper border

It provides attachment to 3 structures from anterior to posterior
1. *Genioglossus muscle*
2. *Hyoepiglottic ligament*
3. *Thyrohyoid membrane.*

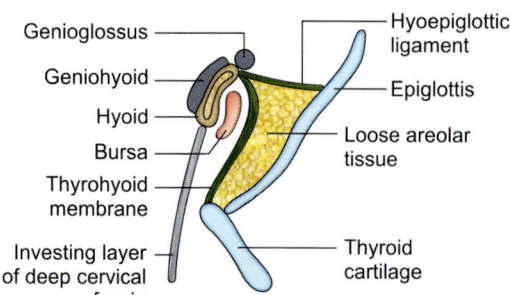

Fig. 22.4: Sectional view of hyoid

b. Lower border

Two muscles are mainly attached to this border on each side of midline from medial to lateral.

1. *Sternohyoid*
2. *Omohyoid*

C. Ends

1. Each end continues posteriorly as greater cornu.
2. Lesser cornu projects upwards at the junction of the body and greater cornu.

II. GREATER CORNUA (SINGULAR: GREATER CORNU)

Greater cronu has two surfaces (upper and lower), two borders (medial and lateral) and a tubercle (at the posterior end).

A. Surfaces

a. Upper surface

It has following attachments from medial to lateral.

1. *Middle constrictor*—along the whole length.
2. *Hyoglossus*—along the whole length.
3. *Stylohyoid muscle*—at the junction of lesser and greater cornua.
4. *Fibrous loop of digastric muscle*—lateral to attachment of stylohyoid muscle.

b. Lower surface

Fibroareolar tissue separates this surface from the thyrohyoid membrane.

B. Borders

a. Medial border

It receives attachment of *thyrohyoid membrane*.

b. Lateral border

Thyrohyoid muscle is attached to this border anteriorly.

III. LESSER CORNUA (SINGULAR: LESSER CORNU)

1. It is a small conical projection attached to the bone at the junction of the body and greater cornu by fibrous tissue.
2. It may form a synovial joint with the greater cornu.
3. It has following attachments:
   i. *Stylohyoid ligament* at the tip.
   ii. *Middle constrictor*—posterolaterally.

OSSIFICATION

1. The hyoid ossifies from ventral portions of the cartilages of 2nd and 3rd arches.
2. Lesser cornua and upper part of the body are developed from the 2nd arch.
3. Greater cornua and lower part of the body are developed from 3rd arch.
4. *Appearance of centres*—6 centres of ossification appear, 2 for body and 1 for each cornu, as follows:

   • Greater cornu: Just before birth

   • Body: Just after birth

   • Lesser cornu: Puberty

5. The cartilage at the tip of each greater cornu persists up to 3rd decade.

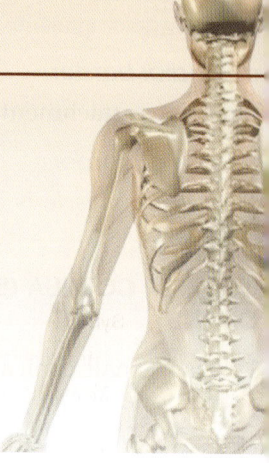

Mandible

TERMINOLOGY

The word 'mandible' is derived from Greek word *mandere* which means to masticate or chew. The Latin word *mandibula* means lower jaw.

PECULIARITIES (Fig. 23.1)

1. It is a U-shaped bone.
2. It is also called 'lower facial skeleton'.
3. Mandible is the largest and strongest bone of the face.
4. It forms the skeleton of lower jaw.

FEATURES AND ATTACHMENTS

The mandible has a body and two rami.

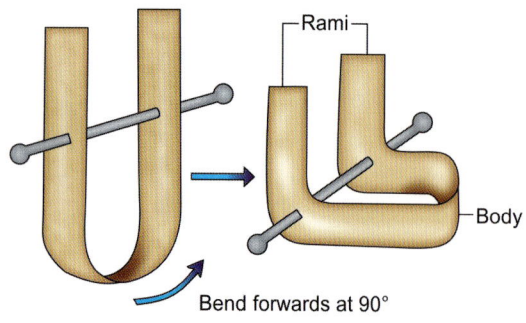

Fig. 23.1: Resemblance of mandible with 'U'

I. BODY

It is shaped like a horseshoe and has 2 surfaces (external and internal) and 2 borders (upper and lower).

A. Surfaces

a. External surface (Figs 23.2 and 23.3)

It has following features:

1. Symphysis menti

It is a faint ridge on the upper part of midline indicating the fusion of two halves of mandible.

2. Mental protuberance

It is triangular area in the lower part of midline. The upper angle of triangle marks the lower end of symphysis menti.

3. Mental tubercles

The lower angles of the triangular mental protuberance are marked by tubercles called mental tubercles.

Note: *Remember that mental protuberance is characteristic of human jaw.*

4. Mental foramen

It is located below the 2nd premolar or junction between two premolar teeth. Mental nerve and vessels pass through it.

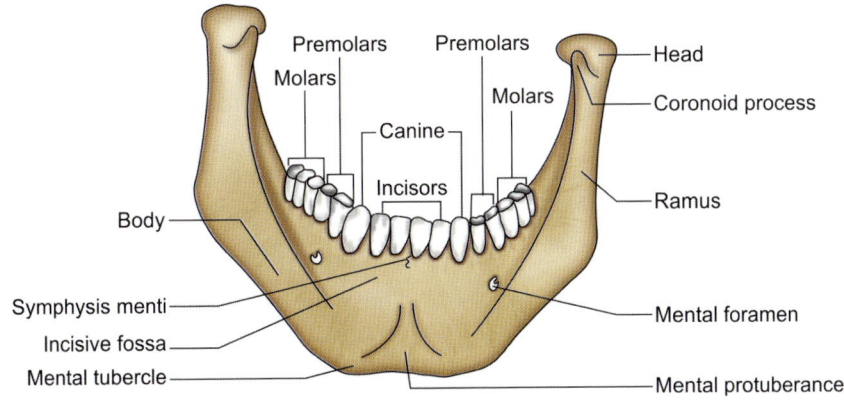

Premolars   Premolars
Molars
Head
Coronoid process
Molars
Canine
Ramus
Incisors
Body
Symphysis menti
Incisive fossa
Mental tubercle
Mental foramen
Mental protuberance

Fig. 23.2: Mandible: Anterior view

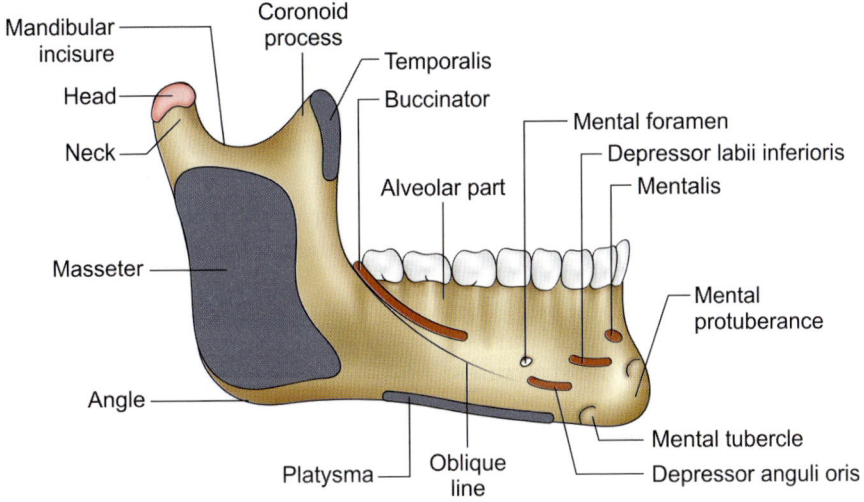

Mandibular incisure
Coronoid process
Head
Temporalis
Neck
Buccinator
Mental foramen
Depressor labii inferioris
Mentalis
Alveolar part
Masseter
Mental protuberance
Angle
Mental tubercle
Platysma
Oblique line
Depressor anguli oris

Fig. 23.3: Right half of mandible: External aspect

5. Incisive fossa

It is a shallow fossa below the incisor teeth. *Mentalis* and *orbicularis oris* originate from this fossa.

6. Oblique line

It is continuation of anterior border of ramus on the external surface of body. It is a faint ridge. It runs downwards and forwards to reach mental tubercle. Following muscles are attached to it from anterior to posterior:

    i. *Depressor labii inferioris.*

    ii. *Depressor anguli oris.*

    iii. *Buccinator (below the molar teeth).*

Note: *Junction of body and ramus is marked by the courses of facial artery and facial vein (Fig. 23.4).*

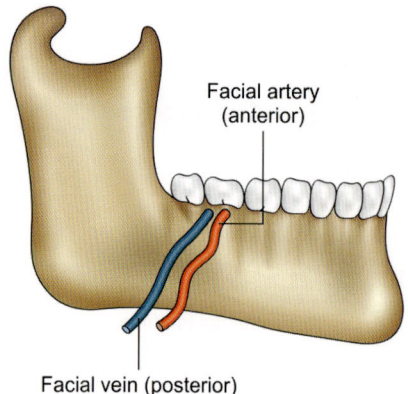

Facial artery
(anterior)

Facial vein (posterior)

Fig. 23.4: Junction of body and ramus of mandible

b. Internal surface (Figs 23.5 and 23.6)

It has following features:

1. Mylohyoid line

It is an oblique ridge. It extends downwards and forwards from behind the 3rd molar tooth (1 cm below the alveolar border) to midline near the lower border between digastric fossae. *Mylohyoid muscle* is attached to it.

2. Submandibular fossa

It is present below the posterior part of mylohyoid line. It lodges following structures:

   i. Submandibular salivary gland.

   ii. Facial artery.

   iii. *Submandibular lymph nodes.*

3. Sublingual fossa

It is an area above the anterior part of mylohyoid line. It lodges the *sublingual salivary gland.*

4. Genial tubercles

These are irregular elevations on either side of midline just above the anterior ends of mylohyoid lines. Upper genial tubercle provides attachment to *genioglossus muscle* while lower genial tubercle gives origin to *geniohyoid muscle.*

> **Note:** *Genial tubercles are for genial muscles, since the tongue is higher as compared to the hyoid bone, the upper tubercle is for genioglossus and lower is for geniohyoid.*

5. Attachment of superior constrictor of pharynx

Superior constrictor originates from the area above the posterior end of mylohyoid line.

6. Attachment of pterygomandibular raphe

This raphe is attached to inner surface of body in continuation with the origin of superior constrictor just behind the 3rd molar tooth.

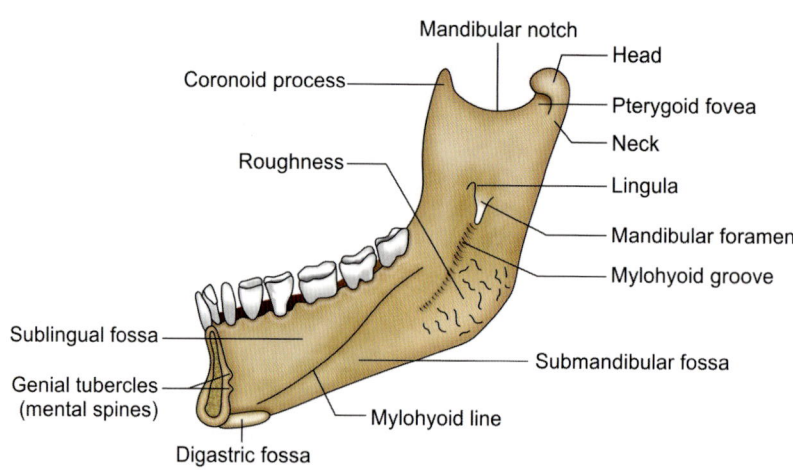

Coronoid process

Roughness

Mandibular notch

Head

Pterygoid fovea

Neck

Lingula

Mandibular foramen

Mylohyoid groove

Sublingual fossa

Genial tubercles
(mental spines)

Digastric fossa

Mylohyoid line

Submandibular fossa

Fig. 23.5: Right half of mandible: Internal aspect

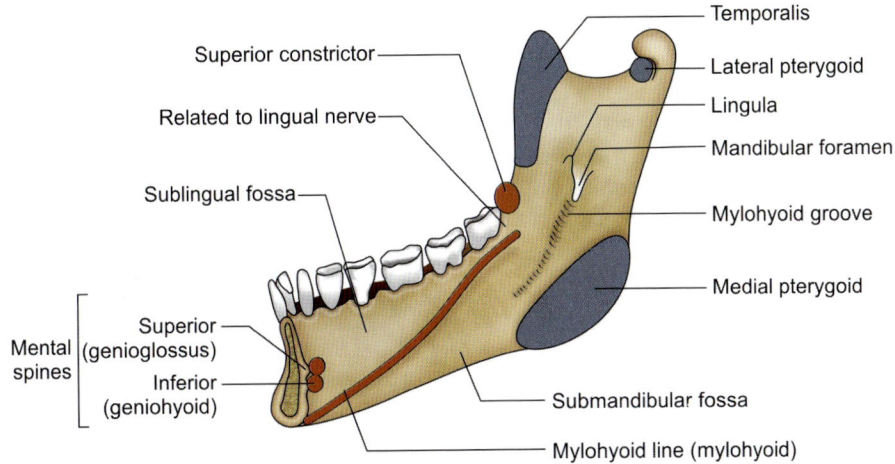

Fig. 23.6: Right half of mandible: Internal aspect

7. Relation of lingual nerve

Lingual nerve is related to mandible between the origin of superior constrictor and posterior end of mylohyoid line.

B. Borders

a. Upper border (Fig. 23.7)

1. It is also called alveolar part of mandible.
2. It is hollowed out by sixteen sockets for the roots of permanent teeth.
3. The sockets vary in size and depth.
4. The sockets may be single or subdivided by septa according to the teeth which they contain.

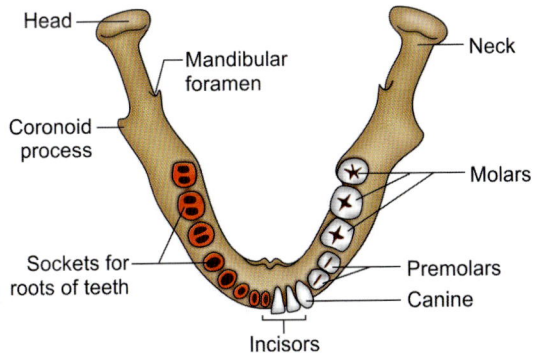

Fig. 23.7: Alveolar part of mandible: Superior view

b. Lower border

1. It is also called the *base* of mandible.
2. *Digastric fossa* is a depression at its anterior (mesial) end on each side of the midline. It receives attachment of *anterior belly of digastric*.
3. *Investing layer of deep cervical fascia* is attached to the whole length of the base.
4. *Platysma* is inserted to the lower border near the outer surface.

II. RAMUS

Ramus of mandible has 2 surfaces (lateral and medial), 4 borders (upper, lower, anterior and posterior) and two processes (coronoid and condylar).

A. Surfaces

a. Lateral surface (Fig. 23.3)

1. A small posterosuperior area is related to *parotid gland*.
2. Remaining major area provides attachment to *masseter*.

Note: *Remember, house of Prime Minister is located on the lateral area. P stands for Parotid and M stands for Masseter.*

b. Medial surface (Figs 23.5 and 23.6)

1. *Mandibular foramen and canal:* Mandibular foramen is located a little above the centre of medial surface. It leads into mandibular canal which curves downwards and forwards into the body, to open on the external surface at the mental foramen. *Inferior alveolar nerve and vessels* enter the mandibular canal through the mandibular foramen.
2. *Lingula:* It is a tongue-shaped projection near the anterior margin of mandibular foramen. *Sphenomandibular ligament* is attached to the lingula.
3. *Mylohyoid groove:* It begins at the lower end of mandibular foramen behind the lingula and continues downwards and forwards to reach the inner surface of body. *Mylohyoid nerve* and *vessels* occupy the mylohyoid groove.
4. Medial surface of ramus between mylo-hyoid groove and angle of mandible is marked by ridges. This area is meant for the attachment of *medial pterygoid.*
5. Area in front of mylohyoid groove is related to *lingual nerve.*

B. Borders

a. Upper border

1. It is thin.
2. It forms *mandibular notch* or *incisure.*
3. *Masseteric nerve* and *vessels* cross the mandibular notch.

b. Lower border

1. It is backward continuation of base of mandible.
2. It meets with the posterior border of ramus to form *angle of mandible.*

c. Anterior border

1. It is continuous above with the coronoid process and below with alveolar border of body.
2. *Temporalis* muscle is inserted on this border and adjoining medial surface.

d. Posterior border

1. It is continuous above with the condylar process.
2. It meets with the lower border to form *angle of mandible.*
3. It is related to *parotid gland.*

C. Processes

a. Coronoid process

1. It is triangular upward projection from the anterosuperior part of ramus.
2. Its anterior border is continuous with the anterior border of the ramus and its posterior border bounds the mandibular notch.
3. *Temporalis muscle* gets inserted on the medial surface, apex and margins of coronoid process.

b. Condylar process

It is an upward projection from the postero-superior part of ramus. It consists of an upper part (*head*) and a lower part (*neck*).

i. Head

1. It is side to side expanded part of condylar process.
2. It articulates with the temporal bone to form *temporomandibular joint.*

ii. Neck

1. It is constricted part below the head.
2. It provides attachment to *capsule* in its upper part.
3. *Lateral ligament of temporomandibular joint* is attached to its lateral part.
4. *Pterygoid fovea* is a depression on its anterior aspect. *Lateral pterygoid muscle* is inserted on the pterygoid fovea.
5. Medially the neck is related to *auriculo-temporal nerve* above and *maxillary artery* below.

OSSIFICATION

1. Mandible is intramembranous as well as endochondral in origin.
2. The membrane involved is the mesenchymal sheath on the lateral aspect of both Meckel's cartilages. A centre appears on each side in this sheath during 7th week of intrauterine life.
3. Cartilages contributing to the mandible are as follows:
   i. *Anterior ends of Meckel's cartilages*
      These are invaded by bone from parent centres at 10th week of intrauterine life.
   ii. *Coronoid cartilages*
      These appear at 10th week of intrauterine life and disappear before birth.
   iii. *Condylar cartilages*
      These appear at 10th week of intrauterine life and persist till 3rd decade.
   iv. *Cartilaginous nodules*
      One or two of these nodules appear on each side of the symphysis menti at about 10th week of intrauterine life. These ossify to form mental ossicles at about the 7th month of intrauterine life and fuse with the body at the age of one year.
4. Parts of the mandible which are derived from cartilage, are:

i. Incisive part below the incisor teeth.
ii. Coronoid and condylar processes.
iii. Part of ramus above the mandibular foramen.

Note: *Remember that the names of all the parts of mandible which ossifying from cartilage start with C, i.e. Coronoid process, Condylar process, Cranial part of ramus and Chin part of body related to Cutting or incisor teeth.*

5. At birth mandible consists of two halves connected at *symphysis menti*. Bony union starts from below upwards during 1st year of age and is completed at the end of 3rd year.

AGE CHANGES IN MANDIBLE

Some of the differentiating features in different age groups are as follows.

I. Children (Fig. 23.8)

1. The body of mandible is more like a shell having sockets for both deciduous and permanent teeth.
2. The angle of mandible measures about 140°.
3. Coronoid process is above the level of condylar process.
4. The mandibular canal and mental foramen are close to the lower border of body.

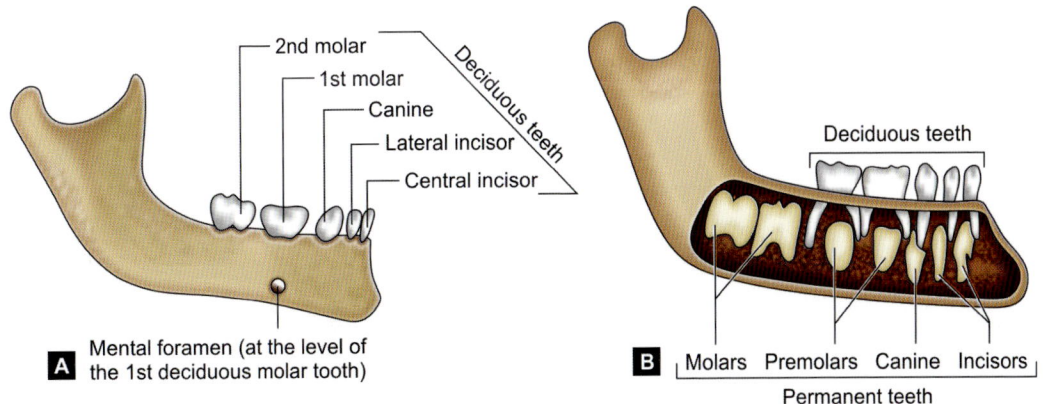

A — 2nd molar / 1st molar / Canine / Lateral incisor / Central incisor — Deciduous teeth — Mental foramen (at the level of the 1st deciduous molar tooth)

B — Deciduous teeth — Molars Premolars Canine Incisors — Permanent teeth

Fig. 23.8: Right lateral view of the mandible of a child between 2 and 6 years. (A) Surface features; (B) Body dissected

II. Adult (Fig. 23.9)

1. The alveolar and subalveolar parts of body are of equal depths.
2. The angle of mandible measures about 110°.
3. Condylar process projects above the level of coronoid process.
4. Mandibular canal runs parallel to the mylohyoid line.
5. The mental foramen is situated midway between upper and lower borders of body.

III. Old age (Fig. 23.10)

1. Loss of teeth is a usual feature.
2. Alveolar part is absorbed.
3. Angle of mandible measures about 140°
4. Neck of mandible is bent backwards making the level of coronoid process higher than condylar process.
5. Mandibular canal and mental foramen are close to the upper border of body.

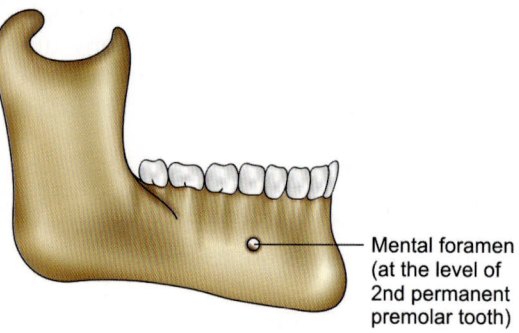

Mental foramen (at the level of 2nd permanent premolar tooth)

Fig. 23.9: Adult mandible: Right lateral view

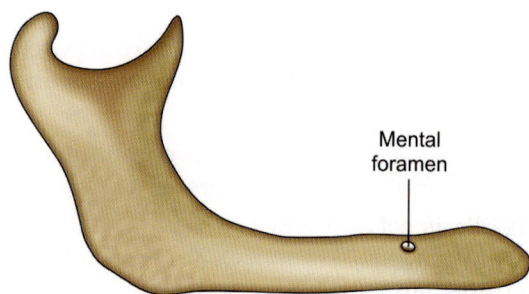

Mental foramen

Fig. 23.10: The mandible at old age. Right lateral view

Maxilla

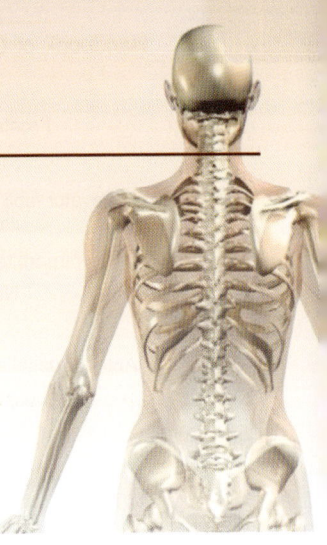

TERMINOLOGY

Maxilla is a Latin word meaning 'cheek' or 'jaw'. The word is commonly used in reference to upper jaw.

LOCATION

1. There are two maxillae which form major part of upper facial skeleton.
2. Whole of the upper jaw is formed by two maxillae.
3. Junction of two maxillae is marked by intermaxillary suture visible in the hard palate and face in midline.

FEATURES AND ATTACHMENTS

Each maxilla consists of a body and four processes (zygomatic, frontal, alveolar and palatine).

I. BODY (Figs 24.1 and 24.2)

It has 4 surfaces (anterior, infratemporal, orbital and nasal).

A. Anterior surface

1. It is directed forwards and laterally.
2. There is a vertical elevation at the site of socket for canine root. This is called *canine eminence.*

3. Medial to canine eminence is a depression called *incisive fossa* which gives origin to *depressor septi.*
4. The anterior surface below the incisive fossa gives attachments to *incisivus superior* and *orbicularis oris.*
5. Just above the incisive fossa there is attachment of *nasalis muscle.*
6. Lateral to canine eminence is another fossa called *canine fossa. Levator anguli oris* originates from the canine fossa.
7. Above the canine fossa is a foramen called *infraorbital foramen.* It transmits *infraorbital nerve and vessels.*
8. Above the infra-orbital foramen is sharp infra-orbital margin which gives origin to *levator labii superioris.*
9. Its upper part is limited medially by a deep notch called *nasal notch.*

B. Infratemporal surface

1. It faces backwards and laterally.
2. It forms anterior wall of *infratemporal fossa.*
3. It shows 2–3 openings of *alveolar canals* which transmit *posterior superior alveolar nerves and vessels.*
4. Its inferoposterior part is marked by *maxillary tuberosity* which articulates with the pyramidal process of palatine bone.

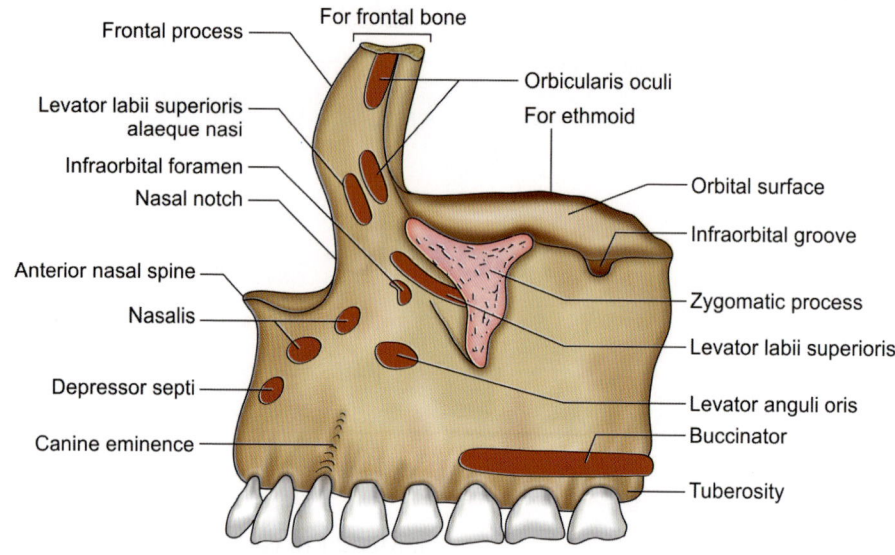

Frontal process

For frontal bone

Levator labii superioris alaeque nasi

Orbicularis oculi

For ethmoid

Infraorbital foramen

Nasal notch

Orbital surface

Infraorbital groove

Anterior nasal spine

Nasalis

Zygomatic process

Levator labii superioris

Depressor septi

Levator anguli oris

Buccinator

Canine eminence

Tuberosity

Fig. 24.1: Left maxilla: Lateral aspect

C. Orbital surface

1. It forms floor of orbit.

2. Running forwards is *infraorbital groove* in the middle of its posterior part. The groove continues with *infra-orbital canal* which opens on the anterior surface as *infraorbital foramen*. It is meant for *infraorbital nerve and vessels*.

3. Anteromedially it gives origin to *inferior oblique muscle*.

4. It has 3 borders (medial, posterior and anterior).

a. Medial border

It is marked anteriorly by *lacrimal notch*. Behind this notch this border provides attachments to lacrimal bone, orbital plate of ethmoid and orbital process of palatine bone from before backwards.

b. Posterior border

It forms anterior border of inferior orbital fissure.

c. Anterior border

It contributes to the medial part of infra-orbital margin.

D. Nasal surface (Fig. 24.2)

1. It forms the lateral wall of nasal cavity.

2. A large opening (*maxillary hiatus*) is the most prominent feature of this surface.

3. Maxillary hiatus leads into *maxillary sinus,* a large air space within the body of maxilla.

4. Maxillary hiatus is greatly reduced in size in articulated skull by ethmoid (uncinate process) and lacrimal bone above, inferior concha below and perpendicular plate of palatine bone behind.

5. Below the hiatus this surface forms inferior meatus of nasal cavity.

6. Posterior part of nasal surface has got an *oblique groove* which is converted into *greater palatine canal* by perpendicular plate of palatine bone. Greater palatine nerve and vessels pass through this canal.

7. In front of hiatus is *nasolacrimal groove*. This is converted into *nasolacrimal canal* by lacrimal bone and inferior concha. This canal is meant for *nasolacrimal duct*.

8. An oblique ridge called *conchal crest*, is present in front of nasolacrimal groove. It articulates with inferior concha.

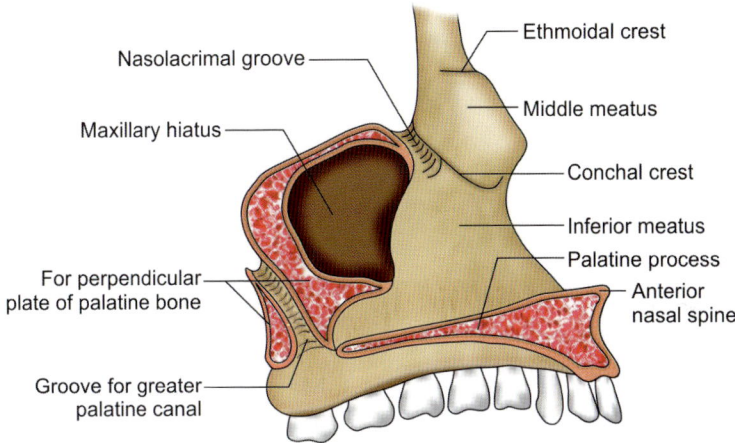

Nasolacrimal groove
Maxillary hiatus
For perpendicular plate of palatine bone
Groove for greater palatine canal

Ethmoidal crest
Middle meatus
Conchal crest
Inferior meatus
Palatine process
Anterior nasal spine

Fig. 24.2: Left maxilla: Medial aspect

I. PROCESSES

A. Zygomatic process

It has three surfaces, anterior, posterior and superior. The latter is rough for articulation with zygomatic bone.

B. Frontal process

It possesses an upper end, 2 surfaces (lateral and medial) and 2 borders (anterior and posterior).

a. Upper end

It articulates with the nasal notch of frontal bone.

b. Surfaces

i. Lateral surface (Fig. 24.1)

1. It has a vertical ridge (*anterior lacrimal crest*) in the middle for the attachment of *medial palpebral ligament*.
2. Area in front of crest gives attachments to *orbicularis oculi* and *levator labii superioris alaeque nasi*.
3. Area behind the lacrimal crest contributes to the anterior half of lacrimal groove.

ii. Medial surface (Fig. 24.2)

1. It has got a horizontal ridge (*ethmoidal crest*) in its middle. It articulates with middle nasal concha.
2. A roughened area above the crest articulates with ethmoid to complete anterior ethmoidal air cells.
3. The area below the ethmoidal crest forms *atrium* of middle meatus.

c. Borders

i. Anterior border

It articulates with nasal bone.

ii. Posterior border

It articulates with lacrimal bone.

C. Alveolar process

1. It is arched lower border of body.
2. It has sockets for upper teeth.
3. *Buccinator* originates from the posterior part of outer surface over the sockets for permanent molars roots.

D. Palatine process

It is a horizontal bracket like projection from the lower part of medial surface of body. It forms anterior 3/4th of hard palate. It has two surfaces (superior and inferior) and three borders (medial, posterior and lateral).

a. Surfaces

i. Superior surface

1. It is concave and smooth.
2. It forms floor of nasal cavity.

ii. Inferior surface

1. It has *depressions* for palatine glands.
2. It has several *nutrient foramina* for nutrient vessels.
3. *Greater palatine groove* for greater palatine nerve and vessels is present in its postero-lateral part.
4. When two maxillae meet, *incisive fossa* is noticed behind the incisor teeth.
5. *Incisive canal* is communication between incisive fossa and nasal cavity. It transmits *greater palatine artery* and *nasopalatine nerve*.

b. Borders

i. Medial border

1. It meets with the similar border of opposite maxilla to form *intermaxillary suture*.
2. This border is raised into a ridge called *nasal crest*. Nasal crests of two sides enclose a groove to receive the vomer.
3. Its anterior end is prolonged and meets with the similar prolongation of opposite side to form *anterior nasal spine*.

ii. Posterior border

It articulates with the anterior border of horizontal plate of palatine bone to form *palatomaxillary suture*.

iii. Lateral border

It fuses with the body.

OSSIFICATION

1. The maxilla is intramembranous in origin.
2. It develops in the mesenchyme just super-ficial to nasal capsule.

3. Three centres of ossification appear:
    i. One centre appears for the main mass just above canine fossa at about 6th week of intrauterine life.
    ii. Two centres appear for os incisivum (premaxillary part).

> **Note:** *Remember that premaxilla is that part of maxilla which holds incisor teeth and is a separate bone in most mammalian upper jaws.*

4. Maxillary sinus appears on the nasal aspect as a groove at about 4th month of intra-uterine life.

AGE CHANGES IN MAXILLA

I. At birth

1. Vertical diameter is lesser than both the transverse and anteroposterior diameters.
2. Body is mainly occupied by sockets for the teeth.
3. Maxillary sinus is seen as a shallow groove on the nasal aspect.

II. Adult

1. Vertical diameter is greater than the transverse and anteroposterior diameters.
2. Maxillary sinus has greatly developed within the body.

III. Old age

1. Due to falling of teeth and resorption of alveolar margin, the vertical diameter is again greatly reduced.
2. Alveolar margin is reduced in thickness at the expense of the labial wall.

MAXILLARY SINUS (ANTRUM OF HIGHMORE)

It is the air space in the body of maxilla. It is pyramidal in shape with base towards nasal cavity and apex towards zygomatic process. Its height and anteroposterior measurements are 1.5 inches each while width is 1 inch only.

Parietal Bone

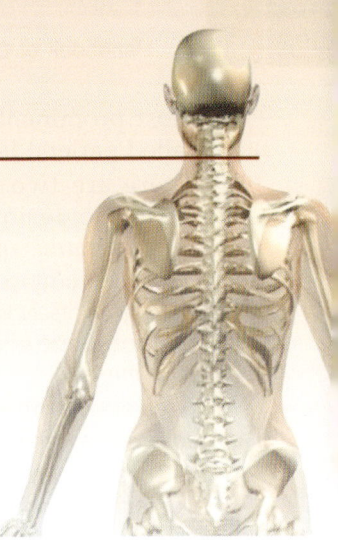

he word parietal is derived from Latin word
aries which means 'wall', because two
parietal bones form large part of walls of
calvaria.

SIDE DETERMINATION

. Keep the bone by the side of your own
   cranial vault in such a way that outer
   surface is convex and inner surface is
   concave.
2. Inferior (squamosal) border is concave.

3. Anteroinferior angle is prominent and has
   got a vascular and narrow groove on its
   inner aspect.
4. The posteroinferior angle has got a shallow
   and wide groove for sigmoid sinus on its
   inner aspect.

FEATURES AND ATTACHMENTS

I. Surfaces

It has two surfaces, external and internal.

A. External surface (Fig. 25.1)

1. It is relatively smooth.

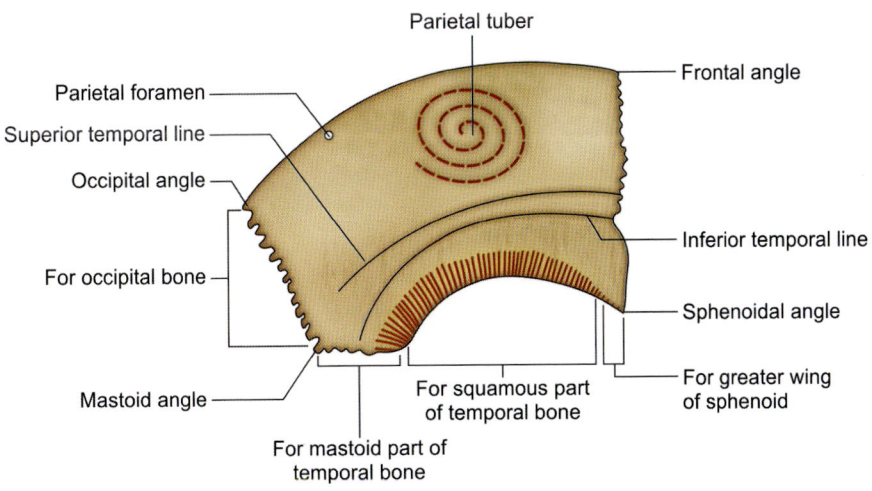

Fig. 25.1: Right parietal bone: External surface

2. Most prominent part of this surface is called parietal *tuberosity* or *eminence*.

3. There are two curved lines running anteroposteriorly. These are called *superior and inferior temporal lines.* Superior temporal line gives attachment to *tempral fascia* while area below inferior temporal line gives attachment to *temporalis muscle.*

4. Area above the superior temporal line is covered by *galea aponeurotica.*

5. A foramen may be present near the posterior part of sagittal border. This is called *parietal foramen.* It transmits *emissary vein.*

B. Internal surface (Fig. 25.2)

1. It is concave and exhibits elevations and depressions for cerebral sulci and gyri respectively.

2. Near the sagittal border there is a longitudinal half groove (to be completed with that of opposite side) for *superior sagittal sinus.* The margins of groove provide attachment to *falx cerebri.*

3. Grooves for the branches of *middle meningeal vessels* are present at the anteroinferior angle and at the middle of the lower border of the bone.

4. Adjacent to groove for superior sagitta sinus there are deep irregular pit (*granular foveolae*) produced by *arachnoi granulations.*

5. The bone is grooved near the postero inferior angle by *sigmoid sinus.*

II. Borders

It has four borders, superior, inferior anterior and posterior.

A. Superior border

1. This is also called sagittal border.

2. It articulates with the similar border o opposite side to form sagittal suture.

B. Inferior border

1. This is also called squamosal border.

2. It articulates with following 3 bones from anterior to posterior:
   i. Greater wing of sphenoid.
   ii. Squamous part of temporal.
   iii. Mastoid portion of temporal.

C. Anterior border

1. This is also called frontal border.

2. It articulates with the frontal bone to form *coronal suture.*

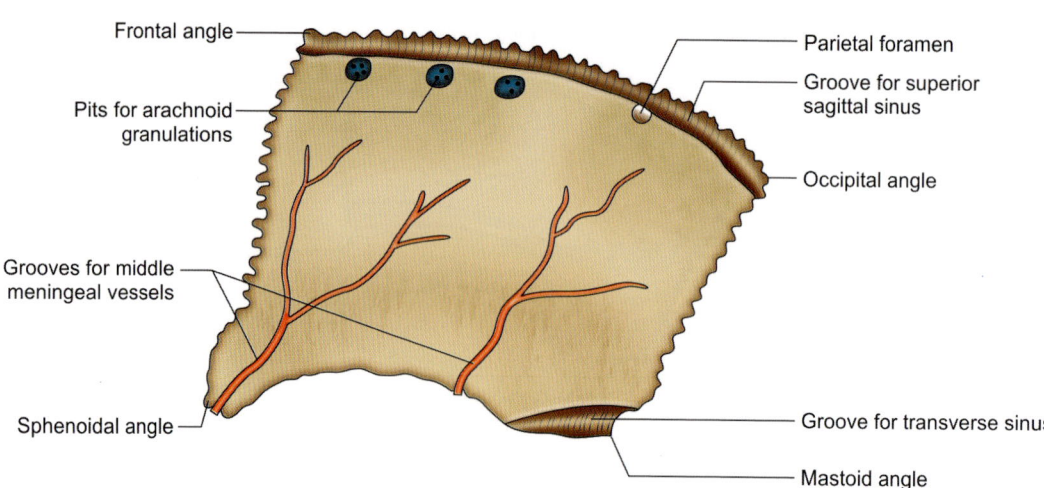

Fig. 25.2: Right parietal bone: Internal surface

. Posterior border

1. This is also called occipital border.
2. It articulates with the squamous part of occipital bone to form *lambdoid suture*.

. Angles

arietal bone has four angles (frontal, phenoidal, occipital and mastoid).

. Frontal angle

. This is also called anterosuperior angle.
. It corresponds to *bregma*, i.e. the junction of coronal and sagittal sutures.

. Sphenoidal angle

1. This is also called anteroinferior angle.
2. It correspsonds to *pterion*, i.e. a small area enclosing four bones (frontal, temporal, parietal and greater wing of sphenoid).

. Occipital angle

1. This is also called posterosuperior angle.
2. It corresponds to *lambda*, i.e. junction of sagittal and lambdoid sutures.

. Mastoid angle

1. This is also called posteroinferior angle.

2. It corresponds to *asterion*, i.e. small area enclosing three bones, parietal, temporal and occipital.

OSSIFICATION

1. Parietal bones ossify in membrane.
2. Each ossifies from two centres which appear at parietal tuberosity at about 7th week of intrauterine life.
3. The centres soon fuse with each other and then the ossification spreads radially.
4. Angles are the parts last to be ossified explaining the existence of a fontanelle at each angle before the ossification is completed.

AGE CHANGES

1. At birth

Temporal lines are present at quite a lower level.

2. Adult

A higher and permanent positions of temporal lines are reached only after the eruption of permanent molar teeth.

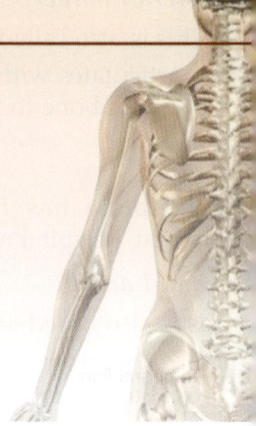

Frontal Bone

TERMINOLOGY

The term 'frontal' is derived from Latin word *frons* which means 'brow' or 'forehead'.

LOCATION

Frontal bone forms the forehead, greater part of the roof of each orbit and most of the floor of anterior cranial fossa.

FEATURES AND ATTACHMENTS

Frontal bone has got a main part (frontal squama) and orbital parts.

I. Frontal squama (main part)

It has got an external surface, right and left temporal surfaces, an internal surface, a nasal part and a margin (parietal or posterior).

A. Surfaces

a. External surface (Figs 26.1 and 26.2)

  i. *Supra-orbital margins*
   1. These are lower limits of external surface on each side.
   2. They form upper borders of the orbital openings.
  ii. *Supra-orbital notch or foramen*
   1. The junction of lateral two-thirds of supra-orbital margin (sharp) with the

medial one-third (rounded) is marke by supra-orbital notch (some time foramen).
   2. This is meant for the passage of *supra-orbital nerve, supra-orbital artery* and *communicating vein* between angula and superior ophthalmic veins.
  iii. *Superciliary arch*

   This is an arched prominence just abov the supra-orbital margin.
  iv. *Glabella*

   It is the median prominence betwee superciliary arches.
  v. *Frontal eminence*
   1. On each side, about 3 cm above th supra-orbital margin, there is a elevated area called frontal eminenc or tuberosity.
   2. It is usually more marked in female.
  vi. *Metopic suture*

   Frontal bone is bilateral in origin and th junction of the two halves is called front. or metopic suture. It remains can be see even in adult in the reigon of glabella.
  vii. *Zygomatic process*
   1. Supra-orbital margin extends laterall on each side into a zygomatic proces
   2. Zygomatic process articulates wit frontal process of zygomatic bone.

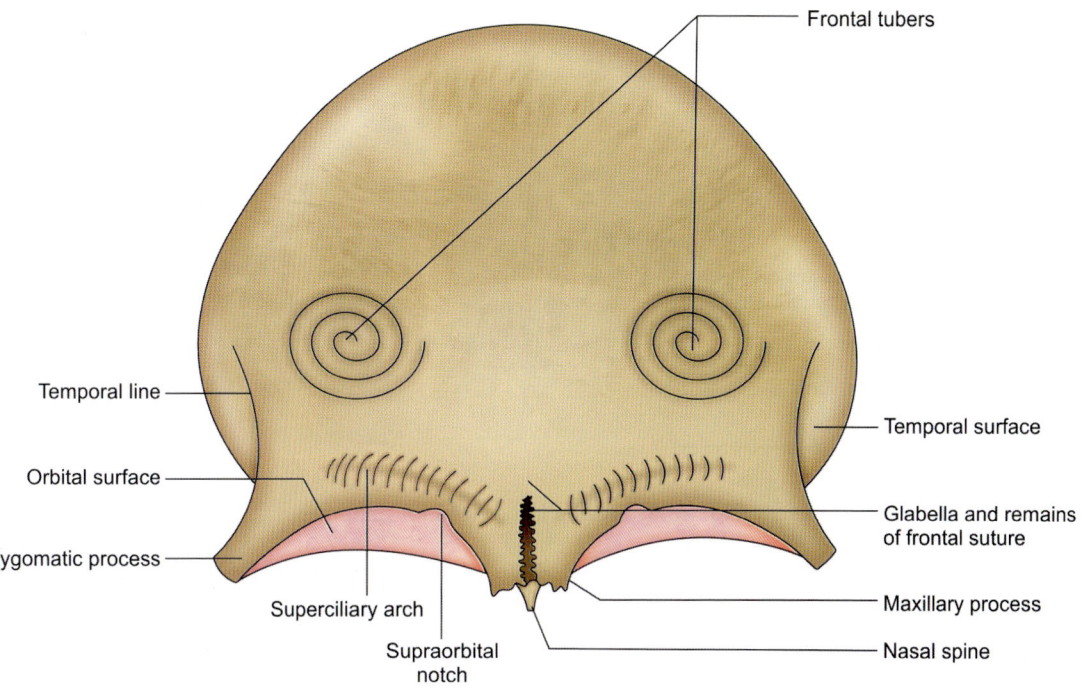

Fig. 26.1: Frontal bone: Anterior aspect

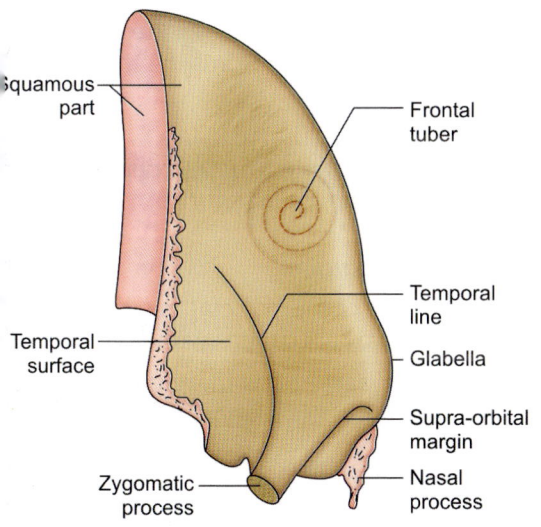

Fig. 26.2: Frontal bone: Right lateral aspect

iii. A line curves upwards and backwards from the zyomatic process. The line soon divides into two lines called *superior and inferior temporal lines.*

b. Temporal surfaces

1. An area on each side below and behind the temporal lines is called temporal surface.

2. It contributes to the anterior part of *temporal fossa* on the lateral aspect of skull (norma lateralis).

3. Superior temporal line gives attachment to *temporal fascia.*

4. Inferior temporal line and temporal surface of frontal bone give origin to *temporalis muscle.*

c. Internal surface (Fig. 26.3)

i. This surface shows depressions and elevations for cerebral gyri and sulci respectively.

ii. *Sagittal sulcus*

1. It is a midline sulcus in the upper part of internal surface.

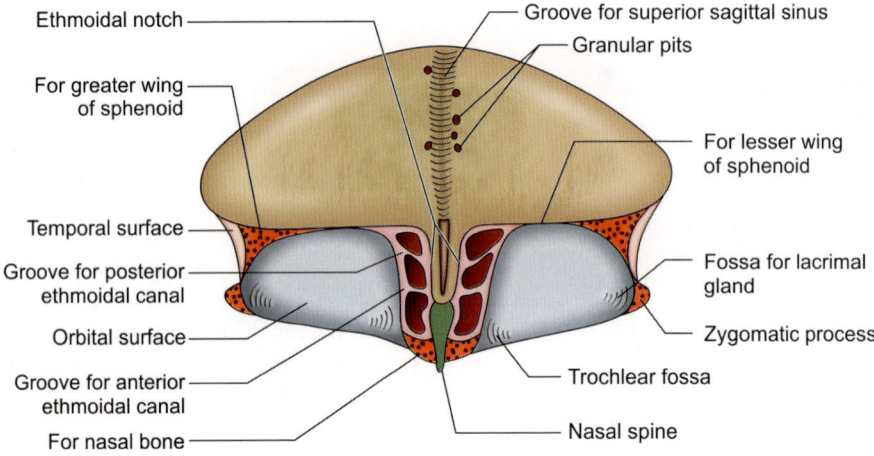

Ethmoidal notch
Groove for superior sagittal sinus
Granular pits
For greater wing of sphenoid
For lesser wing of sphenoid
Temporal surface
Groove for posterior ethmoidal canal
Fossa for lacrimal gland
Orbital surface
Zygomatic process
Groove for anterior ethmoidal canal
Trochlear fossa
For nasal bone
Nasal spine

Fig. 26.3: Frontal bone: Inferior aspect

2. Its margins provide attachments to *falx cerebri*.

3. Sulcus itself lodges *superior sagittal sinus*.

  iii. *Frontal crest*

    1. Margins of sagittal sulcus meet in the midline in the lower part and continue as frontal crest.

    2. This also gives attachment to *falx cerebri*.

  iv. A notch below the frontal crest is converted into *foramen caecum* by articulation with ethmoid bone. An *emissary vein* passing through it connects the vein of nose with superior sagittal sinus.

  v. Several depressions (*granular foveolae*) on each side of sagittal sulcus are produced by *arachnoid granulations*.

B. Nasal part

1. It is a downward projection of frontal bone between two supra-orbital margins.

2. Its lower serrated part is known as *nasal notch*.

3. Each half of the nasal notch articulates with the following three bones from anterior to posterior:

  i. *Nasal bone*.

  ii. *Frontal process of maxilla*.

  iii. *Lacrimal bone*.

4. *Nasal spine* is a midline downward continuation of the nasal part.

5. On each side of nasal spine there is a grooved area which froms the roof of nasal cavity.

6. Nasal spine itself articulates with crest of the nasal bone anteriorly and perpendicular plate of ethmoid posteriorly.

C. Posterior margin

1. This is also called parietal margin because its major part articulates with *parietal bones*.

2. The lower part of this margin is triangular and rough for articulation with *greater wing of sphenoid*.

II. Orbital parts

Orbital parts consist of two triangular laminae (*orbital plates*) separated by a gap called *ethmoidal notch*.

A. Orbital plate

It possesses two surfaces, orbital and internal.

a. Orbital surface

1. It faces downwards.
2. It forms *roof of the orbit*.
3. Its anterolateral part has got a *fossa for the lacrimal gland*.
4. Its anteromedial part (*trochlear fovea*) provides attachment to *fibrocartilaginous pulley* for tendon of superior oblique muscle.

b. Internal surface (Fig. 26.4)

1. It faces upwards.
2. It contributes to anterior cranial fossa.
3. It has impressions for gyri of frontal lobe of cerebral hemisphere.
4. It has grooves for meningeal vessels.

B. Ethmoidal notch (Figs 26.3 and 26.4)

1. It is U-shaped gap occupied by *cribriform plate of ethmoid*.
2. Under surfaces of its lateral margins possess several incomplete air cells which complete the ethmiodal air cells when ethmoid bone is in position.
3. Two grooves on the under surface of each margin are converted into *anterior and posterior ethmoidal canals* by similar grooves on the superior surface of ethmoidal labyrinth. These canals are meant for passages of *anterior and posterior ethmoidal nerves and vessels*.
4. The under surface of the anterior margin of the notch possesses openings for frontal sinuses (one on each side of the nasal spine).

III. Frontal sinus

Each frontal sinus is an irregular cavity of variable size. It is situated between outer and inner tables of frontal bone. They are separated from each other by a bony septum which is usually deviated to one side.

OSSIFICATION

1. Frontal bone ossifies in membrane.
2. Two primary centres appear, one for each half of frontal bone, in the region of frontal tuberosity.
3. Primary centres appear during 8th week of intrauterine life.
4. Ossification extends upwards to form frontal squama, backwards to form orbital part and downwards to form nasal part.
5. At birth frontal bone is made up of two halves separated by *frontal* or *metopic suture* (Fig. 26.5).
6. Union between two parts begins at 2nd year and completes at 8th year.

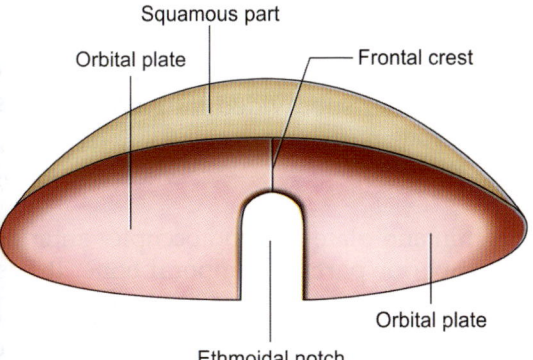

Fig. 26.4: Frontal bone: Superior aspect (diagrammatic)

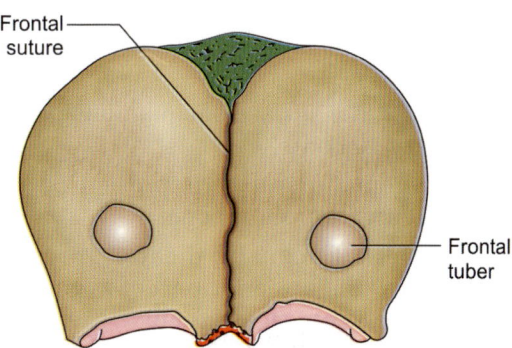

Fig. 26.5: Frontal bone at birth

Temporal Bone

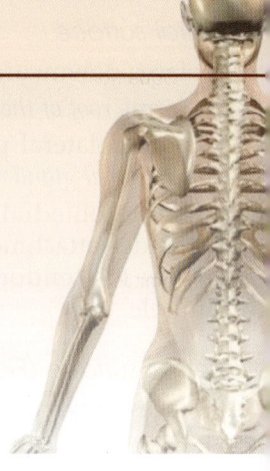

TERMINOLOGY

Temporal bone is so named because of its contribution to temporal region.

SIDE DETERMINATION

I. To distinguish superior and inferior, following features are to be noted:

 1. Thin plate like squamous part is directed upwards and lies in para-sagittal plane.
 2. Styloid and mastoid processes occupy the lower part of the bone and are directed downwards.

II. To distinguish external and internal aspects, one should consider following features:

 1. The outer surface of squamous part is very smooth.
 2. Zygomatic process is present on the external aspect of bone.
 3. External acoustic meatus (present below the posterior part of zygomatic process) opens externally.
 4. Apex of petrous temporal is directed medially and a little forwards.

III. To distinguish anterior from posterior, following criteria should be taken into account:

 1. Zygomatic process is directed forwards.
 2. Mandibular fossa and external acoustic meatus are present below the posterior part of zygomatic process. Relatively, mandibular fossa is anterior to external acoustic meatus.

FEATURES AND ATTACHMENTS

Morphologically temporal bone is divided into four parts.

 1. Squamous part.
 2. Petromastoid part.
 3. Tympanic part.
 4. Styloid process.

For descriptive purpose, the petromastoid part is further subdivided into mastoid part and petrous part.

I. Squamous part

It is thin and plate-like and occupies anterior and superior parts of temporal bone. It has two surfaces (temporal and cerebral) and two borders (superior and anteroinferior).

A. Surfaces

a. Temporal surface (Fig. 27.1)

 1. It is outer surface.
 2. It is smooth and slightly convex.

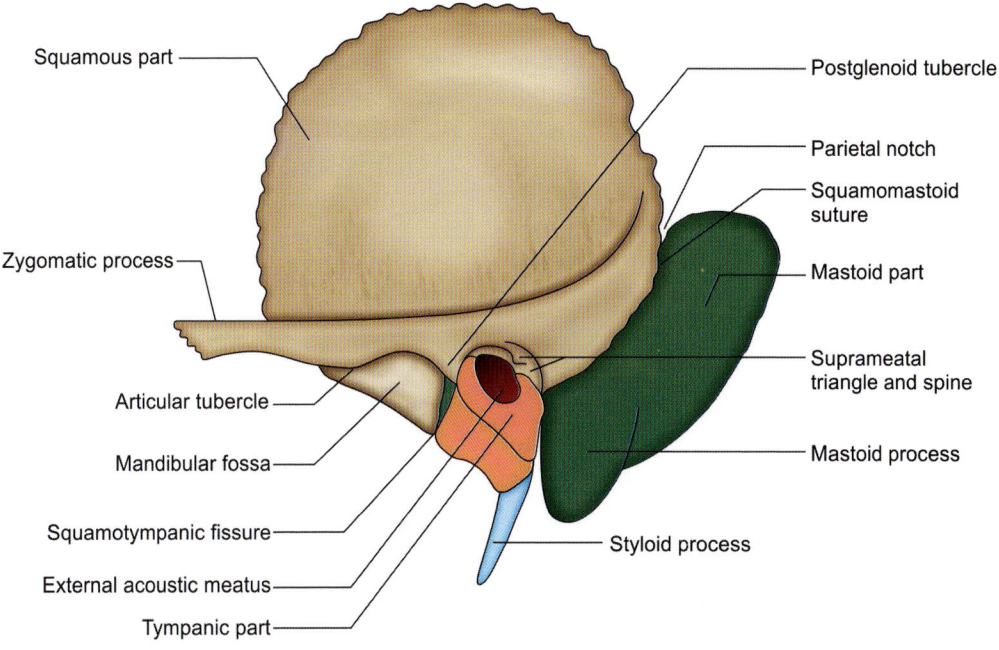

Squamous part

Postglenoid tubercle

Parietal notch

Squamomastoid suture

Zygomatic process

Mastoid part

Articular tubercle

Suprameatal triangle and spine

Mandibular fossa

Mastoid process

Squamotympanic fissure

Styloid process

External acoustic meatus

Tympanic part

Fig. 27.1: Left temporal bone: External aspect

3. It contributes to the temporal fossa meant for the origin of *temporalis muscle*.

4. *Middle temporal artery* grooves the surface, just above the external acoustic meatus.

5. *Supramastoid crest* runs backwards and upwards across its posterior part. Temporal fascia is attached to this crest.

6. *Squamomastoid suture* marks the junction between squamous and mastoid parts. It is situated 1.5 cm below the supra-mastoid crest.

7. Macewen's triangle (suprameatal triangle) (Fig. 27.2)

   i. It is a triangular depression postero-superior to external acoustic meatus.

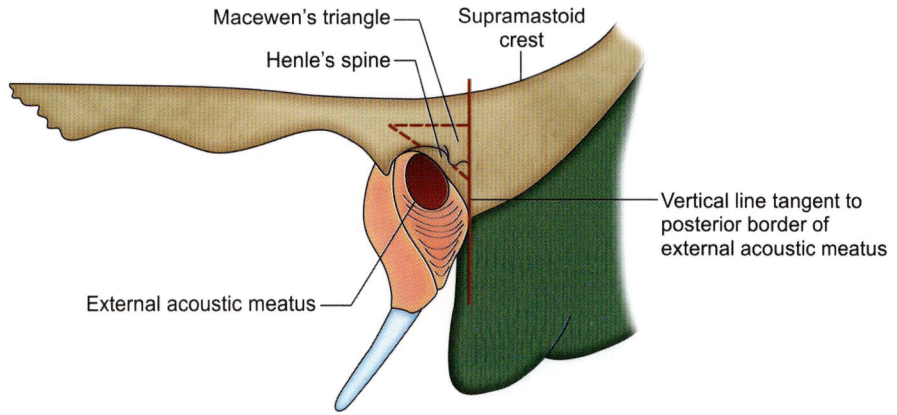

Macewen's triangle

Supramastoid crest

Henle's spine

Vertical line tangent to posterior border of external acoustic meatus

External acoustic meatus

Fig. 27.2: Macewen's triangle of left side

ii. It is bounded by posterosuperior margin of external acoustic meatus, supramastoid crest and a vertical line tangent to posterior border of external acoustic meatus.

iii. *Spine of Henle* is sharp, spur-like projection in the suprameatal triangle.

iv. Mastoid antrum is situated 12.5 mm deep to the surface of suprameatal triangle in adult.

8. *Zygomatic process*

   i. It is a forward projection from the lower part of temporal surface.

   ii. Its anterior end articulates with the temporal process of zygomatic bone to complete the zygomatic arch or zygoma.

   iii. Anterior part of zygomatic process has two surfaces (lateral and medial) and two borders (superior and inferior). *Masseter* originates from its medial surface and inferior border. *Temporal fascia* is attached to its superior border. Its lateral surface is subcutaneous.

   iv. Its posterior part is triangular having superior and inferior surfaces.

   v. Inferior surface of the posterior part of zygomatic process is bounded by two roots (anterior and posterior) which converge at the *tubercle of the root of zygoma*. Lateral *ligament of temporomandibular joint* is attached to this tubercle.

   vi. Anterior root extends medially from tubercle of the root of zygoma and is also called *articular tubercle*.

9. Mandibular fossa

   i. It is situated behind the articular tubercle.

   ii. Only anterior part of mandibular fossa is articular and contributed by squamous part of temporal bone.

   iii. Articular tubercle and anterior part of mandibular fossa is related to the superior surface of *articular disc* of temporomandibular joint.

iv. Posterior part of mandibular fossa is non-articular and contributed by tympanic part of temporal bone. This part is related to the *parotid gland*.

10. *Squamotympanic fissure*

   i. It is situated in the mandibular fossa and marks the junction of squamous and tympanic parts of temporal bone.

   ii. Medial part of this fissure is divided into *petrosquamous and petrotympanic fissures* by the projection of *tegmen tympani* of petrous part of temporal bone.

   iii. Three structures pass through petrotympanic fissure, i.e. *chorda tympani nerve, anterior tympanic artery* and *anterior ligament of malleus*.

Note: *To remember the structures passing through petrotympanic fissure think of a CAT in which C—Chorda tympani nerve, A—Anterior ligament of malleus and T—Tympanic artery.*

   iv. Petrotympanic fissure leads into middle ear.

b. *Cerebral surface*

   1. It is inner surface.
   2. It is grooved by *middle meningeal vessels*.
   3. It has impressions for sulci and gyri of the temporal lobe of cerebrum.

B. *Borders*

a. *Superior border*

It articulates with parietal bone.

b. *Anteroinferior border*

It articulates with greater wing of sphenoid bone.

II. Mastoid part

It forms the posterior part of the temporal bone. It consists of two surfaces (outer and inner), two borders (superior and posterior) and a downward projecting part called mastoid process.

A. Surfaces

a. Outer surface

1. *Auricularis posterior* and *occipital belly of occipitofrontalis* are attached to this surface.
2. *Mastoid foramen* is an infrequent opening near the posterior border. When present this foramen transmits an *emissary vein* from sigmoid sinus and a *branch from occipital artery*.

b. Inner surface

1. *Sigmoid sulcus* is a deep groove on the inner surface. It is meant for *sigmoid sinus*.
2. *Mastoid foramen* opens in the upper part of sigmoid sulcus.

B. Borders

a. Superior border

It articulates with the occipital bone at *occipitomastoid suture*.

b. Posterior border

It articulates with the occipital bone at *occipitomastoid suture*.

C. Mastoid process

It possesses a lateral and a medial surface.

a. Lateral surface

It gives insertions to following three muscles from above downwards:

1. *Sternomastoid*.
2. *Splenius capitis*.
3. *Longissimus capitis*.

b. Medial surface

1. It is marked by a deep groove called *mastoid notch*, from which originates the *posterior belly of digastric*.
2. *Occipital groove* is observed medial to mastoid notch. This groove lodges the *occipital artery*.

III. Petrous part

Petrous is a Latin word which means strong or rock like. It is strong part of temporal bone and protects internal ear within it. Petrous part is comprised of a base, an apex, three surfaces (anterior, posterior and inferior) and three borders (superior, anterior and posterior).

A. Base

1. It is directed laterally.
2. It fuses with squamous part at petrosquamosal suture which disappears soon after birth.
3. Base also fuses with mastoid part.
4. Base is separated from the squamous and mastoid parts by an air filled space called *mastoid antrum*.

B. Apex

1. It projects medially and slightly forwards.
2. It is situated between greater wing of sphenoid and basilar part of occipital bone.
3. It forms posterolateral boundary of foramen lacerum.
4. It possesses anterior orifice of carotid canal.

C. Surfaces

a. Anterior surface (Fig. 27.3)

1. It contributes to middle cranial fossa.
2. This surface shows following features if one goes from apex to base:
   i. *Trigeminal impression*: It is a depression for trigeminal ganglion adjacent to apex.
   ii. *Roof of internal acoustic meatus*: It is another depressed area behind the ridge.
   iii. *Arcuate eminence*: It is a prominent elevation produced by superior semicircular canal. Its posterior sloping lies over lateral and posterior semicircular canals.

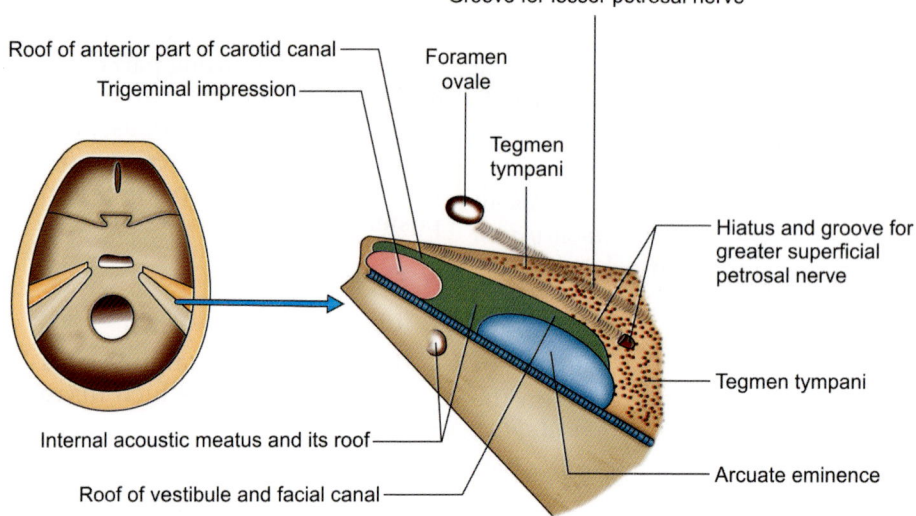

Groove for lesser petrosal nerve

Roof of anterior part of carotid canal

Foramen ovale

Trigeminal impression

Tegmen tympani

Hiatus and groove for greater superficial petrosal nerve

Tegmen tympani

Internal acoustic meatus and its roof

Arcuate eminence

Roof of vestibule and facial canal

Fig.27.3: Anterior surface of petrous part of right temporal bone

3. Area anterolateral to trigeminal impression forms the roof of *anterior part of carotid canal*.

4. Area anterolateral to arcuate eminence forms the roof of vestibule and beginning of *facial canal*.

5. Thin plate of bone between squamous part (cerebral surface) of temporal bone and features described above is called *tegmen tympani*. It forms roof of mastoid antrum, middle ear and canal for tensor tympani from posterior to anterior. Tegmen tympani projects downwards to form lateral walls of canal for tensor tympani and bony Eustachian tube and appears in the squamotympanic fissure.

6. A hiatus (opening) lateral to arcuate eminence leads into a *groove for greater superficial petrosal nerve* which runs towards the foramen lacerum on the tegmen tympani.

7. Lateral to groove for greater superficial petrosal nerve is present a *groove for lesser petrosal nerve* which runs towards the foramen ovale.

b. Posterior surface (Fig. 27.4)

1. It contributes to posterior cranial fossa.

2. *Internal acoustic meatus* is present in the centre of this surface. It transmits *facial and vestibulocochlear nerves* and *labyrinthine vessels*. It is about 1 cm in length.

3. *Fundus* of internal acoustic meatus is a plate of bone at its lateral end. This plate is divided into upper and lower areas by a transverse ridge called *crista falciformis*. The upper area is further divided into anterior and posterior areas by a vertical crest called *Bill's bar*. Anterior area shows *facial canal* for facial nerve. Posterior area is called *superior vestibular* area which presents number of small openings for the nerve fibres supplying utricle and superior and lateral semicircular ducts (Fig. 27.5).

Below the transverse crest, anteriorly is the *cochlear area* (which possesses number of foramina called *tractus spiralis foraminosus*) and posteriorly is the *inferior vestibular* area. Fibres of cochlear nerve

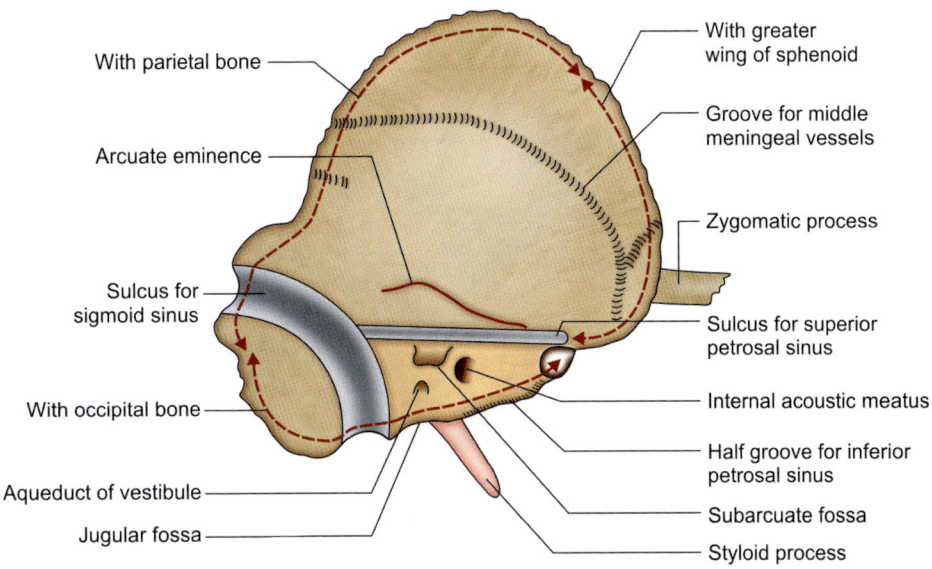

With parietal bone

Arcuate eminence

Sulcus for sigmoid sinus

With occipital bone

Aqueduct of vestibule

Jugular fossa

With greater wing of sphenoid

Groove for middle meningeal vessels

Zygomatic process

Sulcus for superior petrosal sinus

Internal acoustic meatus

Half groove for inferior petrosal sinus

Subarcuate fossa

Styloid process

Fig. 27.4: Left temporal bone: Internal aspect

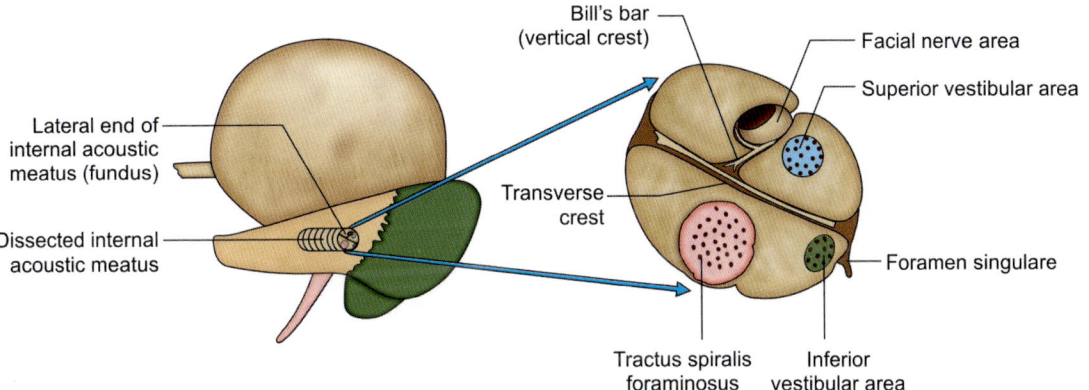

Bill's bar (vertical crest)

Facial nerve area

Superior vestibular area

Lateral end of internal acoustic meatus (fundus)

Dissected internal acoustic meatus

Transverse crest

Foramen singulare

Tractus spiralis foraminosus

Inferior vestibular area

Fig. 27.5: Fundus of right internal acoustic meatus

enter the cochlear area while nerve fibres supplying the saccule enter the inferior vestibular area. Below and behind the inferior vestibular area is *foramen singulare* for the passage of nerve to posterior semicircular duct.

4. A slit behind the internal acoustic meatus leads into *aqueduct of vestibule* which contains saccus and ductus endolymphaticus along with small artery and vein.

5. An irregular depression called *subarcuate fossa* is located above and between the openings of internal acoustic meatus and aqueduct of vestibule. It lodges a process of dura mater.

c. *Inferior surface* (Fig. 27.6)

1. It is rough and triangular.

2. It is divided into four areas from apex to base.

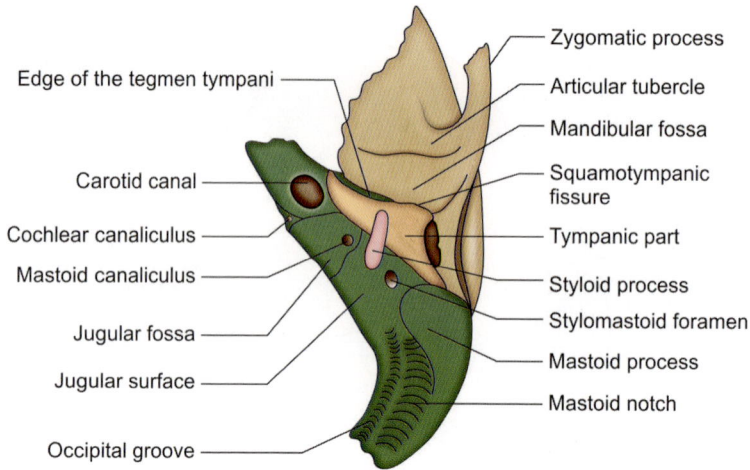

Fig. 27.6: Left temporal bone: Inferior aspect

i. *Quadrilateral area* near the apex provides attachment to *levator palati muscle.*

ii. *Carotid canal* (lower opening) is present behind the quadrilateral area. It transmits *internal carotid artery* along with its *sympathetic* and *venous plexuses.*

iii. *Jugular fossa* is a depression behind the carotid canal. It lodges *superior bulb of internal jugular vein.*

iv. *Jugular surface* is a quadrilateral area behind the jugular fossa. It articulates with jugular process of occipital bone.

3. A triangular depression in front of the medial part of the jugular fossa lodges the *inferior ganglion of glossopharyngeal nerve.* The apex of this triangular depression is marked by an opening leading into *cochlear canaliculus* which is traversed by:

   i. *Perilymphatic duct*

   ii. *Prolongation of dura mater*

   iii. A *vein* from cochlea which drains into internal jugular vein.

4. The *canaliculus for tympanic nerve* (a branch of glossopharyngeal nerve) is situated on the bony ridge between carotid canal and jugular fossa.

5. The *mastoid canaliculus* is present in the lateral wall of jugular fossa. It transmits the *auricular branch of vagus.*

D. Borders

a. Superior border

1. It is grooved by *superior petrosal sinus.*
2. Margins of the groove provide attachment to *tentorium cerebelli.*

b. Anterior border

1. It is divided into medial and lateral parts.
2. Medial part articulates with greater wing of sphenoid.
3. Lateral part joins the squamous part at *petrosquamosal suture* which disappears soon after birth.

c. Posterior border

1. It can be divided into medial and lateral parts.
2. Medial part has got a sulcus which with similar sulcus on the occipital bone forms a *groove for inferior petrosal sinus.*
3. Lateral part is occupied by larger *jugular fossa* laterally and smaller *glossopharyngeal notch* medially. Lateral part forms *anterior boundary of jugular foramen* whose posterior boundary is formed by jugular notch of occipital bone.

IV. Tympanic part

It is curved bony plate situated below the squamous part and in front of mastoid part of temporal bone. It joins the squamous part at *squamotympanic fissure* and mastoid part at *tympanomastoid fissure*. Auricular branch of vagus emerges through the tympanomastoid fissure. Tympanic part has two surfaces (anterior and posterior) and three borders (lateral, upper and lower).

A. Surfaces

a. Anterior surface

1. It forms the posterior nonarticular part of the *mandibular fossa*.
2. It is related to the *parotid gland*.

b. Posterior surface

1. It forms the anterior wall, floor and the lower part of the posterior wall of the *external acoustic meatus*.
2. Its medial end is marked by a groove called *tympanic sulcus*. This sulcus provides attachment to the circumference of the *tympanic membrane*.

B. Borders

a. Lateral border

1. It is free.
2. It continues with cartilaginous part of external acoustic meatus.

b. Upper border

1. Laterally it fuses with the *postglenoid tubercle*.
2. Medially it forms posterior boundary of *petrotympanic fissure*.

c. Lower border

1. Medially it extends up to carotid canal.
2. Laterally it splits to form the veginal process which encloses the root of styloid process.

V. Styloid process

1. Styloid process is divisible into two parts:
   a. **Proximal or tympanohyal part**

It is surrounded by a bony sheath derived from lower border of tympanic part of temporal bone.
   b. **Distal or stylohyal part**

It is visible lower part. It is this part which is described below.

2. Styloid process is a conical projection directed downwards, forwards and slightly medially.
3. It provides attachments to five structures (3 muscles and 2 ligaments):
   i. Medially: *Stylopharyngeus muscle*.
   ii. Anteriorly: *Styloglossus muscle*.
   iii. Posteriorly: *Stylohyoid muscle*.
   iv. Laterally: *Stylomandibular ligament*.
   v. At the tip: *Stylohyoid ligament*.
4. Some important relations are as follows:
   i. It is interposed between two important structures, the *parotid gland* (laterally) and *internal jugular vein* (medially).
   ii. *External carotid* artery crosses the tip of styloid process superficially.
   iii. *Facial nerve* crosses the base of styloid process laterally.
5. *Stylomastoid foramen* is situated behind its base (between it and the mastoid process). Following structures pass through this foramen:
   i. *Facial nerve*.
   ii. *Stylomastoid artery*.

SPACES AND CANALS

I. External acoustic meatus (Fig. 27.7)

1. Bony part of external acoustic meatus is about 16 mm long. This contribution is about 2/3rd of the total length (24 mm).
2. It is directed medially, downwards and slightly forwards.
3. Tympanic part of the temporal bone contributes to its anterior wall, floor and lower part of the posterior wall.
4. Squamous part of the temporal bone forms its roof and upper part of posterior wall.

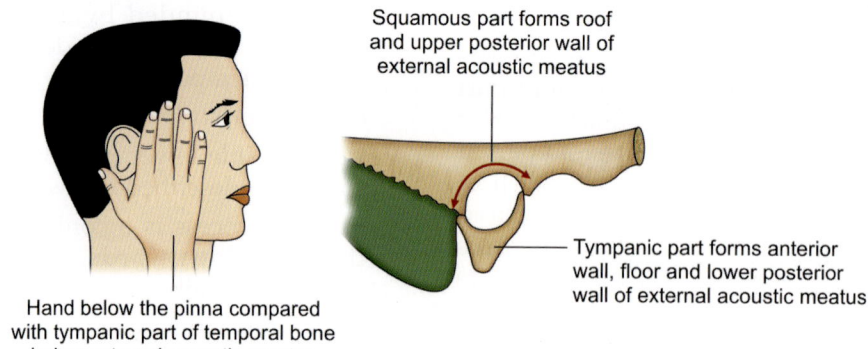

Squamous part forms roof and upper posterior wall of external acoustic meatus

Tympanic part forms anterior wall, floor and lower posterior wall of external acoustic meatus

Hand below the pinna compared with tympanic part of temporal bone below external acoustic meatus

Fig. 27.7: Bony contributions to external acoustic meatus: Right lateral view

II. Middle ear space (tympanic cavity)

A. Parts

Tympanic cavity consists of three parts:

a. *Tympanic cavity proper (mesotympanum):* Opposite the tympanic membrane.

b. *Epitympanic recess (epitympanum):* Above the level of the tympanic membrane.

c. *Hypotympanum:* Below the level of the tympanic membrane.

B. Measurements

1. Vertical diameter: 15 mm.
2. Anteroposterior diameter: 15 mm.
3. Transverse diameters:
   i. Upper part: 6 mm.
   ii. Lower part: 4 mm.
   iii. Opposite the centre of tympanic membrane: 2 mm.

C. Boundaries

a. Roof

It is formed by *tegmen tympani* which separates the middle ear from middle cranial fossa.

b. Floor

It is formed by thin plate of bone which separates the cavity from *superior bulb of internal jugular vein.*

c. *Lateral wall* (Fig. 27.8)

1. It is formed mainly by *tympanic membrane.*
2. Close to circumference for tympanic membrane, there are three small apertures:
   i. *Petrotympanic fissure:* It is located anteriorly.
   ii. *Anterior canaliculus for chorda tympani:* It is located at the medial end of petrotympanic fissure.
   iii. *Posterior canaliculus for chorda tympani:* It is located posteriorly.

d. *Medial wall* (Fig. 27.9)

1. It is the lateral wall of internal ear.
2. It has a rounded elevation called *promontory* produced by the basal turn of cochlea.
3. Promontory is grooved by the nerves of *tympanic plexus.*
4. A depression behind the promontory, the *sinus tympani*, indicates the position of the *ampulla of the posterior semicircular canal.*
5. *Fenestra vestibuli* is a reniform opening posterosuperior to the promontory. It connects the tympanic cavity to the vestibule of internal ear.

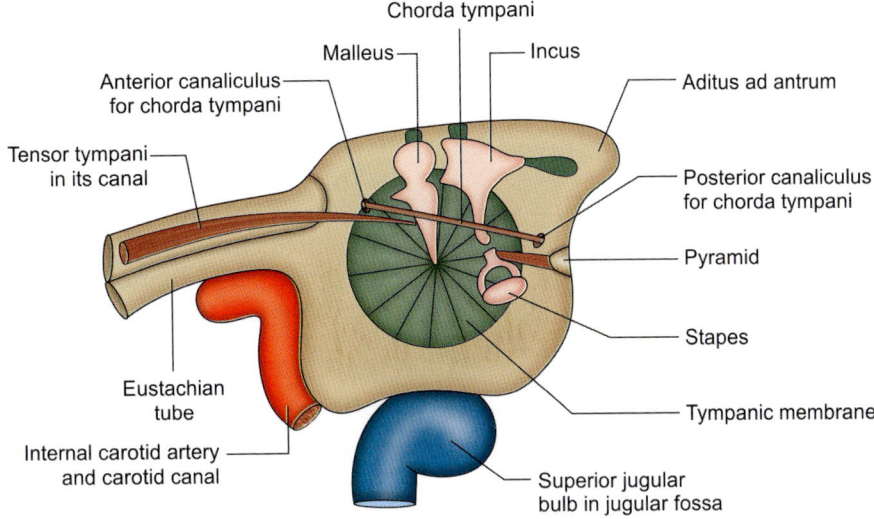

Fig. 27.8: Lateral wall of middle ear of right side

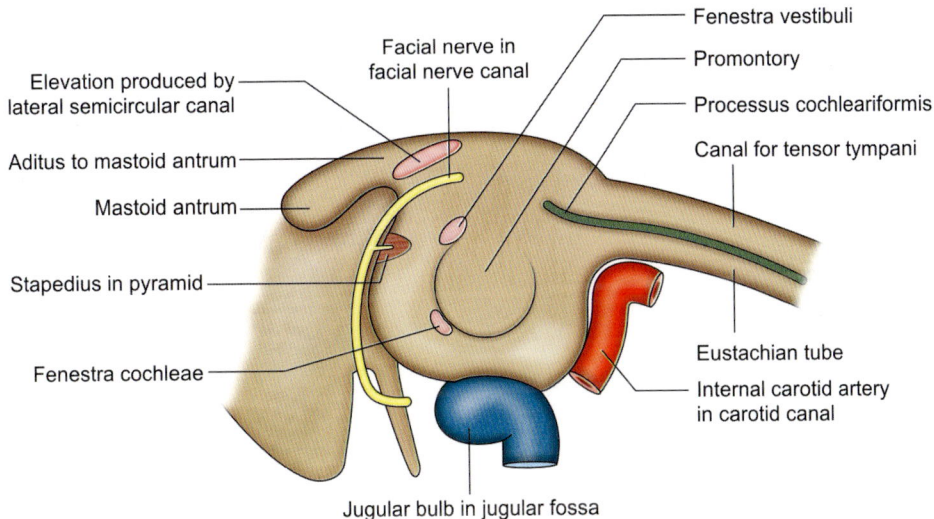

Fig. 27.9: Medial wall of middle ear of the right side

6. *Fenestra cochleae* is a rounded opening in the posteroinferior part of the promontory. It connects the tympanic cavity with the scala tympani of the cochlea.

7. Above and posterior to the fenestra vestibuli there is an elevation produced by *facial nerve canal.*

e. Posterior wall

1. *Aditus to the mastoid antrum* is an opening in the upper part of posterior wall. It connects epitympanic recess with the mastoid antrum.

2. The medial wall of the aditus to mastoid antrum shows an elevation produced by *lateral semicircular canal.*

3. *Facial nerve canal* lies vertically in the posterior wall anterior to which is a *pyramidal eminence* projecting into the middle ear cavity.

4. Pyramidal eminence is occupied by *stapedius muscle*.

5. *Fossa incudis* is a small depression in the postero-inferior part of the epitympanic recess. It contains short process of incus.

f. Anterior wall

1. Its lower part is formed by thin plate of bone which separates middle ear from the *carotid canal*.

2. Its upper part is occupied by two openings. Upper opening leads into *canal for tensor tympani*. The lower opening leads into osseous part of *Eustachian tube*. These two canals are visible from the apex side of petrous temporal at petrosquamosal junction.

3. The septum between the aforementioned canals runs on the medial wall and just above the fenestra vestibuli its posterior end curves laterally to form *processus cochleariformis*.

III. Mastoid antrum

1. It is an air sinus in the petrous part of temporal bone.

2. It is well developed at birth and is almost of adult size.

3. Mastoid antrum is a spherical sinus.

4. In adult the mastoid antrum has a capacity of about 1 ml.

5. *Aditus ad antrum* is an opening in the upper part of anterior wall of mastoid antrum. It connects the antrum with epitympanic recess of middle ear.

6. Roof of antrum is formed by *tegmen tympani*.

7. Posteriorly the antrum is closely related to *sigmoid sinus*.

8. Medial wall is related to posterior semicircular canal.

9. Anteroinferiorly the antrum is related to *canal for facial nerve*.

10. Floor has multiple apertures which connect mastoid antrum with *mastoid air cells*.

11. The lateral wall of antrum corresponds to the *suprameatal triangle*. This wall is 1 mm thick at birth and increases at a rate of 1 mm per year until it reaches the adult thickness of about 12.5 mm.

IV. Mastoid air cells

1. These are very small intercommunicating spaces in the temporal bone continuous with mastoid antrum.

2. At birth neither mastoid air cells nor mastoid process are present. Only after birth mastoid air cells grow out of the mastoid antrum into the mastoid process.

3. The mastoid air cells are mainly seen in the mastoid process, but may extend into the surrounding bones like petrous or squamous parts of temporal bone or even zygomatic bone and jugular process of occipital bone.

4. Some common groups of air cells are as follows (Fig. 27.10):

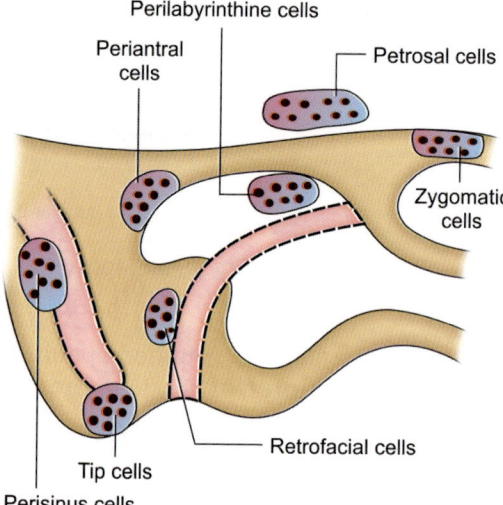

Fig. 27.10: Types of air spaces (air cells) in temporal bone

   i. *Tip cells.*

   ii. *Perisinus cells.*

   iii. *Retrofacial cells.*

   iv. *Periantral cells.*

   v. *Perilabyrinthine cells.*

   vi. *Petrous cells.*

   vii. *Zygomatic cells.*

5. Depending upon the pneumatization, the mastoid process may be of three types (Fig. 27.11):

   i. *Pneumatic or cellular.*

   ii. *Sclerotic or acellular.*

   iii. *Diploeic or mixed.*

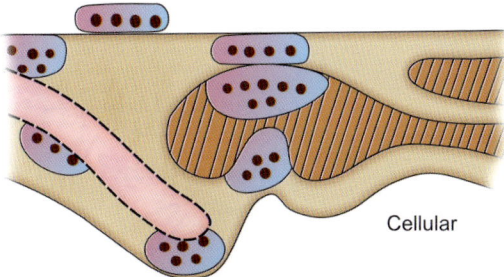

Cellular

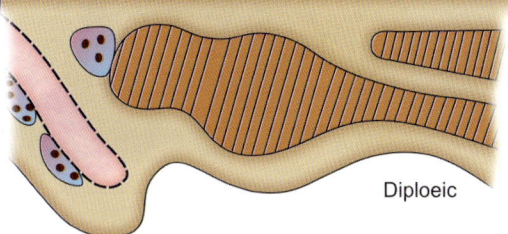

Diploeic

V. Bony labyrinth (osseous labyrinth) (Figs 27.12 and 27.13)

It consists of three parts, vestibule, semicircular canals and cochlea.

A. Vestibule

1. It is the central part of bony labyrinth.

2. In its lateral wall, there is an opening of *fenestra vestibuli* (oval window) occupied by foot plate of stapes in life.

3. Its medial wall corresponds to the fundus of internal acoustic meatus.

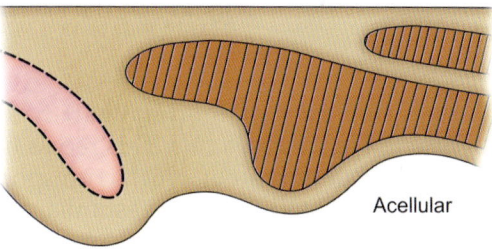

Acellular

Fig. 27.11: Types of mastoid

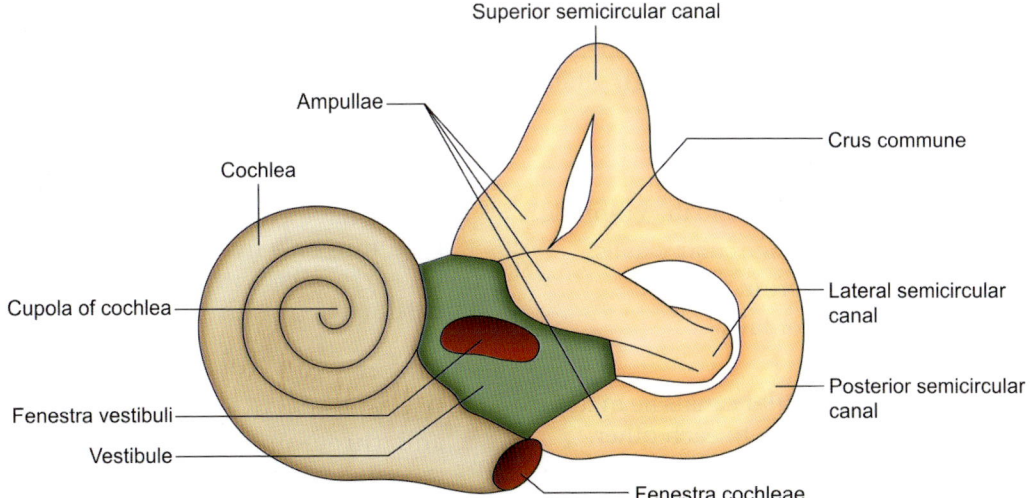

Fig. 27.12: The left bony labyrinth. Lateral aspect

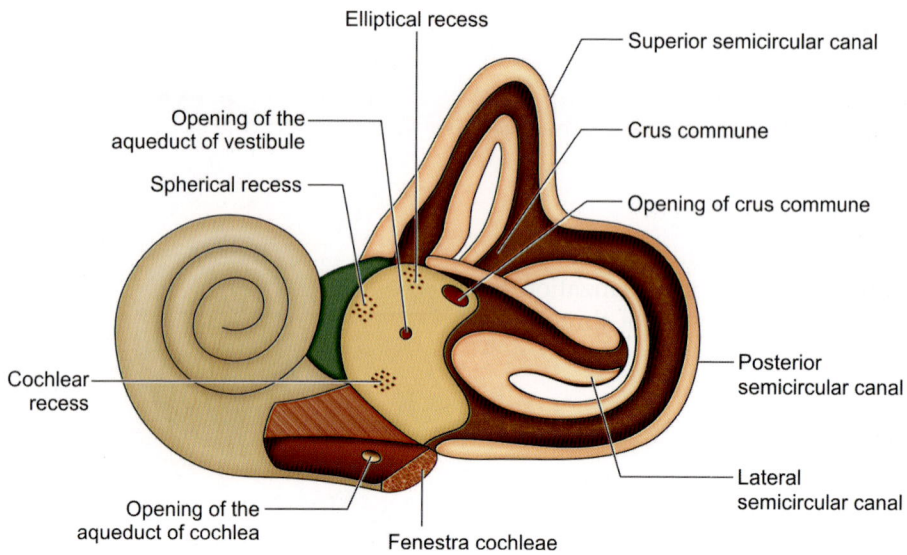

Elliptical recess
Superior semicircular canal
Opening of the aqueduct of vestibule
Crus commune
Spherical recess
Opening of crus commune
Cochlear recess
Posterior semicircular canal
Opening of the aqueduct of cochlea
Lateral semicircular canal
Fenestra cochleae

Fig. 27.13: The interior of the left osseous labyrinth

4. Anterior part of medial wall has a *spherical recess for saccule*. This recess has multiple perforations which correspond to the openings in inferior vestibular area of fundus of internal acoustic meatus.

5. Posterosuperior to spherical recess is an *elliptical recess* which lodges the *utricle*. This recess also has number of foramina which correspond to openings in the superior vestibular area of fundus.

6. Below the elliptical recess is the opening of aqueduct of vestibule through which passes ductus endolymphaticus.

B. Semicircular canals

1. They lie posterosuperior to the vestibule.

2. There are three semicircular canals.

   i. Anterior or superior.

   ii. Lateral or horizontal.

   iii. Posterior.

3. Ipsilateral semicircular canals lie in three planes at right angles to each other.

4. Each canal is about two-thirds of a circle.

5. Superior semicircular canal is placed in a vertical plane perpendicular to the long axis of the petrous bone at about 45° with sagittal plane.

6. Posterior semicircular canal is placed in a vertical plane in the long axis of the petrous bone. This also makes an angle of 45° with sagittal plane.

7. Lateral semicircular canal makes an angle of 30° with horizontal plane. This canal lies horizontally if the head is bent forwards for 30°.

8. One end of each canal is dilated called *ampulla*.

9. Both the ends of each canal open into vestibule. Since non-ampullated ends of superior and posterior semicircular canals have common opening in vestibule, thus only five openings connect the three canals with the cavity of the vestibule.

C. Cochlea

1. It is conical in shape and consists of two and three-quarter spiral turns of a tapering cylindrical canal.

2. The axial bone around which the canal spirals is called as *modiolus*.

3. The basal turn of cochlea produces *promontory* on the medial wall of middle ear.

4. From the modiolus a shelf of bone projects into the canal. Since the shelf follows the spiral path of canal, this is called as *spiral lamina*.

5. The spiral lamina forms a hook-like structure (*called hamulus*) at the apex of modiolus.

6. Basal turn of cochlea shows two holes:

   i. *The fenestra cochleae*

   It is closed in life by *secondary tympanic membrane*.

   ii. *The opening of aqueduct of cochlea*

   It leads downwards to reach the apex of glossopharyngeal notch.

7. Base of modiolus is perforated by spirally arranged foramina. This area corresponds to the cochlear area of the fundus of internal acoustic meatus.

OSSIFICATION

1. Temporal bone ossifies partly in cartilage and partly in membrane.

2. Squamous and tympanic parts ossify in membrane.

3. Petromastoid part and the styloid process ossify in cartilage.

4. **Appearance of centres**

   i. *Squamous part*

   Single centre appears near the root of zygomatic process during 8th week of intrauterine life.

   ii. *Petromastoid part*

   As many as 14 centres may appear in the cartilaginous mass (otic capsule) around developing internal ear during 5th month of intrauterine life. These centres fuse by 6th month of intrauterine life.

   iii. *Tympanic part*

   Single centre appears during 12th week of intrauterine life. At birth, a tympanic ring represents the tympanic part.

   iv. *Styloid process*

   It develops from cranial end of 2nd arch cartilage. It ossifies from two centres. Centre for tympanohyal appears before birth and for stylohyal appears after birth.

5. **Fusion**

   i. Squamous part fuses with tympanic part just before birth.

   ii. Petromastoid part fuses with the squamous part and tympanohyal during 1st year.

   iii. Stylohyal fuses with the tympanohyal after puberty.

Auditory Ossicles

TERMINOLOGY

There are three ossicles named malleus, incus and stapes.

These names are Latin in origin, the meanings of which are as follows:

Malleus : Hammer

Incus : An anvil

Stapes : A stirrup

Note: *Remember that MIS is situated between tympanic membrane and the oval window where M—Malleus, I—Incus and S—Stapes.*

FEATURES AND ATTACHMENTS
(Fig. 28.1)

I. Malleus

It consists of head, neck and handle.

A. Head

1. It is large upper end of the bone.
2. It is located within the epitympanic recess.
3. Its posterior surface articulates with the body of incus.

B. Neck

1. It is the constricted part below the head.
2. Its medial surface is crossed by *chorda tympani nerve.*

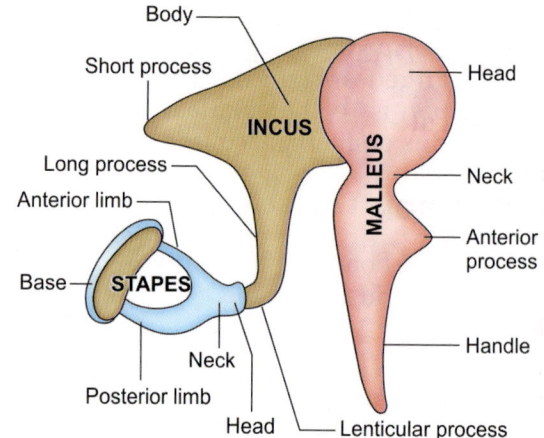

Fig. 28.1: Ossicles of the right ear: Lateral aspect

C. Handle

1. It is lower elongated part of malleus.
2. It is embedded in the tympanic membrane and moves with it.
3. Its upper end (root) shows following features:

   i. A slight projection on the medial aspect provides attachment to *tendon of tensor tympani.*

   ii. *Anterior process* projects forwards. *Anterior ligament of malleus* is attached to it. This ligament extends into the petrotympanic fissure.

iii. *Lateral process* projects laterally from where extend anterior and posterior malleolar folds to the ends of tympanic sulcus.

II. Incus

It has a large body and two processes (long and short).

A. Body

1. It is cubical in shape.
2. Its anterior surface is concave and articulates with head of malleus.

B. Processes

a. Long process

1. It projects downwards parallel to handle of malleus.
2. Its lower end (*lenticular process*) bears an articular surface on the medial aspect for articulation with the head of stapes.

b. Short process

1. It is directed backwards.
2. It is attached by a ligament to the fossa incudis just below the aditus.

III. Stapes

It has a head, a neck, two limbs (anterior and posterior) and a foot plate (base).

A. Head

1. It is rounded
2. It articulates with the long process of incus.

B. Neck

1. It is constricted part adjacent to head.
2. *Tendon of stapedius* is attached to its posterior surface.

C. Limbs (crura)

1. Anterior and posterior limbs diverges from the neck.
2. These two limbs are attached to the foot plate.

D. Foot plate (base)

1. It is oval in shape.
2. It fits into the fenestra vestibuli.

OSSIFICATION

1. Malleus and incus develop from the dorsal end of Meckel's cartilage.
2. Stapes develops from the dorsal end of hyoid arch cartilage.
3. Malleus ossifies by two centres:
    i. One endochondral centre near the neck.
    ii. One centre for anterior process appears in dense connective tissue.
    Appearance
    4th month of intrauterine life.
    Fusion
    6th month of intrauterine life.
4. Incus ossifies by single endochondral centre in the upper part of long process. This centre appears at 4th month of intrauterine life.
5. Stapes ossifies by single endochondral centre which appears in the base at 4th month of intrauterine life.
6. At birth the auditory ossicles are of almost adult size.

FUNCTIONS

1. Malleus functions as a lever as it is attached to the tympanic membrane.
2. The base of stapes is considerably smaller than the tympanic membrane. Due to this fact, the vibratory force of the stapes is about 10 times that of tympanic membrane. Thus, the auditory ossicles increase the force but decrease the amplitude of vibrations transmitted from tympanic membrane.

Occipital Bone

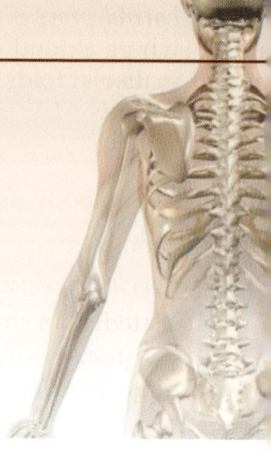

TERMINOLOGY

Word 'occipital' is derived from Greek words *ob* (meaning back) and *cipit* (meaning head). Hence, referred to the back of head.

LOCATION

Occipital bone occupies the posterior part of skull and plays major role in the formation of posterior cranial fossa.

FEATURES AND ATTACHMENTS

The largest foramen of the skull called *foramen magnum*, is located in the occipital bone. The components of occipital bone are better described in relation to this foramen. It consists of 1 *basilar part* (above and in front of foramen magnum), 2 *lateral parts* (lateral to foramen magnum) and 1 *squamous part* (above and behind the foramen magnum).

I. Foramen magnum

1. It is located in the floor of posterior cranial fossa.
2. It provides a communication between posterior cranial fossa and vertebral canal.
3. Its margins provide attachments to following structures:

   i. Anterior margin: *Anterior atlanto-occipital membrane.*
   ii. Posterior margin: *Posterior atlanto-occipital membrane.*
   iii. Lateral margins: *Alar ligament.*

4. Structures passing through the foramen magnum are as follows.

A. Anterior part

   i. *Apical ligament of dens.*
   ii. *Superior longitudinal band of cruciform ligament.*
   iii. *Membrana tectoria.*

B. Posterior part

   i. *Medulla oblongata.*
   ii. *Meninges.*
   iii. *Spinal roots of accessory nerves.*
   iv. *Meningeal branches of upper cervical nerves (c_{1-3})*
   v. *Vertebral arteries.*
   vi. *Sympathetic plexuses around vertebral arteries.*
   vii. *Anterior and posterior spinal arteries.*

II. Basilar part

It extends upwards and forwards to meet the body of sphenoid. Before 25 years of age, a growth cartilage intervenes between sphenoid and basilar part of occipital bone but after this period the two bones fuse. Basilar part has got two surfaces (superior and inferior) and two lateral margins.

a. Superior surface

1. It is smooth.
2. It forms *clivus* with the body of sphenoid.
3. It is related to *medulla oblongata*.
4. Its lower part receives attachments of following structures from above downwards:
   i. Membrana tectoria.
   ii. Superior longitudinal band of cruciform ligament.
   iii. Apical ligament of dens.
5. Its lateral margins are grooved by *inferior petrosal sinuses*.

b. Inferior surface

1. Its middle is marked by a tubercle called *pharyngeal tubercle*. This tubercle is approximately 1 cm anterior to foramen magnum. Attached to this tubercle is the upper part of pharyngeal raphe (*pharyngeal ligament*).
2. Anterolateral to pharyngeal tubercle is the area for *longus capitis.*
3. Posterolateral to pharyngeal tubercle (just in front of condyle) is the attachment of *rectus capitis anterior.*

c. Lateral margins

These are rough and articulate with petrous parts of the temporal bones.

III. Lateral parts (right and left)

Each can be divided into broader medial portion (adjacent to foramen magnum) and narrower lateral portion (jugular process).

A. Medial portion

a. Inferior surface

1. It is marked by an articular *occipital condyle.*

2. The articular surface of occiptal condyle is oval and convex to articulate with concave superior articular process of atlas.
3. Occipital condyle is located lateral to anterior half of foramen magnum.
4. Behind the condyle is *condylar fossa* which may have *condylar canal* for emissary vein from sigmoid sinus.
5. Lateral to anterior part of condyle is the outer opening of *hypoglossal canal.*

b. Medial aspect

1. It has got a *tubercle* and a *foramen*.
2. The *tubercle* is situated on the medial aspect of condyle and provides attachment to *alar ligament*.
3. The foramen located just above the tubercle forms the inner opening of *hypoglossal canal.*
4. Following structures pass through hypoglossal canal:
   i. *Hypoglossal nerve.*
   ii. Meningeal branch of ascending pharyngeal artery.

c. Superior surface

1. It is marked by an oval eminence called *jugular tubercle.*
2. Jugular tubercle overlies the hypoglossal canal.
3. The posterior part of jugular tubercle often presents a shallow groove for IX, X and XI cranial nerves.

B. Jugular process

1. Its lateral end presents a rough area which joins the jugular surface of temporal bone by a growth cartilage. The cartilage ossifies at the age of 25 years.
2. Its anterior margin is notched and completes the *jugular foramen* with similar notch on the posterior border of petrous part of temporal bone.
3. Its superior surface is marked by a deep groove which lodges terminal part of *sigmoid sinus.*

4. Its inferior surface provides attachment to *rectus capitis lateralis.*

IV. Squamous part

It has two surfaces (external and internal), 3 angles (1 superior and 2 lateral) and 4 borders (2 lambdoid and 2 mastoid).

A. Surfaces

a. External surface (Figs 29.1 and 29.2)

1. The middle of the external surface is marked by a projection called *external occipital protuberance.*

2. Two lines extend laterally on each side from external occipital protuberance.

   i. A superior faint line is called *highest nuchal line.* This provides attachment to *occipital belly of occipitofrontalis.*

   ii. An inferior well defined line is called *superior nuchal line.* This receives attachments of *trapezius* and *sternomastoid* in its medial and lateral parts respectively.

3. A midline ridge extends from the external occipital protuberance to foramen magnum. This is called *external occipital crest.* It gives attachment to *ligamentum nuchae.*

4. Running laterally on each side from the middle of external occipital crest is another ridge called *inferior nuchal line.*

5. There are two muscles attached between superior and inferior nuchal lines on both the sides, i.e. *semispinalis capitis* (medially) and *obliquus capitis superior* (laterally).

6. Similarly, there are two muscles attached to each side of midline below the inferior nuchal line, i.e. *rectus capitis posterior major* (laterally) and *rectus capitis posterior minor* (medially).

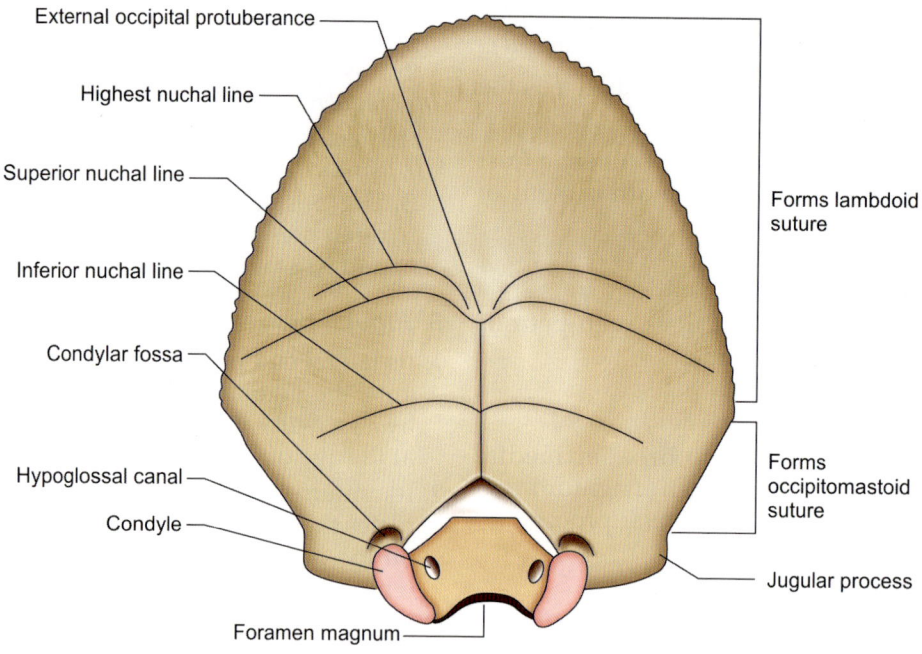

Fig. 29.1: Occipital bone: Posterior aspect

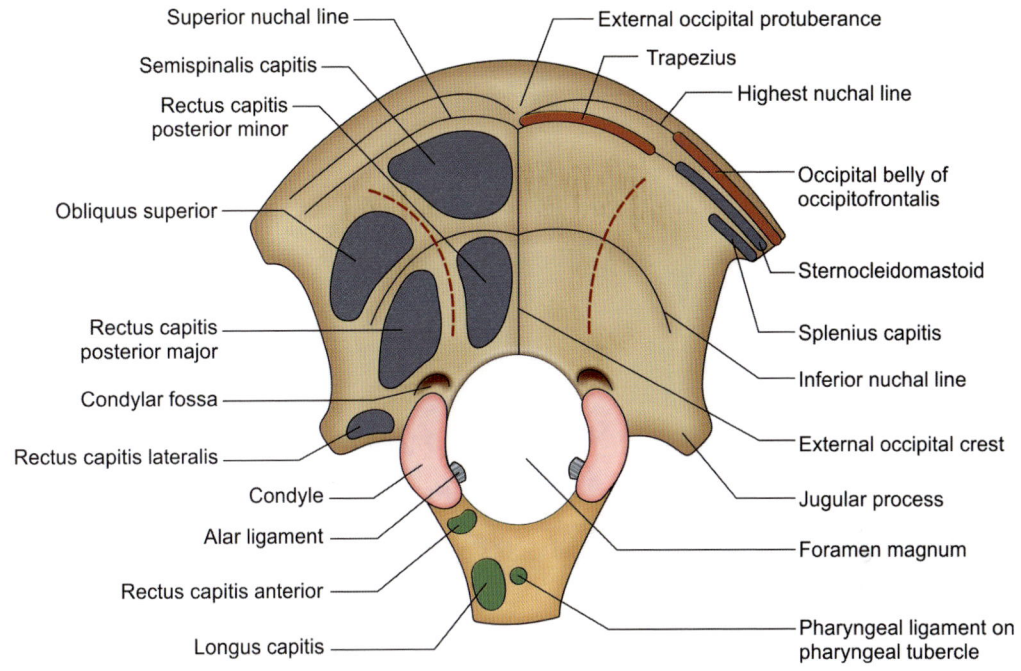

Fig. 29.2: Occipital bone: Inferior aspect

Note: *Remember that the rectus capitis muscles are named after their relations with occipital condyle. The one lying anterior to condyle is rectus capitis anterior. The muscle lying lateral to condyle is called rectus capitis lateralis. Rectus capitis posterior will naturally be located behind the condyle. Since the latter muscle is two in number, these are further qualified by adding 'major' and 'minor' to their names.*

It is interesting to note that rectus capitis anterior, lateralis and posterior are attached to three components of occipital bone, i.e. basilar part, lateral part and squamous part respectively.

b. Internal surface (Fig. 29.3)

1. Its middle is marked by an elevation called *internal occipital protuberance* which corresponds with the external occipital protuberance on the external surface.

2. Four grooves diverge from the internal occipital protuberance, one upwards, one downwards and two laterally whose margins provide attachments to *falx cerebri, falx cerebelli* and *tentorium cerebelli* respectively.

3. The groove running upwards is produced by *superior sagittal sinus*.

4. The groove running downwards is occupied by *occipital sinus*.

5. The groove extending laterally is produced by corresponding *transverse sinus*.

6. The internal surface is marked by a depression in the midline near the posterior margin of foramen magnum. This is *vermian fossa* related to inferior vermis of cerebellum.

7. Midline elevation extending from internal occipital protuberance to posterior margin of foramen magnum is called *internal occipital crest*. *Falx cerebelli* is attached to it.

8. On each side of internal occipital crest a hallow is related to *cerebellar hemisphere*.

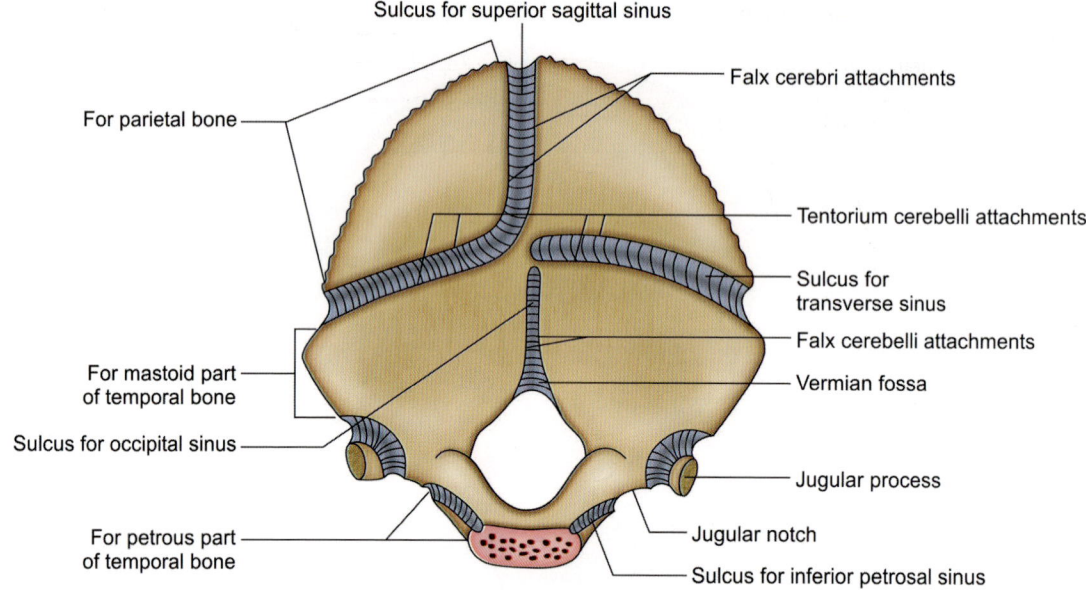

Sulcus for superior sagittal sinus

Falx cerebri attachments

For parietal bone

Tentorium cerebelli attachments

Sulcus for transverse sinus

Falx cerebelli attachments

For mastoid part of temporal bone

Vermian fossa

Sulcus for occipital sinus

Jugular process

For petrous part of temporal bone

Jugular notch

Sulcus for inferior petrosal sinus

Fig. 29.3: Occipital bone: Internal aspect

9. Internal surface above the grooves for transverse sinuses is related to *occipital lobes of cerebrum*.

B. Angles

a. *Superior angle* reaches lambda which during intrauterine life is membranous (*posterior fontanelle*).

b. *Lateral angle* on each side meets with mastoid part of corresponding temporal bone to form *asterion*.

C. Borders

a. Lambdoid border

It extends on each side from superior angle to lateral angle and articulates with posterior margin of corresponding parietal bone to form *lambdoid suture*.

b. Mastoid border

It extends on each side from lateral angle to jugular process and articulates with mastoid part of corresponding temporal bone to form occipitomastoid suture.

OSSIFICATION

I. Origin

1. Part of the occipital bone above the highest nuchal line develops in membrane.
2. Rest of the occipital bone ossifies in cartilage.

II. Appearance of centres

Usually seven centres appear at 8th week of intrauterine life as follows:

- 4 for squamous part (one for each half of the membranous and cartilaginous parts).
- 2 for lateral parts.
- 1 for basilar part.

III. Fusion

1. Membranous and cartilaginous portions fuse with each other when the baby starts holding neck, i.e. 3rd month.

2. Squamous part fuses with lateral parts when primary dentition completes, i.e. at 2 years.

3. Lateral parts fuse with basilar part when the permanent dentition begins, i.e. at 6 years.

4. Basilar part fuses with sphenoid and lateral part fuses with temporal bone at the age of 25 years.

Note: *Remember, the occipital condyle is contributed partly from lateral part and partly from basilar part of occipital bone.*

Zygomatic Bone

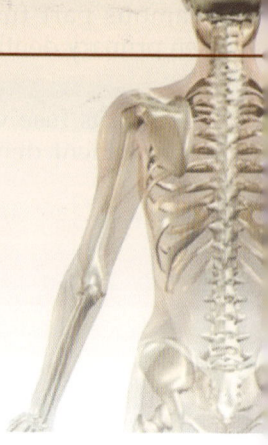

TERMINOLOGY

Term zygomatic is derived from Greek word *zyg* which means 'yoke'. Hence, the zygomatic refers to a bone which is shaped like a yoke uniting the frontal, maxilla and temporal bones.

Zygomatic bone is also called *malar bone* because it forms prominence of the cheek which is called *mala* in Latin.

Term *zygoma* is used by clinicians which includes both 'zygomatic bone' and 'zygomatic arch'. Anatomists use the term 'zygoma' for 'zygomatic arch'.

The term *zygomatic complex* implies to zygomatic bone and other bones adjacent to it, i.e. maxilla and zygomatic process of frontal bone.

LOCATION

Zygomatic bones are present in the upper and lateral parts of face.

FEATURES AND ATTACHMENTS

Each zygomatic bone has three surfaces (lateral, temporal and orbital), five borders (anterosuperior, anteroinferior, posterosuperior, posteroinferior and posteromedial) and two processes (frontal and temporal).

I. Surfaces

A. Lateral surface (Fig. 30.1)

1. It is convex.

2. *Zygomaticofacial foramen* is present near the orbital (anterosuperior) border. It transmits *zygomaticofacial nerve and vessels*.

3. Area below the zygomaticofacial foramen give origin to two muscles:
   i. *Zygomaticus major* (posteriorly)
   ii. *Zygomaticus minor* (anteriorly).

B. Temporal surface (Fig. 30.2)

1. Its anterior part is rough for articulation with maxilla.

2. Its posterior larger part is smooth and forms anterior boundary of temporal fossa.

3. Close to posteroinferior border, this surface provides attachment to *masseter muscle*.

4. *Zygomaticotemporal foramen* present on this surface transmits *zygomaticotemporal nerve and vessels*.

C. Orbital surface

1. It partly contributes to the lateral wall and floor of the orbit.

2. It possesses *zygomatico-orbital foramina* which transmit:
   i. *Zygomaticotemporal and zygomaticofacial nerves.*
   ii. *Zygomatic branches of lacrimal artery.*

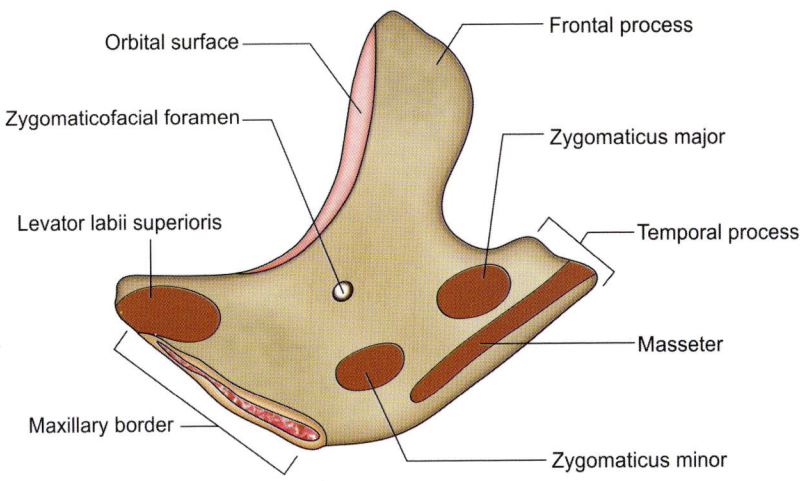

Fig. 30.1: Left zygomatic bone: Lateral aspect

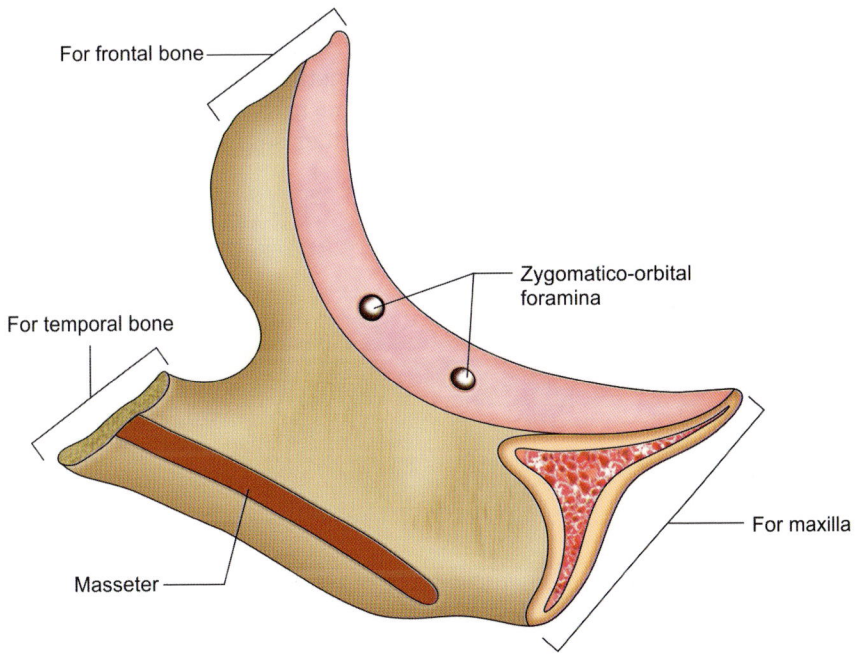

Fig. 30.2: Left zygomatic bone: Medial aspect

II. Borders

A. Anterosuperior border

1. This is also called *orbital border*.
2. It provides attachement to *orbital septum*.

B. Anteroinferior border

1. This is also called *maxillary border*.
2. *Levator labii superioris* arises partly from this border near the orbital border.

C. Posterosuperior border

1. It is also called *temporal border*.
2. *Temporal fascia* is attached to this border.

D. Posteroinferior border

Masseter muscle originates from this border.

E. Posteromedial border

It articulates with the greater wing of sphenoid above and maxilla below.

III. Processes

A. Frontal process

1. It articulates with the zygomatic process of frontal bone (to form *fronto-zygomatic suture*) superiorly and greater wing of sphenoid bone posteriorly.
2. *Whitnall's tubercle* is present on its orbital aspect about 1 cm below the fronto-zygomatic suture. Following structures are attached to this tubercle:

   i. *Lateral check ligament.*
   ii. *Lateral palpebral ligament.*
   iii. *Suspensory ligament of eyeball.*
   iv. *Aponeurosis of levator palpebrae supe rioris.*

B. Temporal process

1. It is directed backwards.
2. It articulates with zygomatic process o temporal bone to complete *zygomatic arch*.
3. Its inferior margin and medial surface provide attachment to *masseter muscle*.

OSSIFICATION

1. Zygomatic bone ossifies in membrane.
2. Usually single centre appears at the age o 8th week of intrauterine life.
3. Sometimes a horizontal suture divides the bone into an upper larger and a lower smaller segments.

Nasal Bone

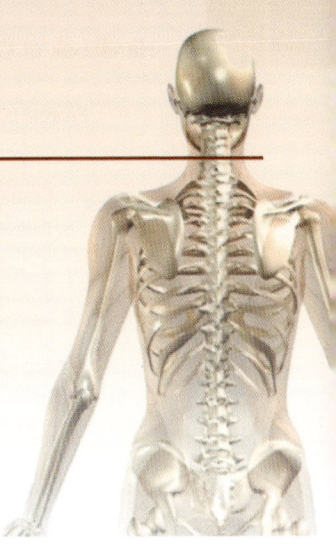

TERMINOLOGY

Nasal bone is so named because of its location. It forms the bridge of the nose.

LOCATION

Two nasal bones meet with each other in midline in the upper part of external nose. They are located below the nasal part of frontal bone and between the frontal processes of maxillae.

FEATURES AND ATTACHMENTS

Each nasal bone has got two surfaces (external and internal) and four borders (superior, inferior, lateral and medial).

I. Surfaces

A. External surface (Fig. 31.1)

1. It is convex from side to side.
2. It is covered by *procerus* and *nasalis* muscles.
3. A foramen in the centre (*vascular foramen*) allows the transmission of a small vein.

B. Internal surface (Fig. 31.2)

1. It is concave from side to side
2. It presents a *vertical groove* for the *anterior ethmoidal nerve*.

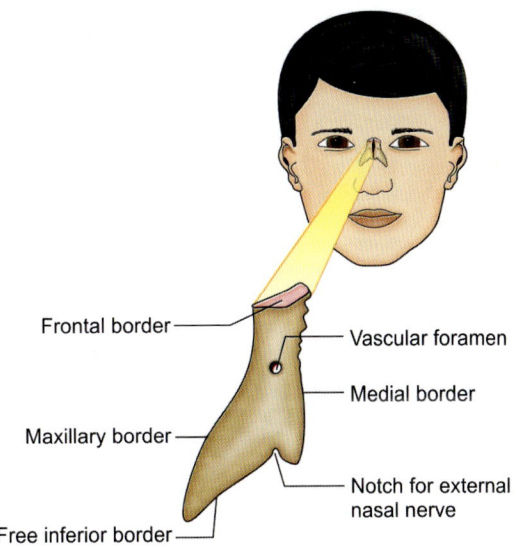

Frontal border

Vascular foramen

Medial border

Maxillary border

Notch for external nasal nerve

Free inferior border

Fig. 31.1: Right nasal bone: External surface

II. Borders

A. Superior border

1. It is serrated.
2. It articulates with nasal part of frontal bone.

B. Inferior border

1. It is notched for the passage of *external nasal nerve*.
2. It is continuous with the lateral nasal cartilage.

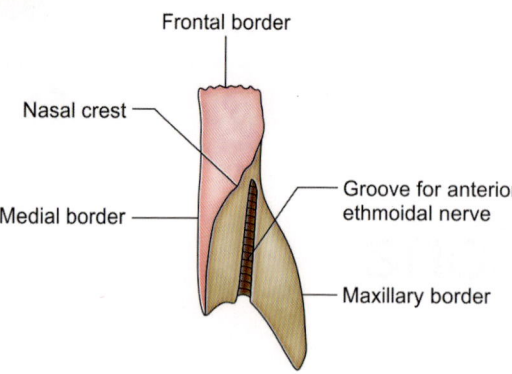

Fig. 31.2: Right nasal bone: Internal surface

C. Lateral border

It articulates with frontal process of maxilla.

D. Medial border

1. It is thick above than below.

2. It articulates with opposite nasal bone (to form internasal suture) and prolonged behind as nasal crest.

3. Nasal crest articulates with following structures from above downwards:

   i. Nasal spine of frontal bone.

   ii. Perpendicular plate of ethmoid.

   iii. Septal cartilage.

OSSIFICATION

1. Nasal bone ossifies in membrane overlying the anterior part of cartilaginous nasal capsule

2. Centre of ossification appears in its middle during 3rd month of intrauterine life.

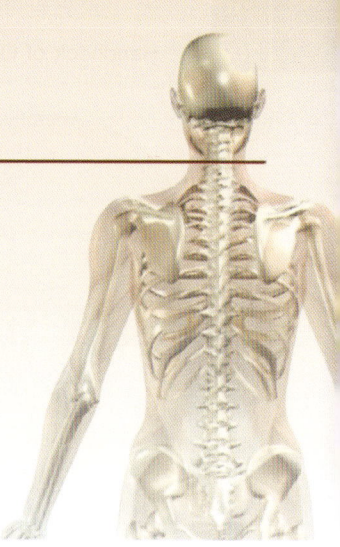

CHAPTER
32

Lacrimal Bone

TERMINOLOGY

'Lacrimal' is a Latin word which means 'tear'. The bone is so named because of its relation with the tear sac.

PECULIARITIES

1. It is most fragile amongst the cranial bones.
2. It is the smallest of the cranial bones.

LOCATION

1. There are two lacrimal bones.
2. Each lacrimal bone is located in the anterior part of the medial wall of orbit.
3. It also contributes to the middle meatus of nose.

FEATURES AND ATTACHMENTS

Lacrimal bone is rectangular in shape. It has two surfaces (medial and lateral) and four borders (anterior, posterior, superior and inferior).

Surfaces

A. Medial surface (Fig. 32.1)

1. It is also called nasal surface.
2. Its anteroinferior part contributes partly to the middle meatus of nose.

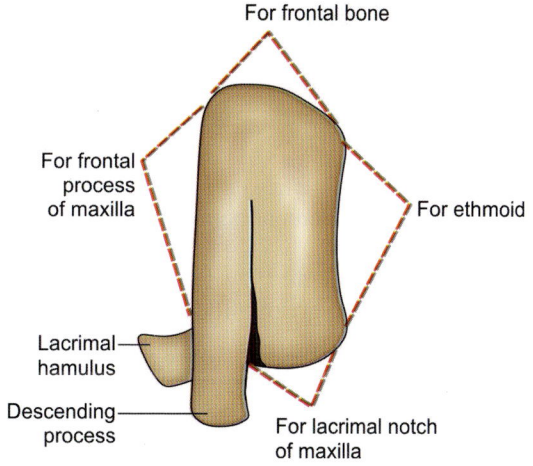

Fig. 32.1: Right lacrimal bone: Medial surface

3. Its posterosuperior part articulates with the ethmoid and completes few anterior ethmoidal air cells.

B. Lateral surface (Fig. 32.2)

1. It is also known as the orbital surface.
2. It is divided into anterior and posterior parts by a vertical crest called *posterior lacrimal crest*.
3. The anterior part is grooved and forms posterior half of the floor of the *lacrimal groove*. Anterior half of the lacrimal

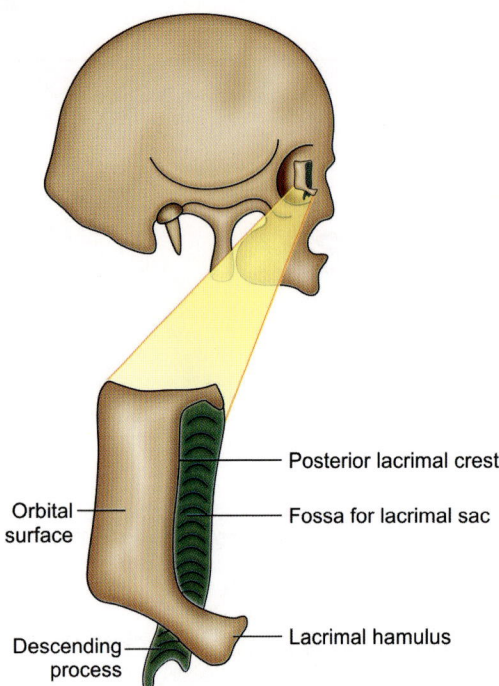

Posterior lacrimal crest

Orbital surface

Fossa for lacrimal sac

Descending process

Lacrimal hamulus

Fig. 32.2: Right lacrimal bone: Lateral surface

groove is formed by frontal process of maxilla. The groove lodges *lacrimal sac.*

4. Portion behind the posterior lacrimal crest is smooth and forms part of medial wall of orbit.

5. Lower end of posterior lacrimal crest projects forwards as *lacrimal hamulus.* It articulates with maxilla to complete the *upper end of nasolacrimal canal.*

6. Posterior lacrimal crest provides attachment to *lacrimal fascia.*

7. The crest and small area of lateral surface immediately behind it give origin to *lacrimal part of orbicularis oculi muscle.*

8. The medial wall of groove project downwards as *descending process.* This process articulates with the lips of nasolacrimal groove of the maxilla and lacrimal process of inferior concha to complete the bony canal for nasolacrimal duct.

II. Borders

A. Anterior border

It articulates with the frontal process of maxilla.

B. Posterior border

It articulates with the orbital plate of ethmoid

C. Superior border

It articulates with the nasal notch of frontal bone.

D. Inferior border

It articulates with the orbital surface of maxilla.

OSSIFICATION

1. Lacrimal bone ossifies in membrane.

2. Single centre of ossification appears in the mesenchyme around the cartilaginous nasal capsule.

3. The centre appears at about 12th week of intrauterine life.

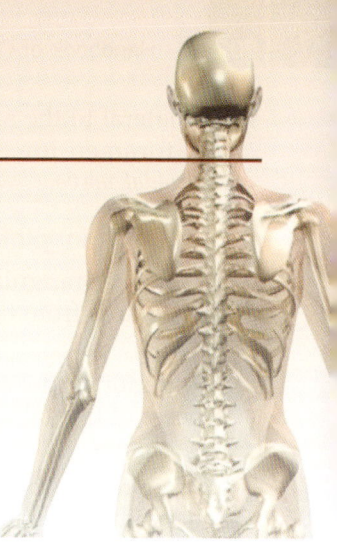

CHAPTER
33

Ethmoid Bone

TERMINOLOGY

'Ethmoid' is a Greek word which means 'sieve-like'. Ethmoid is so named because it possesses a perforated (sieve-like) plate called cribriform plate.

LOCATION

Single ethmoid bone is situated in the anterior part of the base of the cranium between the orbits. It forms part of the medial wall of the orbits and part of the bony septum, roofs and lateral walls of the nasal cavities.

FEATURES AND ATTACHMENTS

Ethmoid bone consists of a cribriform plate, a perpendicular plate and two lateral masses called labyrinths.

Cribriform plate (Fig. 33.1)

1. It is the median part of the superior surface of ethmoid.
2. It contributes to the median portion of anterior cranial fossa (anterior part of the interior of base of skull).
3. It occupies the ethmoidal notch of the frontal bone.
4. It possesses a median triangular upward projection called *crista galli* (named because

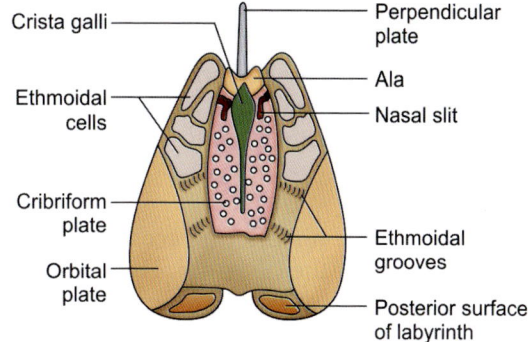

Fig. 33.1: Ethmoid: Superior aspect

of its resemblance to crown of a cock, zoological name of which is *Gallus domesticus*).

5. Posterior sloping border of the crista galli gives attachment to *falx cerebri*.
6. Anterior border of the crista galli has two alae which articulate with frontal bone to complete *foramen caecum. Emissary vein* passes through this foramen.
7. On each side of the crista galli, the cribriform plate shows a number of perforations through which pass about *15–20 filaments of the olfactory nerve*. This part is also related to olfactory bulb superiorly.
8. Just lateral to anterior part of crista galli there is a slit-like passage for a *process of dura mater*.

201

9. Just lateral to the anterior end of slit there is a foramen for the passage of *anterior ethmoidal nerve.*

II. Perpendicular plate (Fig. 33.2)

1. It is a quadrangular flat plate projecting downwards from the midline of cribriform plate.

2. Its anterior border articulates with the nasal process of frontal bone and the crest of the nasal bones.

3. Its posterior border articulates with sphenoidal crest above and vomer below.

4. Its superior border is attached to the cribriform plate.

5. Its inferior border receives the attachment of septal cartilage.

6. Its surfaces are mainly smooth except in the upper parts where there are grooves for filaments of olfactory nerves.

III. Labyrinths

Large number of air filled spaces (*ethmoidal air cells*) constitute the labyrinth. These air cells are divisible into anterior, middle and posterior *ethmoidal sinuses* by bony plates. Many of these air cells open on the surface and completed only when articulating with the adjacent bones. Each labyrinth may be considered to have six surfaces.

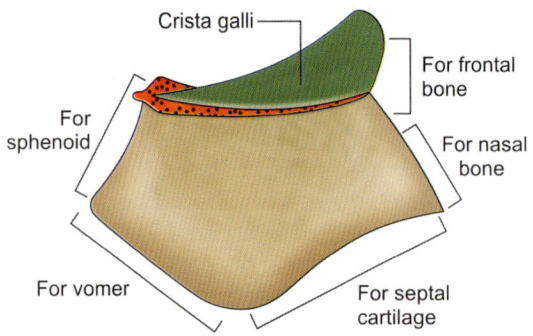

Fig. 33.2: Perpendicular plate of ethmoid: Right lateral aspect

A. Upper surface

1. It has several open air cells which are completed only after articulation with edges of ethmoidal notch.

2. It has two grooves which are converted into anterior and posterior ethmoida canals by articulation with frontal bone

B. Lower surface

It articulates with upper part of the nasa surface of maxilla to complete the ethmoida air cells from below.

C. Anterior surface

It possesses half cut air sinuses which are completed by the frontal process of maxilla and lacrimal bone.

D. Posterior surface (Fig. 33.3)

It articulates with sphenoidal concha and orbital process of palatine bone to complete the posterior ethmoidal sinus.

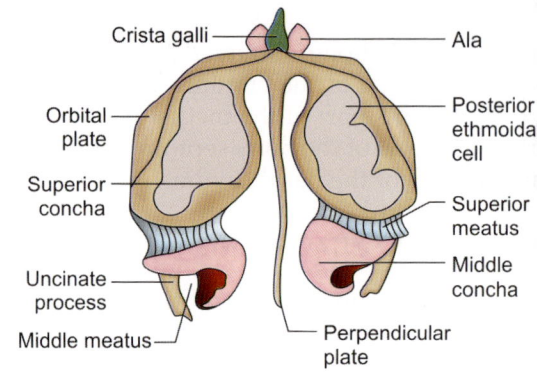

Fig. 33.3: Ethmoid: Posterior aspect

E. Lateral surface (Fig. 33.4)

1. It is thin and smooth plate called *orbita plate.*

2. It covers the middle and posterior ethmoidal sinuses.

3. It forms large part of medial wall of orbit

4. It is quadrangular in shape and articulates as follows:

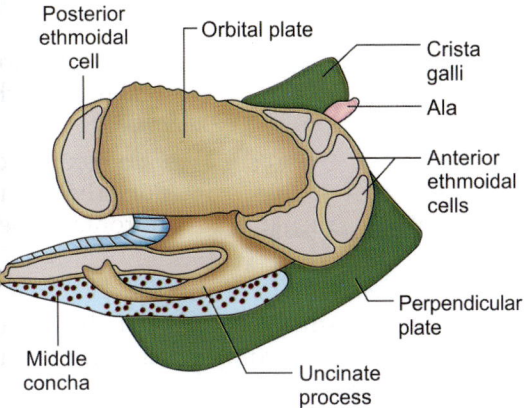

Posterior ethmoidal cell — Orbital plate — Crista galli — Ala — Anterior ethmoidal cells — Perpendicular plate — Uncinate process — Middle concha

Fig. 33.4: Ethmoid: Right lateral aspect

i. Superiorly with orbital plate of frontal bone.

ii. Inferiorly with the maxilla and orbital process of palatine bone.

iii. Anteriorly with lacrimal bone.

iv. Posteriorly with sphenoid bone.

E. Medial surface

1. It forms part of the lateral wall of corresponding half of nasal cavity.

2. Its upper part is marked by numerous vertical grooves which lodge filaments of olfactory nerve.

3. Its posterior part is marked by an anteroposterior fissure called *superior meatus*.

4. Posterior ethmoidal sinus opens into superior meatus.

5. Superior meatus is bounded above by a curved plate called *superior nasal concha*.

6. Below and in front of superior meatus is another curved plate of bone called *middle nasal concha*.

7. Lateral surface of middle concha is concave and forms medial wall of *middle meatus*.

8. Lateral wall of middle meatus is marked by a swelling produced by middle ethmoidal air cells. This swelling is called *bulla ethmoidalis*.

9. Middle ethmoidal sinus opens on the surface of bulla or immediately above it.

10. A thin bar of bone called *uncinate process* projects downwards and backwards from the anterior part of the labyrinth.

11. The curved gap between uncinate process and bulla is called *hiatus semilunaris*.

12. The upper end of hiatus semilunaris is continuous with a curved canal called *ethmoidal infundibulum*.

13. Anterior ethmoidal sinus opens into the infundibulum.

14. In 50% cases the infundibulum continues superiorly as *frontonasal duct* to reach the frontal sinus.

OSSIFICATION

1. At the age of 3rd month of intrauterine life the walls of nasal cavity are marked by a cartilaginous framework called *cartilaginous nasal capsule*.

2. Cartilaginous nasal capsule consists of two lateral regions and a median nasal part.

3. Single centre appears for each labyrinth in the lateral region of nasal capsule at about 5th month of intrauterine life.

4. Perpendicular plate and crista galli ossify from single centre which appears in the median septal part of nasal capsule at the age of 1st year after birth.

5. The labyrinths fuse with perpendicular plate in the region of cribriform plate at about 2 years of age.

6. The ethmoid air cells begin to develop during intrauterine life and are present in the form of narrow pouches at birth.

Inferior Nasal Concha

TERMINOLOGY

'Concha' is a Latin word which means 'shell'. Conchae (superior, middle and inferior) are bracket like projections of thin (like egg shell) bones from lateral wall of nose.

LOCATION

Inferior concha is an independent bone whose long axis occupies the whole length of the lower part of the lateral wall of each half of nasal cavity.

FEATURES AND ATTACHMENTS

Each inferior concha has two ends (anterior and posterior), two surfaces (medial and lateral) and two borders (superior and inferior).

I. Ends

A. Anterior end

It is pointed and directed forwards.

B. Posterior end

It directed backwards and is more pointed and tapering.

II. Surfaces

A. Medial surface (Fig. 34.1)

1. It is convex.

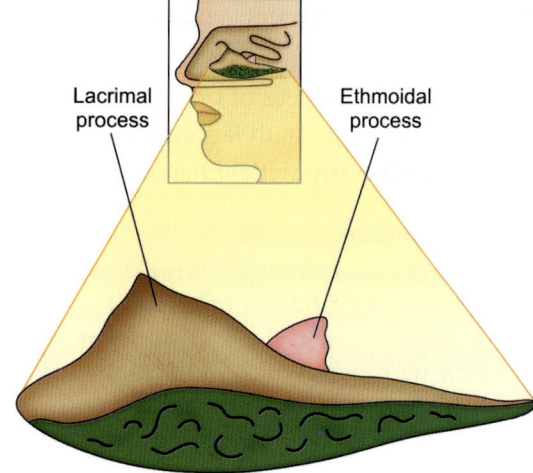

Fig. 34.1: Right inferior concha: Medial aspect

2. It has numerous apertures and grooves for vessels.

B. Lateral surface (Fig. 34.2)

1. It is concave.
2. It forms medial wall of the inferior meatus of nose.

III. Borders

A. Superior border

1. It is thin and irregular.
2. It is divided into three parts:

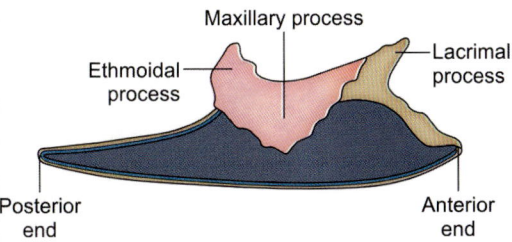

Maxillary process

Ethmoidal process

Lacrimal process

Posterior end

Anterior end

Fig. 34.2: Right inferior concha: Lateral aspect

a. Anterior part

This articulates with conchal crest of maxilla.

b. Posterior part

This articulates with conchal crest of palatine bone.

c. Middle region

This part possesses three processes which are as follows from anterior to posterior:

i. *Lacrimal process*

It is an upward projection to articulate with the descending process of lacrimal bone.

ii. *Maxillary process*

It is a curved downward projection which articulates with nasal surface of maxilla and lower part of anterior border of perpendicular plate of palatine bone.

iii. *Ethmoidal process*

It is an upward projection to articulate with uncinate process of ethmoid.

B. Inferior border

1. It is free.
2. It is thick.

OSSIFICATION

1. It develops from the lowest part of lateral region of the cartilaginous nasal capsule.
2. The centre of ossification appears during the 5th month of intrauterine life.

Vomer

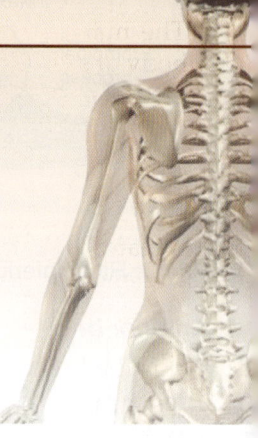

TERMINOLOGY

'Vomer' is a Latin word. The term is used for the thin plate of bone between the nostrils.

LOCATION

Vomer forms the posteroinferior part of the septum of nose (Fig. 35.1).

FEATURES AND ATTACHMENTS

Vomer has got two surfaces (right and left) and four borders (superior, inferior, anterior and posterior).

I. Surfaces

1. It has small grooves for vessels.
2. A large groove runs downwards and forwards. This is meant for *nasopalatine nerve and vessels*.

II. Borders

A. Superior border

1. It is thick.
2. Two lateral projections (*alae*) enclose a deep furrow which fits over the rostrum of sphenoid.

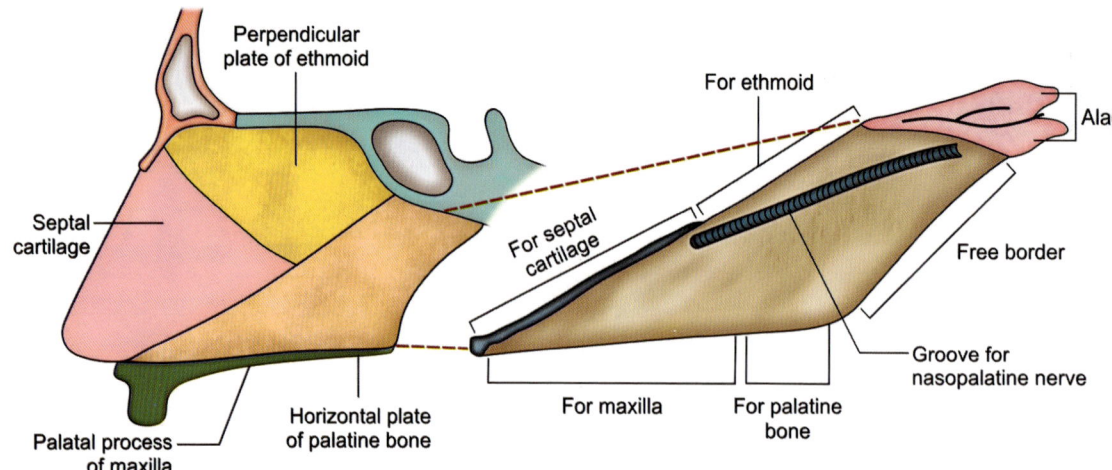

Perpendicular plate of ethmoid

For ethmoid

Alae

Septal cartilage

For septal cartilage

Free border

Groove for nasopalatine nerve

Palatal process of maxilla

Horizontal plate of palatine bone

For maxilla

For palatine bone

Fig. 35.1: Vomer. Left view

3. The margin of ala intervenes between body of sphenoid and vaginal process of medial pterygoid plate. Under surface of the ala forms *vomerovaginal canal* with vaginal process (Fig. 35.2).

B. Inferior border

It articulates with nasal crest formed by the maxillae and palatine bones.

C. Anterior border

1. It is the longest border.
2. Its upper half articulates with the posterior border of the perpendicular plate of ethmoid bone.
3. Its lower half is attached to septal cartilage.

D. Posterior border

1. It is free.
2. It is situated between two posterior nasal apertures (*choanae*).

OSSIFICATION

1. Vomer develops by ossification of membrane covering the median septal part of the cartilaginous nasal capsule.
2. One centre of ossification appears on each side of the cartilage at about 8th week of intrauterine life giving rise to two bony plates separated by a cartilage.
3. Two bony plates fuse with each other in the lower part at about 12th week of intrauterine life.
4. The cartilaginous plate is gradually absorbed allowing the fusion of two bony plates which proceeds upwards from below. Fusion is completed at puberty.

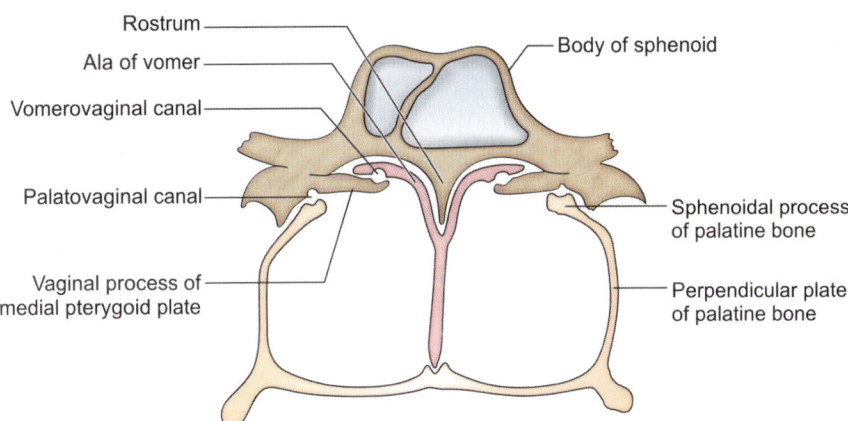

Fig. 35.2: Vomerovaginal and palatovaginal canals

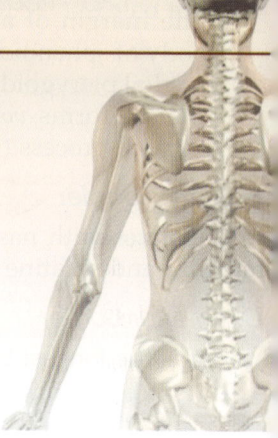

Sphenoid Bone

TERMINOLOGY

'Sphenoid' is derived from Greek word *sphen* which means 'a wedge'. The bone is so named because it is wedged between the frontal bone in front and occipital bone behind.

ANATOMICAL POSITION

1. Hypophyseal fossa faces upwards.
2. Pterygoid processes descend vertically downwards.
3. Openings of sphenoidal sinuses are directed forwards.

ARTICULATIONS

Sphenoid is a key bone in the cranial skeleton as it articulates with following eight bones:

1. Frontal
2. Parietal
3. Temporal
4. Occipital
5. Vomer
6. Zygomatic
7. Palatine
8. Ethmoid

SHAPE

Sphenoid resembles a 'bat' with its wings stretched out.

FEATURES AND ATTACHMENTS

Sphenoid consists of a central body, four wings (2 greater and 2 lesser) and two pterygoid processes (right and left).

I. Body

It has six surfaces (superior, inferior, anterior, posterior and 2 lateral) and a pair of air-filled cavities (sphenoidal sinuses).

A. Surfaces

a. Superior (cerebral) surface (Fig. 36.1)

It shows following features from anterior to posterior.

  i. *Jugum sphenoidale*
    1. It is smooth.
    2. It articulates with posterior margin of cribriform plate.
    3. It is related on each side to gyrus rectus of cerebral hemisphere and olfactory tract.
  ii. *Sulcus chiasmatis*
    1. It is a transverse groove behind the jugum sphenoidale.

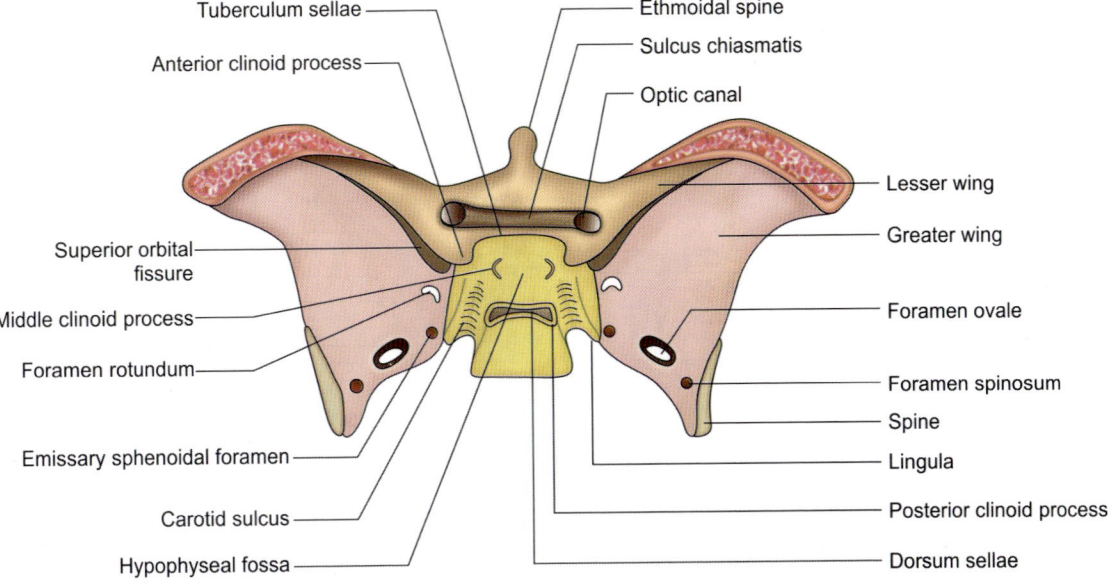

Fig. 36.1: Sphenoid bone: Superior aspect

2. *Optic chiasma* lies just above it.

3. It leads laterally into *optic canal.*

iii. *Tuberculum sellae*

It is an elevation just behind the sulcus chiasmatis.

iv. *Sella turcica*

1. It is a depressed area behind the tuberculum sellae.

2. *Hypophyseal fossa* is the deepest part of the sella turcica. It lodges *pituitary gland.*

3. Anterior part of sella turcica is bounded on each side by an elevation called *middle clinoid process.*

v. *Dorsum sellae*

It is a square plate of bone behind the sella turcica.

vi. *Posterior clinoid process*

1. Superior angles of dorsum sellae project laterally into *posterior clinoid processes.*

2. Attached margin of *tentorium cerebelli* is attached to this process on each side.

vii. *Upper part of clivus*

1. It is sloping behind the dorsum sellae.

2. It is formed by the posterior parts of body and dorsum sellae.

3. It supports the pons.

b. *Posterior surface* (Fig. 36.2)

1. It is rough.

2. It articulates with the basilar part of occipital bone.

c. *Anterior and inferior surfaces* (Fig. 36.3)

1. Midline of the anterior surface is marked by a triangular crest called *sphenoidal crest.*

2. Sphenoidal crest articulates with the upper part of the posterior border of perpendicular plate of ethmoid.

3. The midline of the inferior surface is marked by a triangular spine called *sphenoidal rostrum.* It fits into the groove between the alae of vomer.

4. Both anterior and inferior surfaces of the body on either side of midline, are

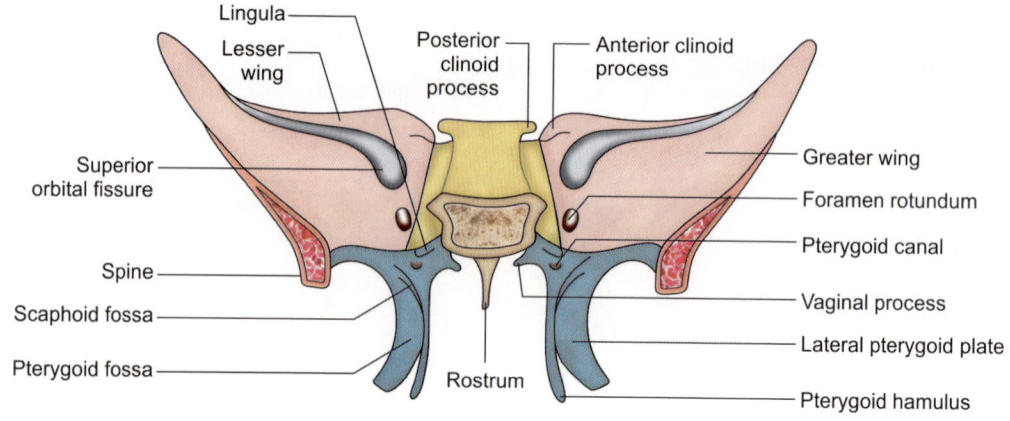

Fig. 36.2: Sphenoid bone : Posterior aspect

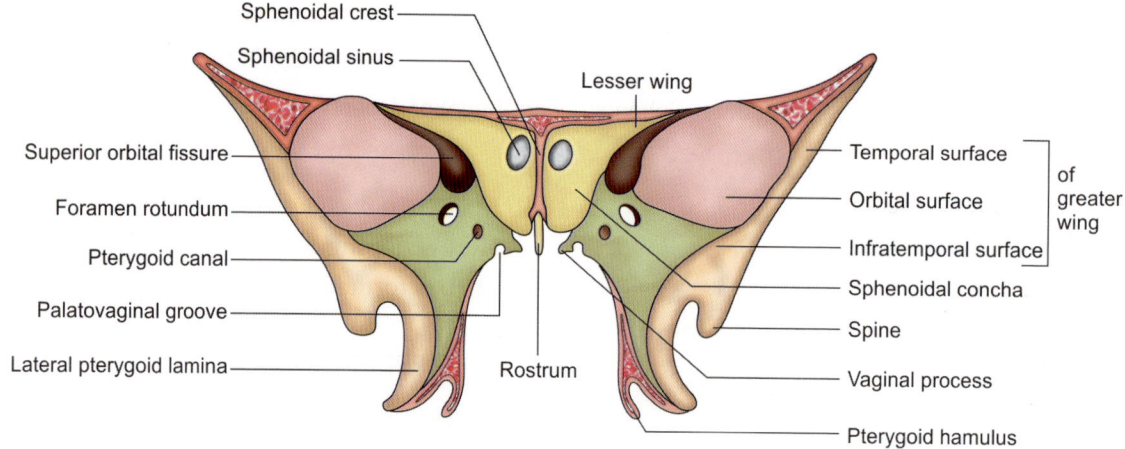

Fig. 36.3: Sphenoid bone: Anterior aspect

occupied by a thin plate of bone called *sphenoidal concha.*

5. Each sphenoidal concha consists of an anterior part which is vertical and quadrangular and a posterior part which is horizontal and triangular.

i. *Anterior part*

It consists of an upper and lateral depressed area which completes the posterior ethmoidal sinus and articulates below with the orbital process of palatine bone. Its lower and medial part forms part of the roof of the nasal cavity and is perforated above by the round opening through which sphenoidal sinus communicates with sphenoethmoidal recess of nasal cavity.

ii. *Posterior part*

It forms part of the roof of nasal cavity and completes the *sphenopalatine foramen.*

d. *Lateral surface*

1. Its lower part unites with the greater wing and medial pterygoid plate.

2. Its upper part is marked by *carotid sulcus* which lodges internal caroid artery and cavernous sinus.

3. The lateral margin of the carotid sulcus at its posterior end, projects backwards into tongue shaped *lingula*.

4. Lingula lies just above the posterior opening of *pterygoid canal*.

B. Sphenoidal sinuses

1. These are two large air spaces present in the body of sphenoid.

2. The two sinuses are separated by a septum and are rarely symmetrical.

3. *Relations*

Superiorly – Optic chiasma.

– Pituitary gland.

Laterally – Internal carotid artery.

– Cavernous sinus.

4. *Size*

Vertical height—2 cm (little less than 2 cm)

Transverse breadth—1.8 cm

Anteroposterior depth—2.1 cm (little more than 2 cm).

Note: *For simplification students may consider all the measurements approximately as 2 cm.*

5. Each sinus communicates with the sphenoethmoidal recess.

6. *Development*

i. Sphenoidal sinus starts developing as nasal mucosal evagination during intrauterine life.

ii. These are in the form of minute cavities at birth.

iii. It develops to its adult size in adolescence.

II. Wings

A. Greater wings

There are two greater wings, a right and a left. Each has three surfaces (cerebral, lateral and orbital) and several margins.

a. Surfaces

i. Cerebral surface

It is concave. It forms part of middle cranial fossa. It is related to temporal lobe of cerebrum. It possesses following foramina.

1. *Foramen rotundum*

It is situated in the anteromedial part. *Maxillary nerve* passes through it.

2. *Foramen ovale*

It is situated posterolateral to foramen rotundum. It transmits:

– *Mandibular nerve.*

– *Accessory meningeal artery.*

– *Lesser petrosal nerve.*

– *Emissary vein.*

Note: *Remember, it is the MALE which passes through foramen ovale in which M—Mandibular nerve, A—Accessory meningeal artery, L—Lesser petrosal nerve, E—Emissary vein.*

3. *Emissary sphenoidal foramen*

It is an inconstant foramen present medial to foramen ovale. It transmits *emissary vein.*

4. *Foramen spinosum*

It is lateral to foramen ovale. It transmits:

– *Middle meningeal artery.*

– *Nervus spinosus.*

5. *Canaliculus innominatus*

It is occasionally present between foramen ovale and foramen spinosum. If present, it transmits *lesser petrosal nerve.*

ii. Lateral surface

1. It is convex from above downwards.

2. *Infratemporal crest* is an anteroposterior ridge which divides the lateral surface into an upper *temporal* and a lower *infratemporal* parts.

3. *Temporal surface* forms part of temporal fossa and gives origin to *temporalis muscle*.

4. *Infratemporal surface* forms roof of infratemporal fossa and gives origin to *upper head of lateral pterygoid muscle*. This surface possesses openings of *foramen ovale* and *foramen spinosum*.

5. *Spine of sphenoid* is a projection at the posterior end of lateral surface. It shows following relations and attachments:

   – Tip gives attachment to *spheno-mandibular ligament*.

   – Medially it is related to *chorda tympani nerve* and *auditory tube*.

   – Laterally it is related to *auri-culotemporal nerve*.

iii. Orbital surface

1. It is quadrilateral in shape.

2. It forms posterior part of the lateral wall of orbit.

3. Its upper serrated edge articulates with orbital plate of frontal bone.

4. Its lateral serrated margin articulates with zygomatic bone.

5. Its inferior smooth border forms the posterolateral boundary of *inferior orbital fissure*.

6. Its medial sharp margin constitutes lower boundary of *superior orbital fissure*. A projection from this border provides attachment to *common tendinous ring*.

7. Below the medial end of superior orbital fissure is a depressed area pierced by *foramen rotundum*.

b. Margins

1. The tip of the greater wing is called *parietal margin*. It articulates with sphenoidal angle of parietal bone at pterion.

2. *Posterior margin* of the greater wing extends from body of sphenoid to its spine. Its medial half forms the anterior boundary of foramen lacerum and receives the opening of pterygoid canal. Its lateral half articulates with the petrous temporal.

3. *Lateral margin* extends forwards from spine to the tip of greater wing. This is *also called squamosal margin* because it articulates with the squamous part of temporal bone.

4. Medial to the tip there is a *triangular rough area* for the frontal bone.

5. Anterior angle of the triangular area continues with a serrated margin (lateral margin of orbital surface) which articulates with zygomatic bone.

B. Lesser wings

It is a triangular bone extending laterally from the anterosuperior part of the body. It consists of a tip, two roots (anterior and posterior), two surfaces (superior and inferior) and two borders (anterior and posterior).

a. Tip

i. It is the lateral end of lesser wing.

ii. It is situated near the lateral end of superior orbital fissure.

b. Roots

i. Lesser wing is connected to body by anterior and posterior roots.

ii. The two roots enclose the *optic canal* which transmits *optic nerve* and *oph-thalmic artery*.

c. Surfaces

i. Superior surface

It forms posterior part of the floor of anterior cranial fossa.

ii. Inferior surface

It forms superior boundary of superior orbital fissure and posterior part of the orbital roof.

d. Borders

i. Anterior border

It articulates with the posterior border of the orbital plate of the frontal bone.

ii. Posterior border

1. It is free.
2. Its medial end forms the *anterior clinoid process* to which is attached the free margin of tentorium cerebelli.

C. Superior orbital fissure

1. It is a triangular slit like communication between the orbit and middle cranial fossa.
2. **Boundaries**

   Medial: *Body of sphenoid*

   Apex: *Frontal bone*

   Superior: *Lesser wing of sphenoid.*

   Inferior: *Greater wing of sphenoid.*
3. It transmits the following structures:

   ### a. Structures which enter the orbit

   i. Upper and lower divisions of oculo-motor nerve.

   ii. Trochlear nerve.

   iii. Three branches (lacrimal, frontal and nasociliary) of ophthalmic division of trigeminal nerve.

   iv. Abducent nerve.

   v. Orbital branch of middle meningeal artery.

   vi. Sympathetic filaments.

   ### b. Structures which appear from the orbit

   i. Superior and inferior ophthalmic veins.

   ii. Recurrent meningeal branch of lacrimal artery.

III. Pterygoid processes

1. Pterygoid process on each side descends vertically downwards from the junction of body and greater wing of sphenoid.
2. Each consists of *a lateral and a medial pterygoid plate.*
3. The plates unite anteriorly in the upper part to enclose a fossa called *pterygoid fossa.*

4. The plates are not united in the lower portion to form *pterygoid fissure* which is filled by the pyramidal process of palatine bone.
5. Anterior surface of the pterygoid process forms posterior boundary of *pterygopalatine fossa.* Anterior opening of pterygoid canal is located in this region.

Some details of the two pterygoid plates are as follows:

A. Lateral pterygoid plate

It has two surfaces (lateral and medial) and two borders (anterior and posterior).

a. Surfaces

i. Lateral surface

It forms medial wall of infratemporal fossa and gives origin to *lower head of lateral pterygoid muscle.*

ii. Medial surface

It forms lateral wall of pterygoid fossa which gives origin to *deep head of medial pterygoid muscle.*

b. Borders

i. Anterior border

It forms posterior boundary of *pterygomaxillary fissure.*

ii. Posterior border

It is free.

B. Medial pterygoid plate

It has two surfaces (lateral and medial) and two borders (anterior and posterior).

a. Surfaces

i. Lateral surface

It forms medial wall of pterygoid fossa and is related to *tensor palati muscle.*

ii. Medial surface

1. It forms the lateral wall of corresponding posterior nasal aperture.
2. *Vaginal process* is a thin lamina projecting medially from its upper

part under the body of sphenoid. A groove on its anterior part of under-surface completes the *palatovaginal canal* with sphenoidal process of palatine bone. This canal transmits pharyngeal branch of maxillary artery and pharyngeal branch of pterygopalatine ganglion.

3. Vaginal process articulates medially with ala of vomer and forms *vomer-ovaginal canal* between the two. This canal transmits branches of pharyngeal nerve and vessels.

b. Borders

i. Anterior border

It articulates with the posterior border of perpendicular plate of palatine bone.

ii. Posterior border

1. At its upper end it splits to enclose *scaphoid fossa* which gives origin to *tensor palati muscle*.
2. Its upper end shows a small projection called *pterygoid tubercle* which lies immediately below the posterior end of pterygoid canal.
3. *Pharyngobasilar fascia* is attached to its whole extent while *superior constrictor* arises from its lower part only.
4. A hook like process at its lower end is called *pterygoid hamulus*. Tondon of tensor palati winds round this process. *Superior constrictor and pterygomandibular raphe* are also attached to it.
5. An angular process projecting from the middle of this margin is called *processus tubarius*. Posterior border above this process is called *notch of auditory tube*. This process and notch support the medial end of auditory tube.

OSSIFICATION

1. Sphenoid ossifies partly in membrane and partly in cartilage.

2. Parts ossifying in membrane are as follows:
   i. Greater wings except their roots.
   ii. Pterygoid processes except pterygoid hamuli.
3. Parts ossifying in cartilage are as follows:
   i. Body of sphenoid.
   ii. Lesser wings.
   iii. Sphenoidal conchae.
   iv. Roots of greater wings.
   v. Pterygoid hamuli.
4. From ossification point of view, the sphenoid is divided into presphenoidal and postsphenoidal parts.
   A. Presphenoidal part is comprised of parts lying in front of tuberculum sellae, i.e. anterior part of body, lesser wings and sphenoidal conchae. Two centres appear for each of these components are as follows:
      Anterior body—9th week of intrauterine life.
      Lesser wings—9th week of intrauterine life.
      Conchae—5th month of intrauterine life.
   B. Rest of the sphenoid is included in postsphenoidal part. Two centres appear for each of the following components of the postsphenoidal part.
      Sella turcica—4th month of intrauterine life.
      Lingulae—4th month of intrauterine life.
      Greater wings (including lateral pterygoid plates)—8th week of intrauterine life.
      Medial pterygoid plates—9th week of intrauterine life.
      Hamuli—3rd month of intrauterine life.
5. Fusions of different components of sphenoid take place as follows:
   i. Medial and lateral pterygoid plates fuse with each other at about 6th month of intrauterine life.
   ii. Presphenoidal part of the body fuses with the postsphenoidal part of the body at about 8th month of intrauterine life.

iii. At birth sphenoid is in three parts, a central part consisting of the body and lesser wings and two lateral parts, each consisting of the greater wing and the pterygoid process.

iv. Greater wing fuses with the body at about 1st year.

v. Concha fuses with the ethmoidal labyrinth at about 4th year.

vi. Concha fuses with the body of sphenoid before puberty.

vii. Body of sphenoid fuses with the basilar part of occipital bone at about 25th year.

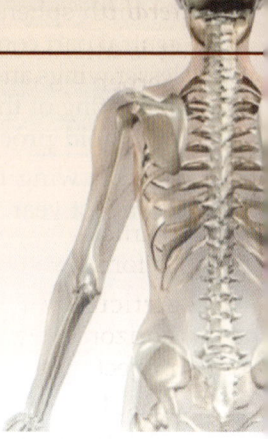

Palatine Bone

TERMINOLOGY

'Palatine' bone is so named because of its contribution to the 'hard palate'. The word 'palate' is derived from 'plate' because it forms 'plate-like' partition between nasal and oral cavities.

LOCATION

Each palatine bone is located between the maxilla and pterygoid process of sphenoid in the posterior part of nasal cavity.

FEATURES AND ATTACHMENTS

Each palatine bone is 'L' shaped in appearance and consists of two plates (horizontal and perpendicular) and three processes (pyramidal, orbital and sphenoidal).

I. Plates

A. Horizontal plate

It projects medially from the lower end of perpendicular plate. It has two surfaces (nasal and palatine) and four borders (anterior, posterior, lateral and medial).

a. Surfaces

i. Nasal surface
1. It faces superiorly.
2. It is concave from side to side.

3. It forms posterior part of the floor of nasal cavity.

ii. Palatine surface
1. It faces inferiorly.
2. With the corresponding surface of the opposite side, it forms posterior 1/4th of the hard palate.
3. Near its posterior border, this surface presents a curved ridge called *palatine crest*. This crest and the area behind it gives attachment to *palatine aponeurosis*.

b. Borders

i. Anterior border
It articulates with the posterior border of palatine process of maxilla to form *palatomaxillary suture*.

ii. Posterior border
1. It is concave.
2. It is free.
3. This gives attachment to *palatine aponeurosis* (the aponeurosis is also attached to palatine crest and the area behind it).
4. Its medial end projects backwards and with that of opposite side forms *posterior nasal spine*. To this spine is attached the *musculus uvulae*.

iii. Lateral border

1. It is attached to the lower border of perpendicular plate.
2. Its lower end is marked by greater palatine groove.

iv. Medial border

1. It articulates with that of opposite bone to form *interpalatine suture*.
2. Articulating medial borders of horizontal plates of two palatine bones project upwards to form *nasal crest*.
3. Nasal crest articulates with the posterior part of lower border of vomer and is continuous anteriorly with the nasal crests of maxillae.

B. Perpendicular plate

It has two surfaces (maxillary and nasal) and four borders (anterior, posterior, superior and inferior).

a. Surfaces

i. Maxillary surface (Fig. 37.1)

1. It faces laterally.
2. Its major part is rough to articulate with the nasal surface of maxilla.

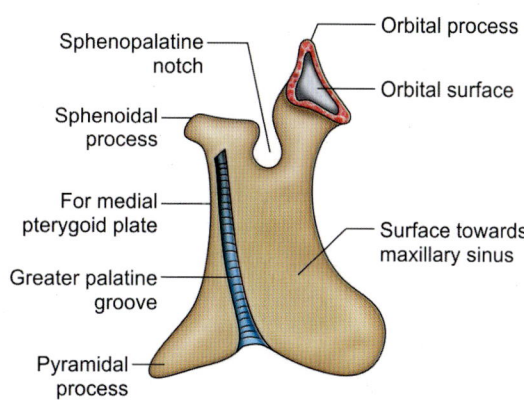

Fig. 37.1: Right palatine bone: Lateral aspect

3. Its upper and posterior part is smooth and forms medial wall of *pterygopalatine fossa*.
4. Its anterior part is also smooth and forms posterior part of medial wall of *maxillary sinus*.
5. Its posterior part shows a vertical groove (*greater palatine groove*) which is converted into *greater palatine canal* by maxilla in articulated skull. *Greater palatine vessels and nerve* pass through greater palatine canal.

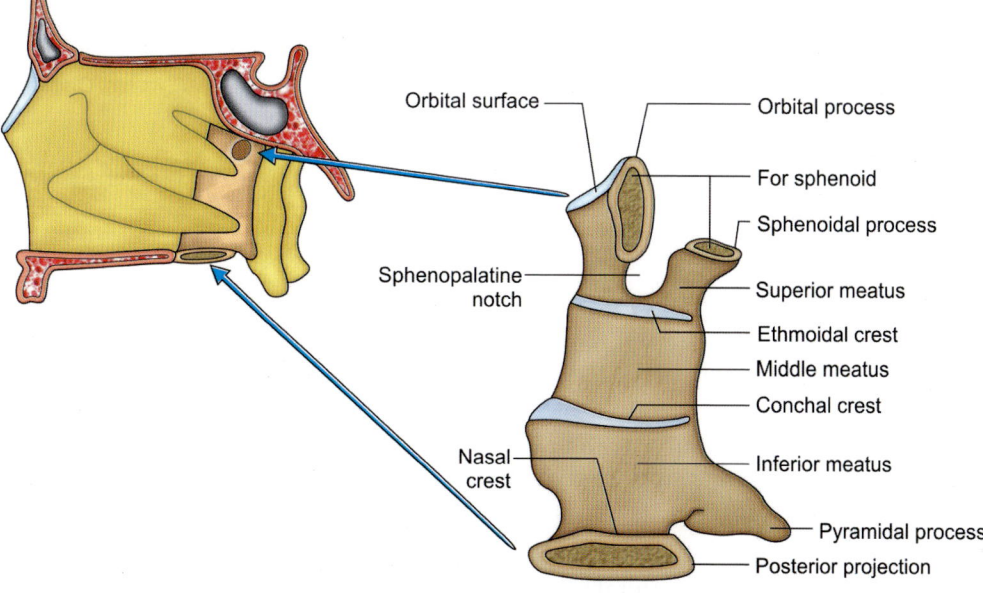

Fig. 37.2: Right palatine bone: Medial aspect

ii. Nasal surface (Fig. 37.2)

1. It faces medially.
2. It has two horizontal crests. The lower crest is called the *conchal crest* because it articulates with the inferior concha. The upper one is named the *ethmoidal crest* because of its articulation with the middle concha of ethmoid.
3. The area below the conchal crest forms *inferior meatus* of nose.
4. The area between the two crests contributes to *middle meatus* of nose.
5. The area above the ethmoidal crest takes part in the formation of *superior meatus* of nose.

b. Borders

i. Anterior border

1. Its lower part articulates with the maxillary process of inferior concha and assists in the formation of medial wall of maxillary sinus.
2. Its upper part forms the posterior boundary of maxillary hiatus.

ii. Posterior border

It articulates with the anterior border of medial pterygoid plate of sphenoid.

iii. Superior border

1. It supports the *orbital process* in front and *sphenoidal process* behind.
2. Between the orbital and sphenoidal processes is the *sphenopalatine notch* which is converted into *sphenopalatine foramen* by the inferior surface of the body of sphenoid.
3. Sphenopalatine foramen is the communication between pterygopalatine fossa and the posterior part of superior meatus of nose.
4. Sphenopalatine foramen transmits *sphenopalatine vessels* and *posterior superior nasal nerves*.

iv. Inferior border

1. It is continuous with the lateral border of horizontal plate.

2. In front of pyramidal process it is marked by lower end of greater palatine groove.

II. Processes (Figs 37.1 to 37.3)

A. Pyramidal process

1. It projects downwards, backwards and laterally from the junction of two plates of palatine bone.
2. It fits into pterygoid fissure of pterygoid process of sphenoid.
3. Its posterior surface completes the lower part of pterygoid fossa.
4. Its lateral surface is rough anteriorly and smooth posteriorly. The rough part articulates with maxillary tuberosity. Smooth part forms the lower part of infratemporal fossa.
5. Its inferior surface presents *lesser palatine foramina* for *lesser palatine nerves and vessels*.

B. Orbital process

It projects upwards and laterally from the anterior part of upper border of perpendicular plate. A constricted neck connects it with the

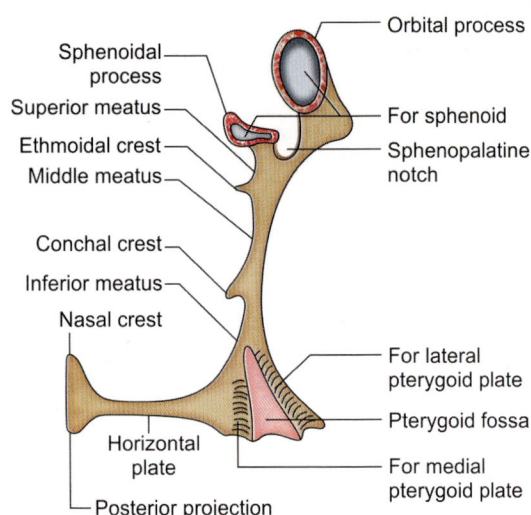

Fig. 37.3: Right palatine bone: Posterior aspect

perpendicular plate. It has three articular surfaces (anterior, posterior and medial) and two non-articular surfaces (superior and lateral)

a. Articular surfaces

i. Anterior surface

It articulates with maxilla.

ii. Posterior surface

It articulates with sphenoidal body.

iii. Medial surface

It articulates with ethmoidal bulla.

b. Non-articular surfaces

i. Superior surface

It forms posterior part of the floor of orbit.

ii. Lateral surface

It forms part of the medial wall of pterygopalatine fossa.

The border between lateral and posterior surfaces is prolonged downwards as anterior boundary of *sphenopalatine notch*.

C. Sphenoidal process

It is directed upwards and medially from the posterior part of upper border of perpendicular plate. It has three surfaces (superior, inferomedial and lateral) and three borders (posterior, anterior and medial).

a. Surfaces

i. Superior surface

1. It articulates with under surface of sphenoidal concha and root of medial pterygoid plate.

2. It is grooved to complete the *palatovaginal canal*.

ii. Inferomedial surface

It contributes to the roof and lateral wall of nasal cavity.

iii. Lateral surface

1. Its posterior part articulates with medial pterygoid plate.

2. Its anterior part contributes to the medial wall of pterygopalatine fossa.

b. Borders

i. Posterior border

It articulates with the vaginal process of medial pterygoid plate.

ii. Anterior border

It forms posterior boundary of *sphenopalatine notch*.

iii. Medial border

It articulates with ala of vomer.

OSSIFICATION

1. Palatine bone ossifies in membrane.
2. Single centre appears in the perpendicular plate during 8th week of intrauterine life.
3. The ossification spreads into the processes and horizontal plate.
4. At birth the height of perpendicular plate is equal to the transverse width of horizontal plate.
5. Length of perpendicular plate becomes double the transverse width of horizontal plate at puberty.

Skull: General Features

INTRODUCTION (Fig. 38.1)

1. Skull is the skeleton of the head.

2. Cranium means skull minus the mandible.

3. Neurocranium is upper part of skull which encloses the brain

4. Calvaria is the upper part of the cranium. It is also called the skull cap.

5. Facial skeleton (viscerocranium) is skull minus the calvaria.

6. Facial skeleton is further divided into upper facial skeleton and lower facial skeleton (mandible).

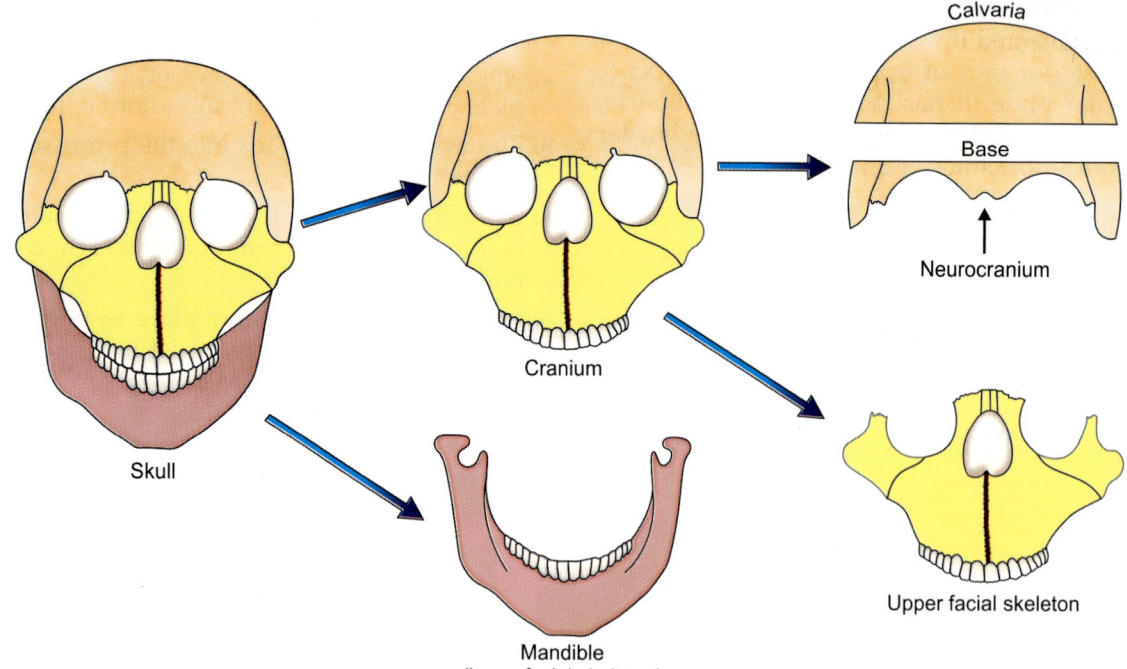

Skull

Cranium

Calvaria

Base

Neurocranium

Mandible
(lower facial skeleton)

Upper facial skeleton

Fig. 38.1: Subdivisions of skull

NEUROCRANIUM

The bones which constitute the neurocranium can be classified as:

A. Paired bones

These include:
  a. Parietal bones.
  b. Temporal bones.

B. Unpaired bones

These include:
  a. Frontal bone.
  b. Occipital bone.
  c. Sphenoid.
  d. Ethmoid.

FACIAL SKELETON (VISCEROCRANIUM OR SPLANCHNOCRANIUM)

It is composed of following bones:

A. Paired bones

These include:
  a. Maxillae.
  b. Zygomatic bones.

  c. Nasal bones.
  d. Lacrimal bones.
  e. Palatine bones.
  f. Inferior conchae.

B. Unpaired bones

These include:
  a. Mandible.
  b. Vomer.

ANATOMICAL POSITION OF SKULL (Fig. 38.2)

Skull can be kept in normal anatomical position by Reid's baseline or Frankfurt's horizontal plane.

A. Reid's baseline

It is a horizontal line formed by the joining of infraorbital margin with the centre of the external acoustic meatus.

B. Frankfurt's horizontal plane

It is marked by the horizontal line joining the infraorbital margin with the upper margin of the external acoustic meatus.

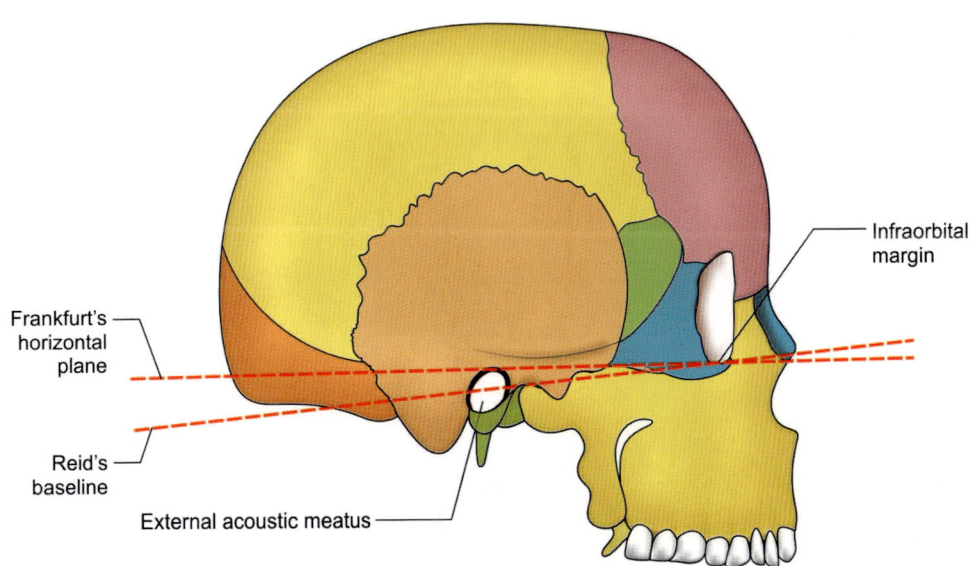

Fig. 38.2: Skull in relation to horizontal planes

Note: *Remember that Reid's starts with 'R' which also stands for 'Round' opening of external acoustic meatus, thus Reid's baseline passes through the rounded external acoustic meatus.*

On the other hand, 'Frankfurt' starts with 'F' which also stands for 'Fly' and anything that has to fly has to be above, therefore, Frankfurt's horizontal plane passes above the external acoustic meatus.

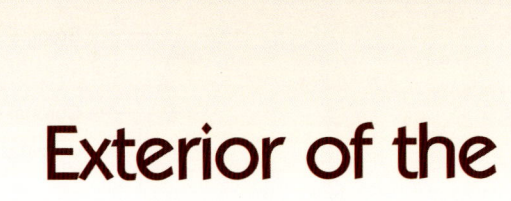

Exterior of the Skull

Different views of skull are considered from the description point of view. These are as follows:

   I. **Norma verticalis:** This is superior view.
  II. **Norma occipitalis:** This is posterior view.
 III. **Norma frontalis:** This is anterior view.
 IV. **Norma lateralis:** This is lateral (side) view.
  V. **Norma basalis:** This is inferior view.

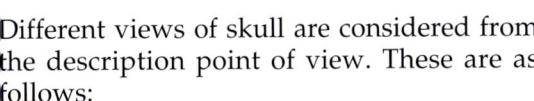

I. NORMA VERTICALIS

Definition

Observation of skull from superior aspect is called norma verticalis.

Shape

Norma verticalis view of skull appears ovoid in shape. It is relatively wider posteriorly.

Bones

The following bones contribute to the norma verticalis:

1. *Frontal bone (frontal squama):* It lies anteriorly.
2. *Occipital bone (squamous part):* It lies posteriorly.
3. *Parietal bones (paired):* These lie on each side of midline.

Junctions of Bones (sutures)

1. Sutures are the immovable joints of skull which are fibrous in nature.
2. In norma verticalis following sutures can be seen:

    i. *Coronal suture*: It is between frontal and parietal bones.

   ii. *Sagittal suture:* It is between the two parietal bones.

 iii. *Lambdoid suture:* It is between occipital and two parietal bones.

Features (Fig. 39.1)

a. Vertex

It is the highest point on sagittal suture.

b. Vault

It is the arched roof of skull.

c. Bregma

1. It is situated at the intersection between coronal and sagittal sutures.
2. Bregma is the site of a membranous gap in the foetal skull. This gap is known as *anterior fontanelle.*
3. Anterior fontanelle closes by 18 months.

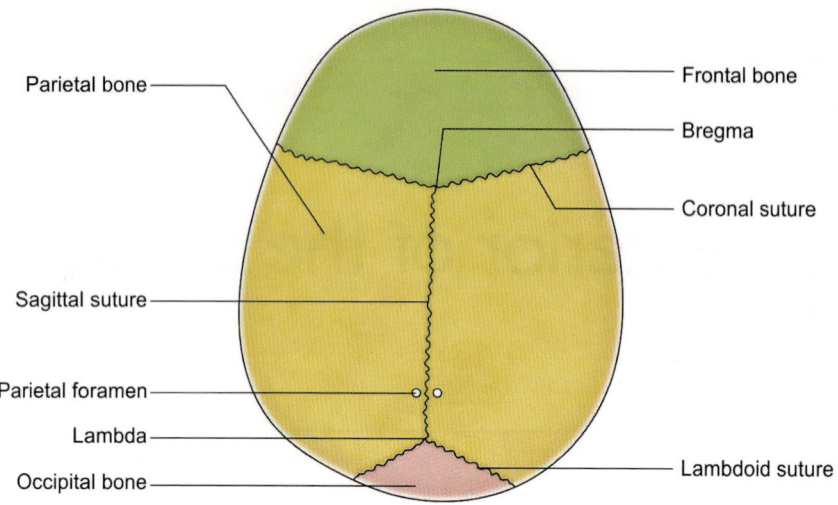

Parietal bone

Frontal bone

Bregma

Coronal suture

Sagittal suture

Parietal foramen

Lambda

Occipital bone

Lambdoid suture

Fig. 39.1: The skull: Norma verticalis

d. Lambda

1. It is situated at the intersection of sagittal and lambdoid sutures.
2. In foetal skull there is a membranous gap at the site of lambda. This gap is known as *posterior fontanelle*.
3. Posterior fontanelle closes by 2–3 months.

e. Parietal foramen

It pierces the parietal bone on each side of midline about 3.5 cm in front of lambda. *Emissary vein* passes through it.

f. Obelion

It is the region on the sagittal suture between two parietal foramina.

g. Parietal eminence

It is the area of maximum convexity of the parietal bone.

h. Temporal lines

1. There are two temporal lines on each side:
   i. *Superior temporal line.*
   ii. *Inferior temporal line.*
2. Both the temporal lines start as single line from the zygomatic process of frontal bone.

3. The two lines arch backwards and upwards and cross the frontal bone, coronal suture and parietal bone.
4. Superior temporal line fades out in the posterior part of parietal bone.
5. *Epicranial aponeourosis* and *temporal fascia* are attached to superior temporal line.
6. Inferior temporal line marks the upper limit of the origin of *temporalis muscle.*

II. NORMA OCCIPITALIS

Definition

When the skull is observed from posterior aspect, it is known as norma occipitalis.

Shape

Norma occipitalis is convex upwards and flat below.

Bones

Following bones contribute to the norma occipitalis.

1. Parietal bones (paired).
2. Squamous part of occipital bone (unpaired).
3. Mastoid parts of temporal bones (paired).

Sutures

a. Posterior part of sagittal suture

b. Lambdoid suture

1. It is between the two parietal bones and the occipital bone.
2. The lower end of lambdoid suture meets with the mastoid portion of temporal bone at a point which forms the junction of *occipitomastoid* and *parietomastoid* sutures.

c. Occipitomastoid suture

It is situated between the occipital bone and the mastoid part of the temporal bone.

d. Parietomastoid suture

It is situated between the parietal bone and the mastoid part of the temporal bone.

Features (Fig. 39.2)

a. External occipital protuberance

1. It is a midline protuberance on the lower part of norma occipitalis.
2. It marks the junction of head and neck posteriorly.
3. *Inion* is the most prominent point of external occipital protuberance.
4. *Trapezius* originates from the upper part of external occipital protuberance.
5. *Ligamentum nuchae* is attached to the lower part of this protuberance.

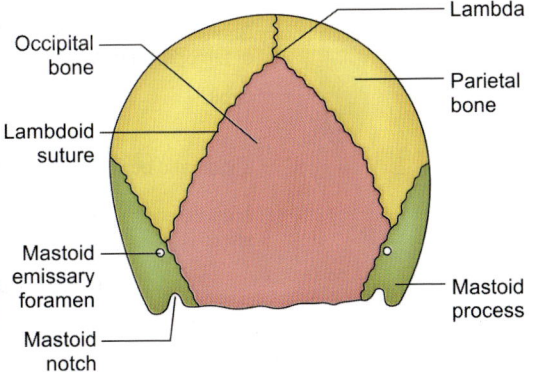

Fig. 39.2: The skull: Norma occipitalis

b. Superior nuchal lines

1. These are curved ridges passing laterally from the external occipital protuberance.
2. These form junction of head and neck posteriorly.
3. *Trapezius* originates from the medial 1/3rd of superior nuchal line.
4. *Sternomastoid* is inserted on the lateral part of superior nuchal line.
5. *Splenius capitis* is also inserted on the lateral part of this line below the attachment of sternomastoid.

c. Highest nuchal lines

1. These are situated about a 'cm' above the superior nuchal lines.
2. *Epicranial aponeurosis* is attached to their medial parts.
3. *Occipital belly of occipitofrontalis* originates on each side from its lateral 2/3rd.

d. Mastoid foramen

1. It is located near the occipitomastoid suture.
2. It opens internally into the sigmoid sulcus.
3. Following structures transverse through it:
   i. *Meningeal branch of occipital artery.*
   ii. *Emissary vein.*

e. Occipital point

1. It is situated in the midline a little above the inion.
2. It is farthest from glabella.

III. NORMA FRONTALIS

Definition

When the skull is observed from the anterior aspect it is known as norma frontalis.

Shape

It is oval in shape being wider above than below.

Bones

Major bones contributing to the surface features of norma frontalis (excluding bones contributing to deeper orbits, nasal cavity and oral cavity) are as follows:

1. Frontal bone (unpaired).
2. Maxillae (paired).
3. Nasal bones (paired).
4. Zygomatic bones (paired).
5. Mandible (unpaired).

Junctions of Bones (Sutures)

a. Junction between zygomatic process of frontal bone and frontal process of zygomatic bone is called *frontozygomatic suture*. It is observed along the lateral margin of orbital opening.

b. Junction between nasal part of frontal bone and frontal process of maxilla (*fronto-maxillary suture*) is observed along the medial margin of orbital opening in its upper part.

c. Junction between nasal part of frontal bone and nasal bones are called *fronto-nasal sutures*.

d. Junction between two nasal bones is a midline suture just above the anterior nasal aperture. This is called *internasal suture*.

e. Junction between maxilla and zygomatic bone (*zygomaticomaxillary suture*) is an oblique suture extending downwards and laterally from the lower border of each orbital opening.

f. Junction between two maxillae is called *intermaxillary suture*. It is a midline suture just below the anterior nasal aperture.

Note: *Intermaxillary suture is also observed in hard palate between palatine processes of two maxillae.*

Features (Fig. 39.3)

A. Three large apertures

One anterior nasal aperture and two orbital openings form the most striking feature of the norma frontalis.

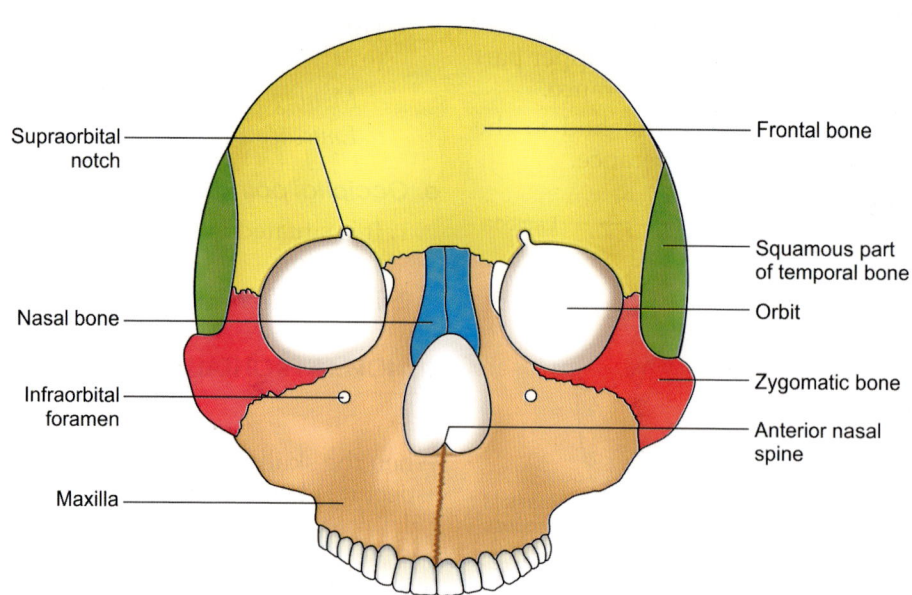

Supraorbital notch — Frontal bone

Nasal bone — Squamous part of temporal bone

— Orbit

Infraorbital foramen — Zygomatic bone

— Anterior nasal spine

Maxilla —

Fig. 39.3: The skull: Norma frontalis

a. Anterior nasal aperture

1. It is a midline aperture.
2. It is piriform in shape and wider below than above.
3. Its upper boundary is formed by lower borders of nasal bones.
4. Its lateral and inferior boundaries are contributed by nasal notches of two maxillae.
5. *Anterior nasal spine* is a sharp projection at the lower margin of nasal aperture, in the midline.
6. *Rhinion* is the lower end of internasal suture.
7. A notch at the inferior border of nasal bone is meant for passage of *external nasal nerve.*
8. Margins of aperture give attachments to the *nasal cartilages.*

b. Orbital openings

Each is present above and lateral to the anterior nasal aperture. It is quadrangular in shape and possesses four margins (supraorbital, infraorbital, lateral and medial).

i. *Supraorbital margin*
1. It is formed by frontal bone.
2. *Supraorbital notch (or foramen)* is situated at the junction of medial 1/3rd (rounded) and lateral 2/3rd (sharp) of supraorbital margin.
3. Supraorbital notch transmits *supraorbital nerve and artery and a communicating vein between angular and superior ophthalmic veins.*

ii. *Infraorbital margin*
It is formed by *maxilla* medially and *zygomatic bone* laterally.

iii. *Lateral orbital margin*
It is formed by the *frontal process* of zygomatic bone below and the *zygomatic process of frontal bone* above.

iv. *Medial orbital margin*
It is formed by the *frontal bone* above and the *lacrimal crest of frontal process of maxilla* below.

B. Frontal region

a. Superciliary arch
It is curved elevation above the medial part of the supraorbital margin.

b. Glabella
It is median elevation between two superciliary arches.

c. Nasion
It is the junction of internasal and frontonasal sutures.

d. Frontal eminence (frontal tuber)
It is rounded elevation above each superciliary arch.

C. Maxillae
Each maxilla shows following features:

a. Infraorbital foramen
1. It is situated about 1 cm below the infraorbital margin.
2. *Infraorbital nerve and vessels* pass through infraorbital foramen.

b. Incisive fossa
It is situated above the incisor teeth.

c. Canine eminence
It is produced by the root of canine tooth.

d. Canine fossa
It is situated just lateral to canine eminence.

e. Frontal process
It is sandwiched between nasal bone and lacrimal bone.

f. Zygomatic process
It articulates with the zygomatic bone.

g. Alveolar process
It bears the sockets for the upper teeth.

D. Zygomatic bones
1. Each bone is situated below and lateral to the orbital opening.

2. It is marked by a foramen called *zygo-maticofacial foramen*.

3. *Zygomaticofacial nerve* traverses the zygomaticofacial foramen.

E. Mandible

It forms the lower facial skeleton. For details of the features please consult the description of individual bone.

Attachments (Fig. 39.4)

A. Nasal bone: *Procerus*

B. Superciliary arch: *Corrugator supercilii*

C. Frontal process of maxilla.

1. *Orbital part of orbicularis oculi (it is also attached to nasal part of frontal bone).*

2. *Medial palpebral ligament.*

3. *Levator babii superioris alaeque nasi.*

D. Between infraorbital margin and infraorbital foramen: *Levator labii superioris.*

E. Below the infraorbital foramen (to canine fossa): *Levator anguli oris.*

F. Zygomatic bone just below the zygomaticofacial foramen: *Zygomaticus minor.*

G. Lateral to zygomaticus minor: *Zygo maticus major*.

H. Adjacent to nasal notch: *Nasalis* (transverse part above and alar part below).

I. Incisive fossa.

Medially: *Depressor septi*

Laterally: *Incisivus labii superioris.*

J. Alveolar process of maxilla opposite to molar teeth: *Buccinator.*

K. Mandible: Please consult the description of individual bone.

IV. NORMA LATERALIS

Definition

When skull is observed from side, it constitutes norma lateralis.

Bones

Following bones can be visualized in this view:

1. Frontal.

2. Parietal.

3. Occipital.

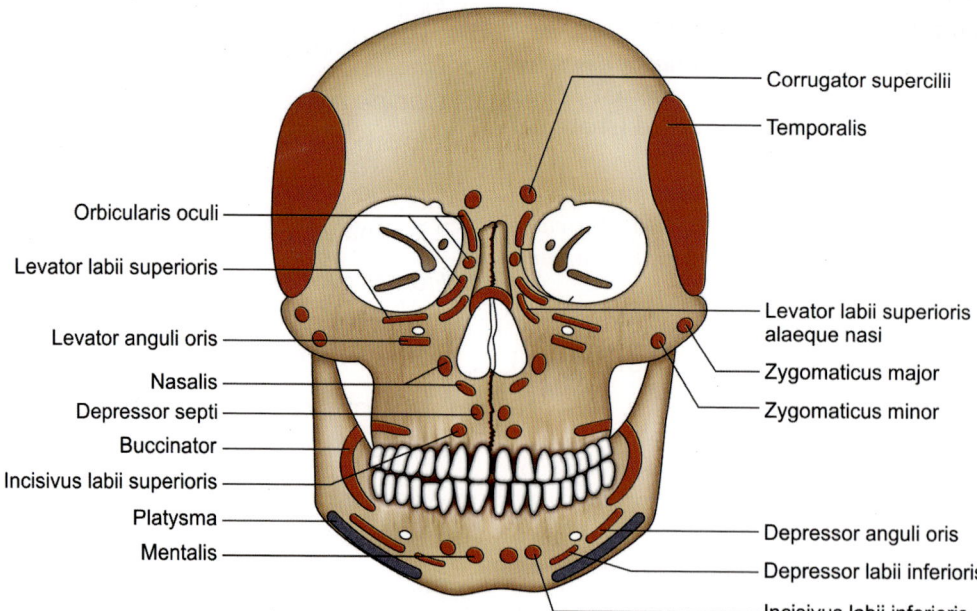

Fig. 39.4: Attachments on skull: Norma frontalis

4. Nasal.

5. Zygomatic.

6. Temporal.

7. Sphenoid.

8. Maxilla.

Features and attachments (Fig. 39.5)

A. Temporal lines

There are two temporal lines, superior and inferior.

a. Superior temporal line

1. It commences at frontal process of zygomatic bone.
2. It arches upwards and backwards across parietal bone.
3. It fades away on temporal bone.
4. *Temporal fasia* is attached to it.

b. Inferior temporal line

1. It commences at the same point.
2. It runs inferior and parallel to the superior temporal line.
3. Posteriorly it curves downwards and forwards on the temporal bone to continue with supramastoid crest.

4. It limits the attachment of *temporalis muscle.*

B. Temporal fossa

i. Boundaries

1. Anteriorly – *Zygomatic bone.*
2. Superiorly – *Superior temporal line.*
3. Posteriorly – *Superior temporal line.*
   – *Supramastoid crest.*
4. Inferiorly – *Zygomatic arch.*

ii. Anterior wall of the fossa is formed by:

1. *Temporal surface of zygomatic bone.*
2. *Greater wing of sphenoid.*
3. *Frontal bone.*

iii. Its floor is formed by following bones:

1. *Frontal.*
2. *Parietal.*
3. *Temporal.*
4. *Greater wing of sphenoid.*

iv. Temporalis muscle is attached to the floor and inferior temporal line.

v. Other contents of fossa are:

1. *Middle temporal artery* (a branch of superficial temporal artery).

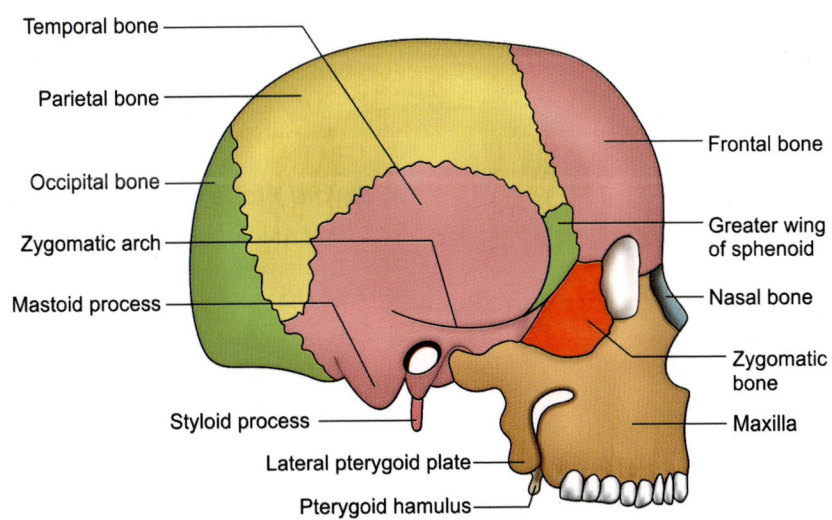

Fig. 39.5: The skull : Norma lateralis

2. *Deep temporal arteries* arising from maxillary artery.

3. *Zygomaticotemporal nerve and a minute artery* appears from the zygomaticotemporal foramen located on the temporal surface of zygomatic bone.

4. *Deep temporal nerves* arising from mandibular nerve.

C. Pterion

1. It is a circular area in the anterior part of temporal fossa which encloses four bones, frontal, parietal, sphenoid and temporal. These four bones form an 'H' shaped suture.

2. It is located 4 cm above the zygomatic arch and 3.5 cm behind the frontozygomatic suture.

3. *Middle meningeal vein, anterior branch of middle meningeal artery* and *stem of the lateral sulcus of brain* lie deep to pterion.

D. Zygomatic arch

1. It is formed by the *temporal process of zygomatic bone* and *zygomatic process of temporal bone.*

2. It has two surfaces (outer and inner) and two borders (upper and lower).

3. Its outer surface is subcutaneous and crossed by following structures from posterior to anterior:
   i. *Auriculotemporal nerve.*
   ii. *Superficial temporal vein.*
   iii. *Superficial temporal artery.*

4. *Masseter* originates from its inner surface and lower border.

5. *Temporal fascia* is attached to its upper border.

6. Posterior end of lower border is marked by *tubercle of root of zygoma.* To this is attached *lateral ligament of temporomandibular joint.*

7. Roots of zygomatic arch diverge from tubercle. Anterior root (*articular tubercle*) passes medially in front of mandibular fossa. Posterior root continues with *supramastoid crest.*

E. External acoustic meatus

1. It is located behind the mandibular fossa below the posterior root of zygoma.

2. Its anterior wall, floor and lower part of posterior wall is formed by the tympanic part while its roof and upper part of posterior wall is contributed by squamous part of temporal bone.

3. Margins of the meatus give attachment to *cartilaginous part of external acoustic meatus.*

F. Macewen's triangle (suprameatal triangle)

1. It is situated posterosuperior to external acoustic meatus.

2. *Spine of Henle (suprameatal spine)* may be present at the anteroinferior part of triangle.

3. Mastoid antrum is situated about 12.5 mm deep to suprameatal triangle.

g. Mastoid process

1. It is a downward projection from the mastoid part of temporal bone.

2. It is present below and behind the external acoustic meatus.

3. The muscles attached to it from anterior to posterior are:
   i. *Sternocleidomastoid.*
   ii. Splenius capitis.
   iii. *Longissimus capitis.*

4. *Posterior belly of digastric* originates from its medial aspect (*digastric notch*).

H. Styloid process

1. It is a slender, elongated projection below the external acoustic meatus and in front of mastoid process.

2. It provides attachments to following five structures:
   i. Anteriorly: *Styloglossus muscle.*
   ii. Posteriorly: *Stylohyoid muscle.*
   iii. Medially: *Stylopharyngeus muscle.*
   iv. Laterally: *Stylomandibular ligament.*
   v. On the tip: *Stylohyoid ligament.*

I. Infratemporal fossa

It is an irregular space below the zygomatic arch.

a. Boundaries

Anterior	: Posterior surface of body of maxilla.
Medial	: Lateral pterygoid plate and pyramidal process of palatine bone.
Lateral	: Ramus of mandible
Roof	: Infratemporal surface of greater wing of sphenoid.

b. Contents

i. Muscles

1. Lateral and medial pterygoids.
2. Temporalis.

ii. Arteries

1. Maxillary artery (Ist and 2nd parts) with its branches.
2. Posterior superior alveolar branch of 3rd part of maxillary artery.

iii. Veins

1. Maxillary vein.
2. Pterygoid venous plexus.
3. Posterior superior alveolar vein.

iv. Nerves

1. Mandibular nerve and its branches.
2. Chorda tympani.
3. Maxillary nerve.
4. Posterior superior alveolar nerve.

c. *Anterior wall* of the fossa shows two to three perforations for the *posterior superior alveolar nerve and vessels.*

d. Junction of anterior and medial walls is marked by a fissure (*pterygomaxillary fissure*) through which it communicates with pterygopalatine fossa.

e. The junction of roof and anterior wall is marked by **lateral part of inferior orbital fissure.**

f. *Foramen ovale* and *foramen supinosum* are present in the **roof of the fossa.**

g. *Lateral part of fossa* communicates with temporal fossa through a gap between zygomatic arch and side of skull.

J. Pterygomaxillary fissure

1. It is a gap which leads into pterygopalatine fossa.
2. *Boundaries*

   Anterior : Maxilla.

   Posterior : Pterygoid process.
3. *Maxillary artery* enters the pterygopalatine fossa through pterygomaxillary fissure.
4. *Maxillary nerve* courses forwards through it from pterygopalatine fossa to enter the orbit through inferior orbital fissure.

K. Pterygopalatine fossa

a. Boundaries

Anterior : Posterior surface of *maxilla.*

Posterior : 1. *Pterygoid process.*
2. *Greater wing of sphenoid.*

Medial : Perpendicular plate of *palatine bone.*

Floor : Fusion of anterior and posterior walls.

b. Communications

The pterygopalatine fossa communicates with:

1. The orbit, through the inferior orbital fissure.
2. The middle cranial fossa, through foramen rotundum.
3. The infratemporal fossa, through pterygomaxillary fissure.
4. The nasal cavity, through palatovaginal canal and sphenopalatine foramen.
5. The foramen lacerum, through pterygoid canal.

c. Contents

1. *Third part of maxillary artery and its branches.*
2. *Maxillary nerve with its branches.*
3. *Pterygopalatine ganglion and its branches.*

V. NORMA BASALIS

Definition

Observation of cranium (skull without mandible) from inferior aspect is called norma basalis.

Boundaries

Anterior : *Incisor teeth.*

Posterior : *Superior nuchal line.*

Lateral (side):

1. *Rest of teeth.*
2. *Zygomatic arch.*
3. *Posterior root of zygoma.*
4. *Mastoid process.*

Subdivisions

For the sake of convenience, norma basalis is divided into anterior, middle and posterior parts. Hard palate and alveolar arch are included in the anterior part. An imaginary horizontal line passing through the anterior margin of foramen magnum separates the posterior part from the middle part of norma basalis.

Features and attachments (Figs 39.6 and 39.7)

A. Anterior part of norma basalis

a. Posterior border of hard palate

1. It forms the junction of anterior and middle parts of norma basalis.
2. *Posterior nasal spine* is a spinous projection from its middle in the median plane.
3. *Musculus uvulae* is attached to posterior nasal spine.

b. Alveolar arch

1. It possesses *sockets for the roots of upper teeth.*
2. Number of sockets depends upon number of roots. There is single socket

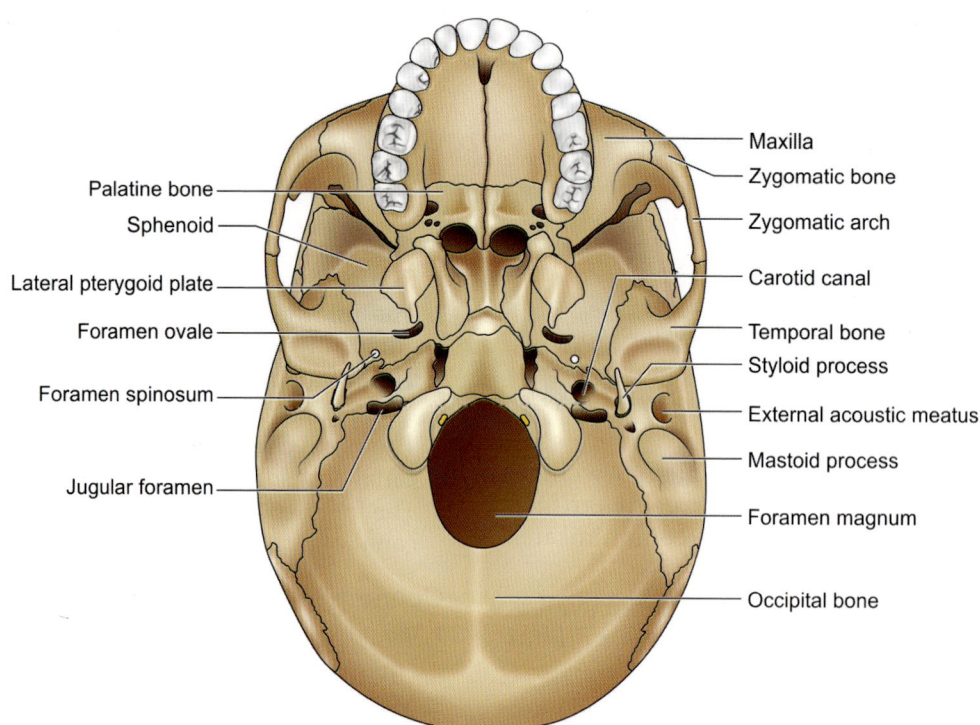

Palatine bone

Sphenoid

Lateral pterygoid plate

Foramen ovale

Foramen spinosum

Jugular foramen

Maxilla

Zygomatic bone

Zygomatic arch

Carotid canal

Temporal bone

Styloid process

External acoustic meatus

Mastoid process

Foramen magnum

Occipital bone

Fig. 39.6: The skull: Norma basalis

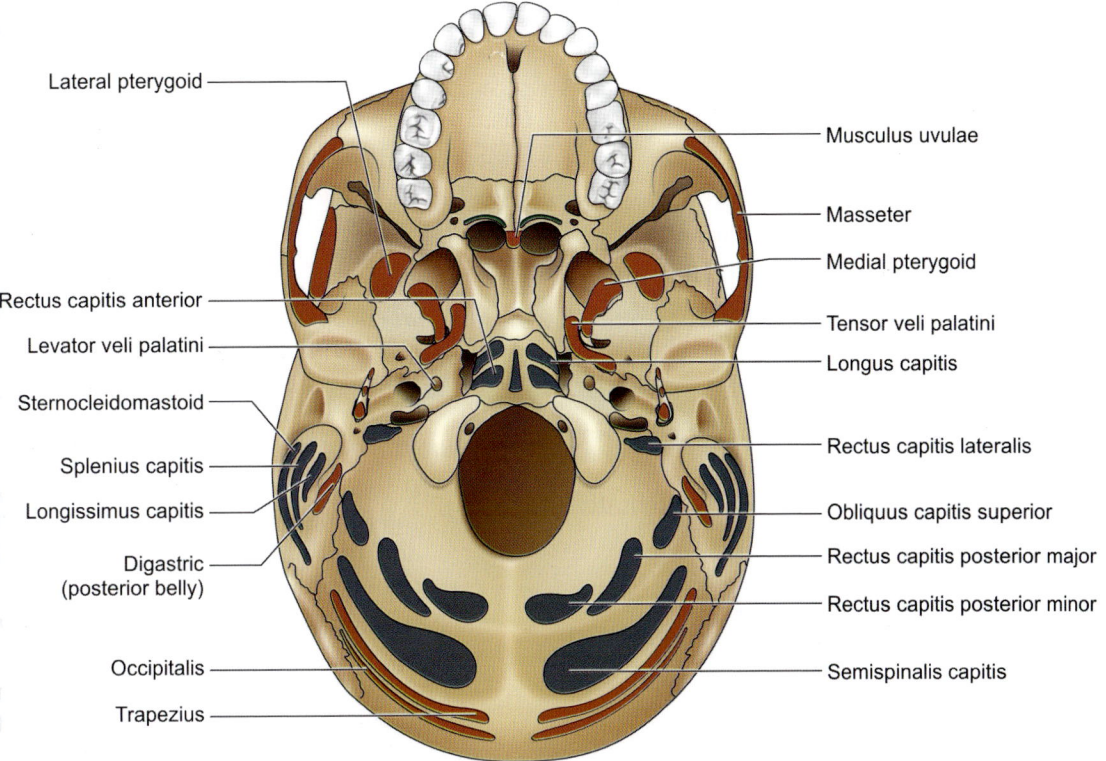

Lateral pterygoid

Rectus capitis anterior

Levator veli palatini

Sternocleidomastoid

Splenius capitis

Longissimus capitis

Digastric
(posterior belly)

Occipitalis

Trapezius

Musculus uvulae

Masseter

Medial pterygoid

Tensor veli palatini

Longus capitis

Rectus capitis lateralis

Obliquus capitis superior

Rectus capitis posterior major

Rectus capitis posterior minor

Semispinalis capitis

Fig. 39.7: The skull: Norma basalis showing muscular attachments

for each of the incisors, canines and premolars. There are three sockets for each of the upper molars.

c. Bones contributing to hard palate

1. *Palatine processes* of *two maxillae* contribute to the anterior 2/3rd of the hard palate.
2. Posterior 1/3rd of the hard palate is formed by the *horizontal plates* of *palatine bones*.
3. Bony palate is marked by several depressions produced by *palatine glands*.

d. Cruciform suture

It is formed by the following three sutures:

 i. *Intermaxillary suture.*

 ii. *Interpalatine suture.*

 iii. *Palatomaxillary sutures.*

e. Incisive fossa

1. It is present anteriorly in the median plane of hard palate.
2. *Incisive foramen* (right and left) pierces its corresponding side.
3. Each incisive foramen is transversed by *nasopalatine nerve* and *greater palatine vessels*.

f. Greater palatine foramen

1. It is present behind the lateral part of palatomaxillary suture.
2. *Greater palatine vessels and nerve* pass through it.
3. A groove observed between greater palatine foramen and incisive fossa is meant for greater palatine vessels.

g. Lesser palatine foramin a

1. These are 1–3 foramina in the pyramidal process of palatine bone and located just

behind the greater palatine foramen on each side.

2. *Lesser palatine nerves and vessels* pass through these foramina.

h. Palatine crest

1. It is a curved ridge observed in the hard palate near its posterior border.

2. *Palatine aponeurosis* is attached to the palatine crest, posterior border of hard palate and the area between the two.

i. Premaxilla

1. It is a triangular piece of maxilla holding four incisor teeth.

2. It is a separate bone in most vertebrates.

B. Middle part of norma basalis

For the sake of convenience it is divided into a median area and two lateral areas (right and left).

a. Median area

i. *Posterior nasal apertures*

These are also known as *choanae*.

ii. *Posterior border of vomer*

It separates two choanae.

iii. *Alae of vomer*

1. These are two bony plates formed by the splitting of vomer superiorly.

2. It articulates with the rostrum of sphenoid.

iv. *Vomerovaginal canal*

1. It is formed between the lateral border of each ala of vomer and the vaginal process of the medial pterygoid plate.

2. It transmits *branches of pharyngeal nerve and vessels*.

v. *Palatovaginal canal*

1. It is a canal between *vaginal process of medial pterygoid plate* and *sphenoidal process of the palatine bone*.

2. This canal leads anteriorly into posterior wall of pterygopalatine fossa.

3. It transmits *pharyngeal branches of pterygopalatine ganglion* and *pharyngeal branches of 3rd part of maxillary artery.*

Note: *Students are invariably confused as to which is the palatovaginal canal and which one is vomerovaginal canal. To differentiate keep in mind that vaginal process of medial pterygoid plate is common to both but as the palatine bone is anterior to medial pterygoid plate the palatovaginal canal is relatively anterior to vomerovaginal canal.*

vi. *Broad bar of bone behind the alae*

1. It is formed by the continuation of inferior surface of body of sphenoid and that of basilar part of occipital bone.

2. It extends up to *foramen magnum.*

3. *Pharyngeal tubercle* is a median elevation just in front of foramen magnum. It is better felt than seen.

4. Pharyngeal tubercle gives attachments to:

• *Highest fibres of superior constrictor.*

• *Pharyngeal raphe.*

5. *Longus capitis* is inserted on the basilar part of occipital bone just lateral to pharyngeal tubercle.

6. *Rectus capitis anterior* is inserted on each side just in front of occipital condyle.

b. Lateral area

i. *Pterygoid processes*

1. Pterygoid processes are located just behind the posterior ends of alveolar arch.

2. Each pterygoid process descends vertically downwards from the junction of body and greater wing of sphenoid.

3. Pterygoid process consists of a lateral and a medial plate.

4. Ptergoid plates unite anteriorly in the upper part to enclose a fossa called *pterygoid fossa*.

5. The lower ununited portions form *pterygoid fissure* which is filled by the pyramidal process of palatine bone.

6. Anterior surface of pterygoid process forms posterior boundary of *pterygopalatine fossa*.

7. Lateral surface of lateral pterygoid plate forms medial wall of *infratemporal fossa* and gives origin to lower head of *lateral pterygoid muscle*.

8. Medial surface of lateral pterygoid plate forms lateral wall of *pterygoid fossa* and gives origin to *deep head of medial pterygoid muscle*.

9. Lateral surface of medial pterygoid plate forms medial wall of pterygoid fossa and is related to *tensor palati* muscle.

10. Medial surface of the medial pterygoid plate forms the lateral wall of corresponding posterior nasal aperture.

11. Posterior border of the medial pterygoid plate shows following features:

   • At its upper end it splits to enclose *scaphoid fossa* which gives origin to *tensor palati* muscle.

   • Its upper end shows a small projection called *pterygoid tubercle* which lies immediately below the posterior end of *pterygoid canal*.

   • *Pharyngobasilar fascia* is attached to its whole extent while *superior constrictor* arises from its lower part only.

   • A hook like process at its lower end is called *pterygoid hamulus*. Tendon of *tensor palati* winds round this process. *Superior constrictor* and *pterygomandibular raphe* are also attached to it.

   • An angular process projecting from the middle of this margin is

called *processus tubarius*. Posterior border above this process is called *notch of auditory tube*. This process and notch support the medial end of *auditory tube*.

ii. *Infratemporal surface of greater wing of sphenoid*

   1. It is pentagonal in shape.

   2. It forms roof of *infratemporal fossa*.

   3. It gives origin to the *upper head of lateral pterygoid muscle*.

   4. It is crossed by *deep temporal* and *masseteric nerves*.

   5. *Spine of sphenoid* is a projection from posteriormost part of infratemporal surface.

   6. *Infratemporal crest* is the lateral limit of infratemporal surface.

   7. From scaphoid fossa to spine of sphenoid, four foramina can be noticed, i.e. *foramen of Vesalius, foramen ovale, canaliculus innominatus* and *foramen spinosum*.

iii. *Foramen ovale*

   1. It is an oval foramen.

   2. It transmits the *mandibular nerve, accessory meningeal artery, lesser petrosal nerve and emissary vein*.

Note: *For remembering the structures passing through foramen ovale remember MALE, in which M—Mandibular nerve, A—Accessory meningeal artery, L—Lesser petrosal nerve and E—Emissary vein.*

iv. *Foramen spinosum*

   1. It is situated near the spine of sphenoid, posterolateral to foramen ovale.

   2. It transmits *middle meningeal artery, nervus spinosus* (meningeal branch of mandibular nerve) and *parietal trunk of middle meningeal vein*.

v. *Foramen of Vesalius (sphenoidal emissary foramen)*

1. It is an infrequently seen foramen between scaphoid fossa and foramen ovale.

2. It transmits an emissary vein connecting cavernous sinus with pterygoid venous plexus.

vi. *Canaliculus innominatus (foramen innominatum)*

1. This is also an infrequently seen foramen between foramen ovale and foramen spinosum.

2. It transmits *lesser petrosal nerve.*

vii. *Spine of sphenoid*

1. It is related laterally to *auriculotemporal nerve* and medially to *chorda tympani nerve* and *Eustachian tube.*

2. *Sphenomandibular ligament* is attached to its tip.

3. Most posterior fibres of *tensor palati* originate from its anterior surface.

viii. *Sulcus tubae*

1. It is a groove between posteromedial margin of infratemporal surface of greater wing of sphenoid and inferior surface the petrous part of temporal bone.

2. *Cartilaginous part of Eustachian tube* (also called auditory tube or pharyngotympanic tube) occupies this sulcus.

ix. *Inferior surface of petrous part of temporal bone*

1. It is located just behind the infratemporal surface of greater wing of sphenoid.

2. Its anteromedial serrated end marks the apex of petrous part.

3. The quadrilateral area near the apex provides attachment to *levator palati muscle.*

4. Lower opening of *carotid canal* is located just behind the quadrilateral area. It *transmits internal carotid artery with its sympathetic and venous plexuses.*

5. Carotid canal runs forwards and medially in petrous part and perforates its apex as upper opening of carotid canal.

x. *Foramen lacerum*

1. It is located between sphenoid and apex of petrous temporal.

2. It is named *lacerum* because of irregular margins.

3. *Carotid canal* and *pterygoid canal* open into it.

4. Only two structures pass through it i.e. *meningeal branch of ascending pharyngeal artery* and *emissary vein.*

5. *Internal carotid artery* traverses its upper part *with its sympathetic and venous plexuses.*

6. *Nerve of pterygoid canal (Vidian nerve)* is formed in its upper part by the union of *greater superficial petrosal and deep petrosal nerves.*

xi. *Tympanic part of temporal bone*

1. It is a triangular bone which occupies the angle between the petrous and squamous parts of temporal bone.

2. Its anterior surface is related to *parotid gland.*

xii. *Squamous part of temporal bone*

Only a small part of squamous part of temporal bone is seen in norma basalis and shows following features from posterior to anterior:

1. Anterior (articular) part of *mandibular fossa.*

2. *Articular tubercle.*

3. Part of the roof of infratemporal fossa.

xiii. *Squamotympanic fissure*

1. It marks the junction of squamous and tympanic parts of temporal bone.

2. Downward edge of tegmen tympani (a part of petrous part of temporal

bone) divides the squamotympanic fissure into *petrotympanic* (posterior) and *petrosquamous* (anterior) *fissures.*

3. *Chorda tympani nerve, anterior tympanic artery* and *anterior ligament of malleus* pass through petroty-mpanic fissure.

C. Posterior part of norma basalis

For the sake of convenience this part can be divided into a median area and two lateral areas (right and left).

a. Median area

It consists of foramen magnum, external occipital crest and external occipital protuberance from anterior to posterior.

i. *Foramen magnum*

1. It is the largest foramen in skull.

2. It is single foramen located in the lowest part of posterior cranial fossa.

3. It is oval in shape.

4. It is the communication between cranial cavity and vertebral canal.

5. *Anterior atlanto-occipital membrane* is attached to its anterior margin.

6. *Posterior atlanto-occipital membrane* is attached to its posterior margin.

7. Lateral margins provide attachments to *alar ligaments.*

8. Following structures pass through its anterior part:

   • *Apical ligament of dens.*

   • *Superior longitudinal band of cruciform ligament.*

   • *Membrana tectoria.*

9. Following structures pass through its posterior part:

   • *Medulla oblongata.*

   • *Meninges.*

   • *Spinal roots of accessory nerves.*

   • *Meningeal branches of upper cervical nerves (C_{1-3}).*

   • *Vertebral arteries.*

   • *Sympathetic plexuses around vertebral arteries.*

   • *Anterior and posterior spinal arteries.*

ii. *External occipital crest*

1. It extends from posterior margin of foramen magnum to external occipital protuberance.

2. Upper margin of *ligamentum nuchae* is attached to it.

iii. *External occipital protuberance*
Trapezius is attached to it superiorly and *ligamentum nuchae* inferiorly.

b. Lateral area

i. *Occipital condyles*

1. These are located lateral to anterior half of foramen magnum.

2. Each is oval and convex to articulate with concave superior articular process of atlas.

ii. *Condylar fossa*

1. It is present just behind the occipital condyle.

2. It may have *condylar canal for emissary vein* from sigmoid sinus.

iii. *Hypoglossal canal*

1. Lateral to anterior part of condyle is the outer opening of hypoglossal canal.

2. It transmits:

   • *Hypoglossal nerve.*

   • *Meningeal branch of ascending phary-ngeal artery.*

   • *Emissary vein from basilar venous plexus.*

iv. *Squamous part of occipital bone*

1. *Superior nuchal line* is a well-defined ridge which extends laterally from external occipital protuberance on each side. Its medial 1/3rd provides origin to *trapezius* while lateral 1/3rd receives insertions of *sternomastoid* (above) and *splenius capitis* (below).

2. Running laterally on each side from the middle of external occipital crest is another ridge called *inferior nuchal line.*

3. A vertical line on each side along with inferior nuchal line divides the region below the superior nuchal line into four areas, each meant for the attachment of a muscle as follows:

- Upper medial area for *semispinalis capitis*.
- Upper lateral area for *obliquus capitis superior*.
- Lower medial area for *rectus capitis posterior minor*.
- Lower lateral area for *rectus capitis posterior major*.

v. *Jugular foramen*

1. It is an interosseous foramen situated between anterior margin of jugular process of occipital bone and posterior margin of petrous part of temporal bone at the petro-occipital suture.

2. It is divided into anterior, middle and posterior parts.

3. 9th, 10th and 11th cranial nerves pass through its middle part.

4. *Inferior petrosal sinus* and *meningeal branch of ascending pharyngeal artery* pass through its anterior part.

5. *Sigmoid sinus* and *meningeal branch of occipital artery* traverse through its posterior part.

6. At its posterior end the anterior wall (petrous temporal) is hollowed out to form the *jugular fossa* which lodges the superior bulb of internal jugular vein.

7. *Mastoid canaliculus* is a minute canal in the lateral wall of jugular fossa which transmits the *auricular branch of vagus*.

8. *Glossopharyngeal notch* is on the posterior border of petrous temporal bone near the medial end of jugular foramen.

9. *Cochlear canaliculus* is located at the apex of glossopharyngeal notch. The *aqueduct of cochlea* opens into the cochlear canaliculus.

10. *Tympanic canaliculus* is present in the ridge between jugular fossa and lower opening of carotid canal. It transmits the *tympanic branch of glossopharyngeal nerve* to middle ear.

vi. *Inferior surface of jugular process of occipital bone*

1. It is the area just lateral to occipital condyle behind the jugular foramen.

2. It provides attachment to *rectus capitis lateralis*.

vii. *Styloid process*

1. It is a conical projection just below the tympanic part of temporal bone.

2. It is directed downwards, forwards and slightly medially.

3. It provides attachments to 3 muscles and 2 ligaments. Three muscles attached to it are *styloglossus* (anteriorly), *stylohyoid* (posteriorly) and *stylopharyngeus* (medially). Two ligaments attached to it are *stylomandibular* (laterally) and *stylohyoid (on the tip)*.

4. It is interposed between *parotid gland* (laterally) and *internal jugular vein* (medially).

5. Two structures cross it superficially, i.e. *facial nerve* (near the base) and *external carotid artery* (near the tip).

viii. *Mastoid process*

1. It is a prominent projection from the temporal bone posterolateral to styloid process.

2. The medial aspect of this process shows a deep groove (*digastric notch*) which provides attachment to *posterior belly of digastric*.

3. Medial to digastric notch, there can be another *groove for occipital artery*.

ix. *Stylomastoid foramen*

1. It is present between styloid and mastoid processes.

2. *Facial nerve* and *stylomastoid artery* pass through this foramen.

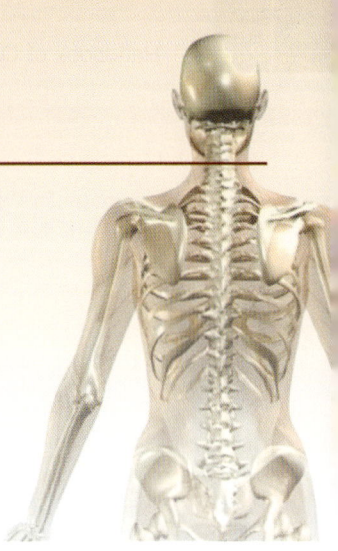

Orbital Cavity

DEFINITION

Orbits are two bony sockets which lodge the eye balls and the associated structures.

SHAPE AND PARTS (Fig. 40.1)

Each orbit is pyramidal in shape having an anterior base (orbital opening), posterior apex and four walls (medial, lateral, roof and floor).

BONY CONTRIBUTIONS (Fig. 40.2)

A. Orbital opening (base)

It consists of four margins (supraorbital, infraorbital, lateral and medial).

a. Supraorbital margin

1. It is formed by the frontal bone.
2. *Supraorbital notch (or foramen)* is situated at the junction of its medial 1/3rd (rounded) and lateral 2/3rd (sharp) parts.
3. Supraorbital notch transmits:
   i. *Supraorbital nerve.*
   ii. *Supraorbital artery.*
   iii. *Communicating vein between angular and superior ophthalmic veins.*

b. Infraorbital margin

It is formed by maxilla medially and zygomatic bone laterally.

c. Lateral orbital margin

It is formed by the frontal process of zygomatic bone below and the zygomatic process of frontal bone above.

d. Medial orbital margin

It is formed by the frontal bone above and the lacrimal crest of frontal process of maxilla below.

B. Apex

1. It forms the posterior end of orbit.
2. It is contributed by sphenoid.
3. Usually the medial end of superior orbital fissure is said to mark the apex.

C. Medial wall

It is formed by the following bones from anterior to posterior:

a. Posterior part of the frontal process of *maxilla.*
b. *Lacrimal bone.*
c. The orbital plate of *ethmoid.*
d. Body of *sphenoid.*

D. Lateral wall

It is contributed by:

a. *Greater wing of sphenoid bone* posteriorly.
b. *Orbital surface of zygomatic bone* and *medial aspect of its frontal process* anteriorly.

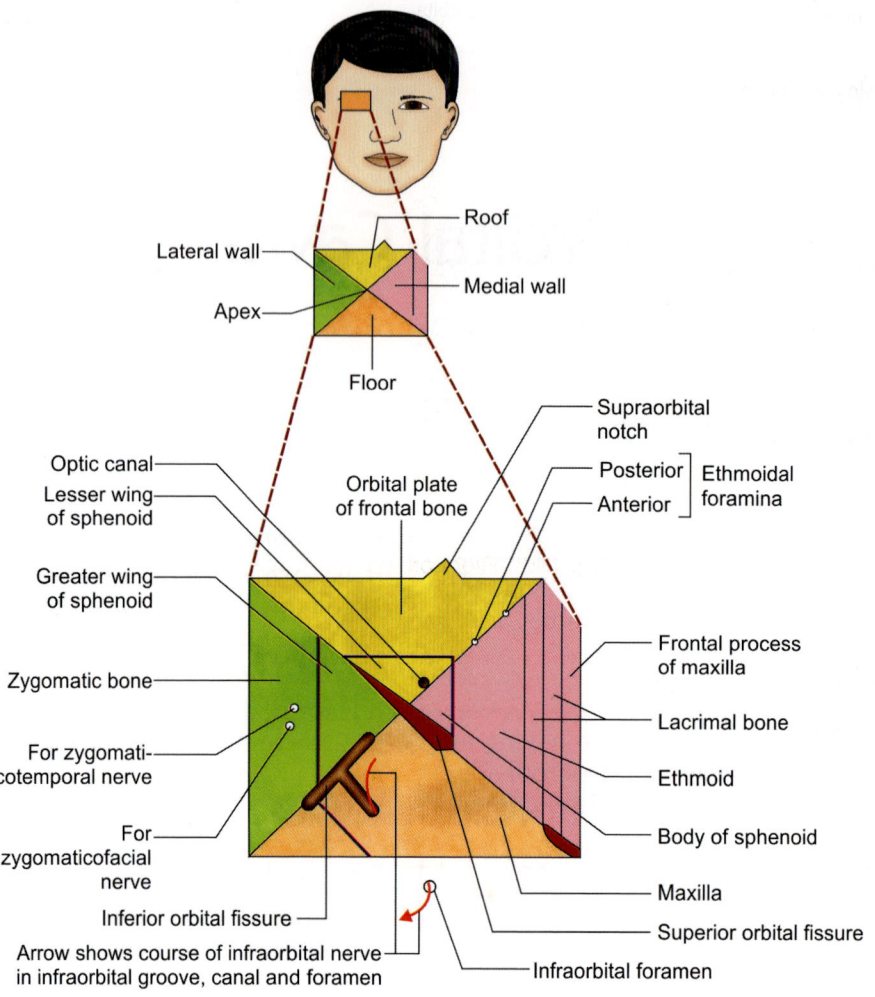

Fig. 40.1: Right orbit: Anterior view

E. Roof

It is formed by:

a. *Orbital plate of frontal bone* anteriorly.

b. *Lesser wing of sphenoid* posteriorly.

F. Floor

It is formed by:

a. *Orbital surface of maxilla* medially. It is the major contribution.

b. *Orbital surface of zygomatic bone.*

c. *Orbital process of palatine bone.* It is an insignificant contribution near the posterior end at the junction of medial wall and floor.

COMMUNICATIONS (Fig. 40.3)

The orbit communicates through several passages with adjacent regions as shown below:

Passages	Adjacent regions
1. Orbital opening	Face
2. Infraorbital canal	Face
3. Optic canal	Middle cranial fossa
4. Superior orbital fissure	Middle cranial fossa
5. Inferior orbital fissure	
a. Medially	Pterygopalatine fossa
b. Laterally	Infratemporal fossa

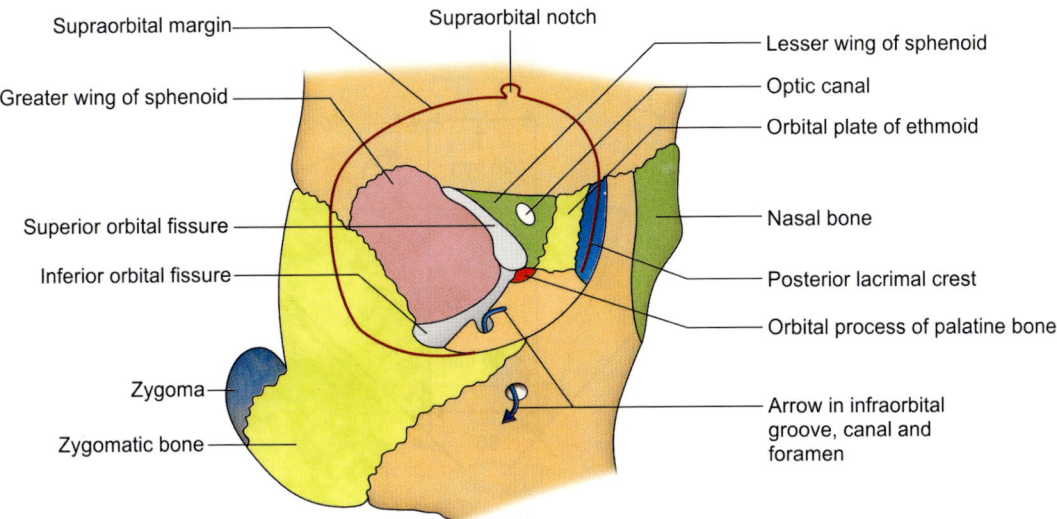

Fig. 40.2: Right orbit: Anterior view

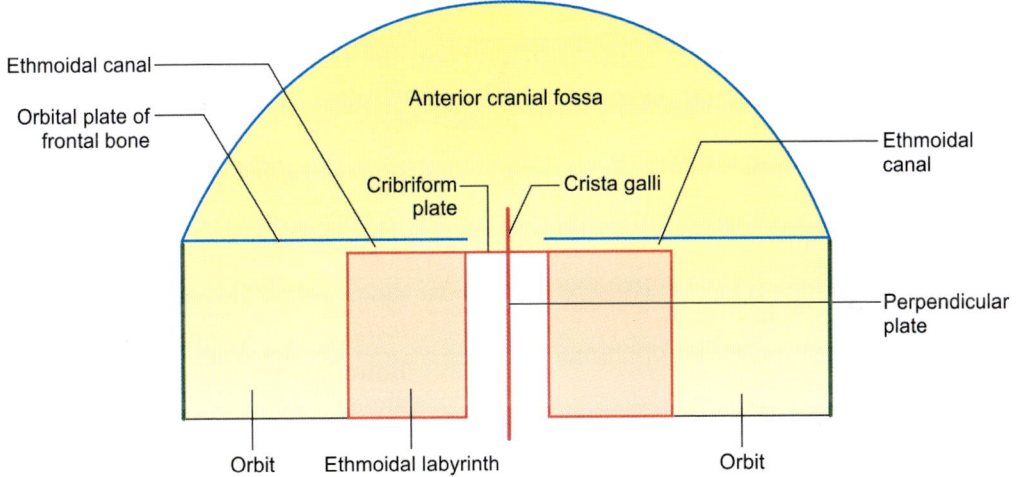

Fig. 40.3: Diagrammatic representation of ethmoidal canal in coronal sectional view

6. Zygomatico-orbital foramina	Face and temporal fossa
7. Anterior and posterior ethmoidal canals	Anterior cranial fossa
8. Nasolacrimal canal	Nasal cavity

MEASUREMENTS (Fig. 40.4)

1. Length of medial wall—50 mm.
2. Length of lateral wall—50 mm.

3. Width of orbital opening, i.e. distance between medial and lateral orbital margins—40 mm
4. Distance between two lateral orbital margins—100 mm
5. Distance between two medial orbital margins—25 mm
6. Angle between two lateral walls—90°
7. Angle between lateral and medial walls of each orbit—45°

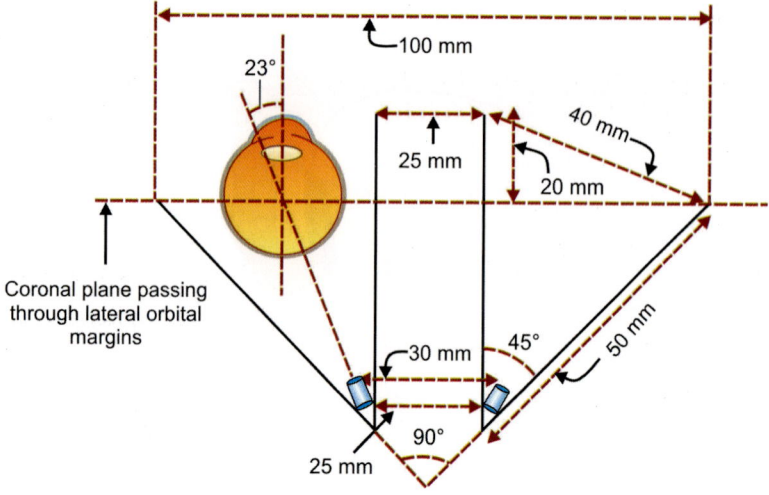

Fig. 40.4: Horizontal sectional view of orbits showing measurements

8. Angle between long axis of orbit and anteroposterior axis of eyeball—23°.
9. Distance between medial orbital margin and coronal plane passing through lateral orbital margins—20 mm.
10. Measurements of optic canal:
    i. Length—3–9 mm
    ii. Diameter—5 mm
    iii. Distance between orbital openings of optic canals—30 mm
    iv. Distance between cranial openings of optic canals—25 mm

FEATURES

1. Anterolateral part of roof is slightly hollowed out to form *fossa for lacrimal gland.*
2. The anteromedial part of roof near the orbital opening is marked by the *trochlear fovea* or *spine* for the attachment of fibrocartilaginous pulley meant for the tendon of superior oblique muscle.
3. *Optic canal* is present at the posterior end of junction of roof and medial wall. *Optic nerve* and *ophthalmic artery* pass through optic canal.

4. The posterior part of the junction of lateral wall and floor is marked by **inferior orbital fissure**. It transmits the following structures:
    i. *Maxillary nerve.*
    ii. *Infraorbital vessels.*
    iii. *Zygomatic nerve.*
    iv. *A branch from inferior ophthalmic vein.*
    v. *Some twigs (orbital branches) from pterygopalatine ganglion.*
    Boundaries of inferior orbital fissure are as follows:
    a. Superiorly: *Greater wing of sphenoid.*
    b. Inferiorly: *Body of maxilla* and *orbital process of palatine bone*
    c. Laterally: *Zygomatic bone.*
5. Maxillary part of the floor is marked by a groove (*infraorbital groove*) in the posterior part. This groove is directed forwards and continues with the *infraorbital canal* in the anterior part of floor and ultimately opens on the face as *infraorbital foramen.* Infraorbital groove, canal and foramen are meant for the passage of infraorbital nerve and vessels.

6. In the anterior part of medial wall, the posterior part of frontal process of maxilla (behind the anterior lacrimal crest) and anterior part of lacrimal bone (anterior to posterior lacrimal crest) form a vertical fossa called *lacrimal fossa*. This fossa continues down with the beginning of *nasolacrimal canal*. The fossa and canal are meant for *lacrimal sac* and *nasolacrimal duct* respectively.

7. *Anterior lacrimal crest* provides attachments to:
   i. *Lacrimal fascia.*
   ii. *Medial palpebral ligament.*
   iii. *Orbicularis oculi.*

8. *Posterior lacrimal crest* gives attachments to:
   i. *Lacrimal fascia.*
   ii. *Lacrimal part of orbicularis oculi.*

9. The junction of orbital plate of frontal bone (roof) and orbital plate of ethmoid (medial wall) shows two openings which lead into *anterior and posterior ethmoidal canals*. These transmit corresponding *ethmoidal nerves and vessels.*

10. Orbital surface of zygomatic bone in the lateral wall possesses *zygomatico-orbital foramina* meant for the passage of *zygomaticotemporal* and *zygomaticofacial nerves* and *zygomatic branches of lacrimal artery.*

11. **Superior orbital fissure**
   A. *Location*
      It is located at the junction of roof and lateral wall of orbit.
   B. *Shape*
      It is triangular in shape with base medially and apex laterally.
   C. *Communication*
      It connects orbit with middle cranial fossa.
   D. *Boundaries*
      i. Medial: *Body of sphenoid bone.*
      ii. Apex: *Frontal bone.*
      iii. Superior: *Lesser wing of sphenoid.*
      iv. Inferior: *Greater wing of sphenoid.*
   E. *Common annular tendon*
      The lower margin of fissure presents a bony projection for the attachment of common tendinous ring (common annular tendon) for the attachment of recti of eyeball.
   F. *Structures passing through*
      Common annular tendon divides the fissure into three compartments for the passage of number of structures as shown below:
      a. Lateral part
         i. *Lacrimal nerve.*
         ii. *Frontal nerve.*
         iii. *Trochlear nerve.*
         iv. *Superior ophthalmic vein.*
         v. *Meningeal branch of lacrimal artery.*
         vi. *Orbital branch of middle meningeal artery.*
      b. Part within tendinous ring
         i. *Upper and lower divisions of the oculomotor nerve.*
         ii. *Nasociliary nerve.*
         iii. *Abducent nerve.*
      c. Part below the tendinous ring
         i. *Inferior ophthalmic vein*
         ii. *Sympathetic twigs.*

12. The lateral wall of orbit near the lateral orbital margin presents an ill-defined *Whitnall's tubercle*. It is located on the orbital surface of frontal process of zygomatic bone about 1 cm below the frontozygomatic suture. Following structures are attached to this tubercle:
   i. *Lateral palapebral ligament.*
   ii. *Lateral check ligament.*
   iii. *Suspensory ligament of eyeball.*
   iv. *Aponeurosis of levator palpebrae superioris.*

Nasal Cavity

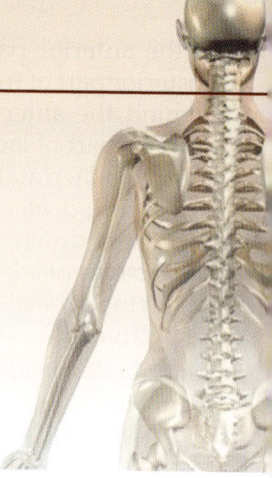

Nasal cavity is the beginning of respiratory system. It is divided into right and left halves by a midline partition called *nasal septum*. To study the cavity, a sagittal section of skull is considered in which one-half of the skull shows *lateral wall of nasal cavity* and the second half shows *nasal septum*.

FEATURES

Each half of the nasal cavity consists of a roof, floor, medial wall and lateral wall.

I. Roof

It has anterior and posterior slopings and middle horizontal part.

A. Anterior sloping

It is formed by the *nasal bone* and *nasal spine* of the frontal bone.

B. Posterior sloping

1. It is formed by the following bones from anterior to posterior:
   i. Anterior surface of *body of sphenoid*.
   ii. *Ala of vomer*.
   iii. *Sphenoidal process of palatine bone*.
2. It possesses *opening of sphenoidal sinus*.

C. Middle horizontal part

1. It is formed by the *cribriform plate* of *ethmoid bone*.

2. Number of foramina in it provide passages for *filaments of olfactory nerve*.
3. One of these perforations in its anterior part transmits *anterior ethmoidal nerve and vessels*.

II. Floor

1. It is formed by the superior surface of bony palate, i.e. *palatine process of maxilla* and *horizontal plate of palatine bone*.
2. Anteriorly near the septum a small *infundibular opening* leads into *incisive canal*.
3. *Nasopalatine nerve* and *greater palatine* vessels traverse the incisive canal.

III. Medial wall (Fig. 41.1)

1. It is formed by bony septum in a dried skull.
2. Posteroinferior part of the bony septum is contributed by *vomer*.
3. Its anterosuperior part is formed by *perpendicular plate of ethmoid*.
4. *Nasal crest* (below), *sphenoidal crest* and *rostrum* (above and behind) provide minor contributions to bony septum.
5. A groove on each side of vomer descends downwards and forwards towards incisive canal. It lodges nasopalatine nerve.

IV. Lateral wall (Fig. 41.2)

1. This is very irregular.
2. This is marked by three bracket like projections which run anteroposteriorly

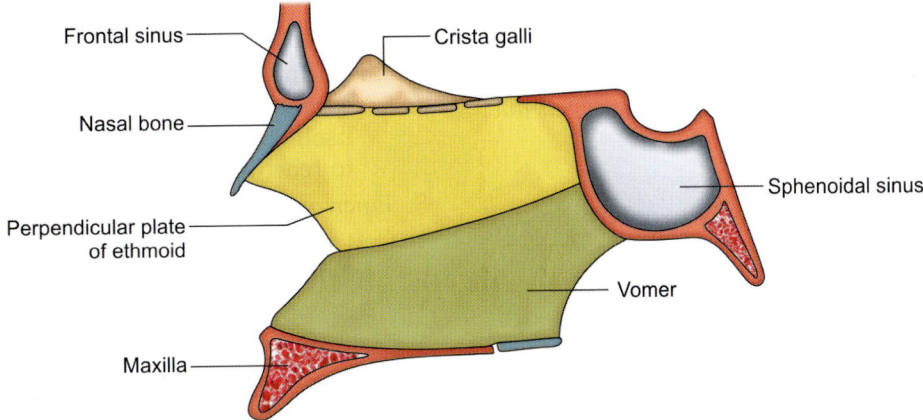

Fig. 41.1: Left surface of bony nasal septum

and lie one above the other. These projections are named from above downwards, *superior, middle and inferior conchae.*

3. Each concha forms medial wall and roof of corresponding meatus. Therefore, there are three *meatuses, superior, middle and inferior.*

4. The part of the lateral wall above the superior concha is called *sphenoethmoidal recess.*

5. Main bony contributions in the lateral wall are as follows:

   i. Below and in front: *Nasal surface of maxilla.*

   ii. Behind: *Perpendicular plate of palatine bone.*

   iii. Above: *Ethmoidal labyrinth* (with superior and middle conchae).

   iv. Below: *Inferior concha* (an independent bone).

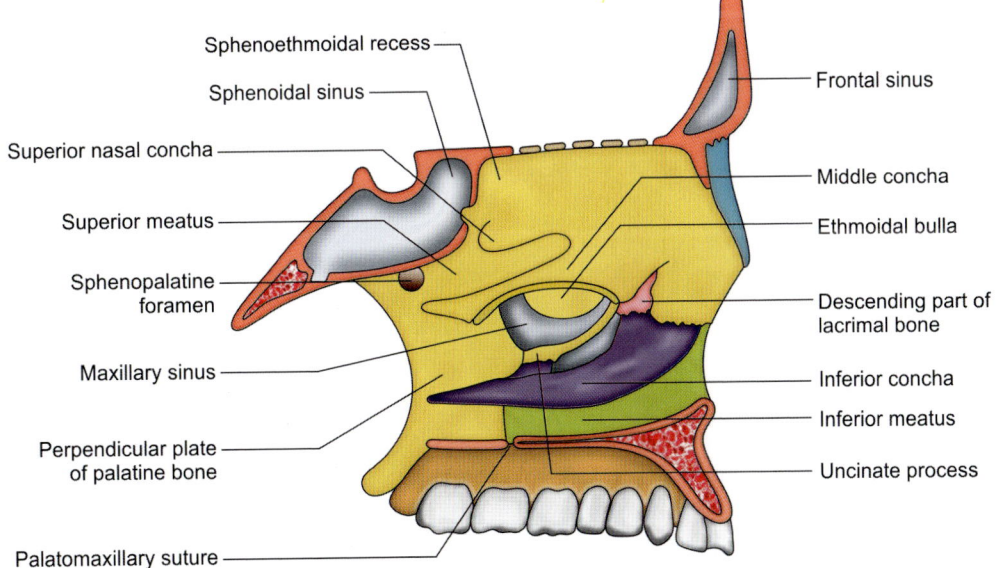

Fig. 41.2: Lateral wall of left nasal cavity

6. *Inferior meatus*

　a. It lies below and lateral to inferior concha.

　b. It receives *opening of nasolacrimal duct* in its anterior part.

7. *Middle meatus*

　i. It is situated between middle and inferior conchae.

　ii. A rounded elevation in its upper part is called *ethmoidal bulla* produced by middle ethmoidal air cells.

　iii. On the surface or just above the bulla is the *opening of middle ethmoidal sinus.*

　iv. Behind the bulla is the *opening of maxillary* sinus.

　v. Anteroinferior to bulla is a curved, thin bony projection called *uncinate process of ethmoid.*

　vi. Uncinate process passes backwards and encloses a curved gap between it and bulla. This gap is called *hiatus semilunaris.*

　vii. Upper end of hiatus semilunaris continues with *ethmoidal infundibulum.*

　viii. Infundibulum of ethmoid receives *opening of anterior ethmoidal sinus* and itself continues up as *frontonasal duct* to reach the frontal sinus.

8. *Superior meatus*

　i. It is situated between superior and middle conchae.

　ii. *Opening of posterior ethmoidal sinus* is located in the superior meatus.

9. *Sphenoethmoidal recess*

　i. It is situated between roof and superior concha.

　ii. It receives the *opening of sphenoidal air sinus.*

10. *Sphenopalatine foramen*

　i. It is located just behind the superior concha.

　ii. It transmits *sphenopalatine artery* and *nasal branches of pterygopalatine ganglion.*

Interior of the Cranial Vault

DEFINITION

It is the internal surface of the skull cap.

SHAPE

This is ovoid like norma verticalis.

BONES

Same bones contribute to this part which were observed in norma verticalis, i.e.

1. Frontal bone, anteriorly.
2. Occipital bone, posteriorly
3. Parietal bones, on each side.

SUTURES

Sutures correspond with those observed in norma verticalis which are as follows:
1. *Coronal suture,* between frontal and parietal bones.
2. *Sagittal suture,* between two parietal bones.
3. *Lambdoid suture,* between parietal and occipital bones.

FEATURES (Fig. 42.1)

  A. *Frontal crest*
    1. It is a midline crest seen at its anterior part.
    2. *Falx cerebri* is attached to it.

  B. *Sagittal sulcus*
    1. It is an anteroposterior groove in the median plane.
    2. It is narrow anteriorly but widens posteriorly.
    3. It contains superior *sagittal sinus.*
    4. *Falx cerebri* is attached to its margins.

  C. *Bregma and lambda*

    These mark the junctions of sagittal suture with coronal and lambdoid sutures respectively (see norma verticalis).

  D. *Parietal foramen*

    It pierces the parietal bone on each side of midline about 3.5 cm in front of lambda. Emissary vein passes through it.

  E. *Granular foveolae*
    1. These are irregular depressions on each side of sagittal sulcus.
    2. These are produced by *arachnoid granulations.*
    3. These are deep and more abundant in aged skull.

  F. *Grooves for meningeal vessels*
    1. Grooves for anterior (frontal) twigs of middle meningeal vessels are located just behind the coronal suture.

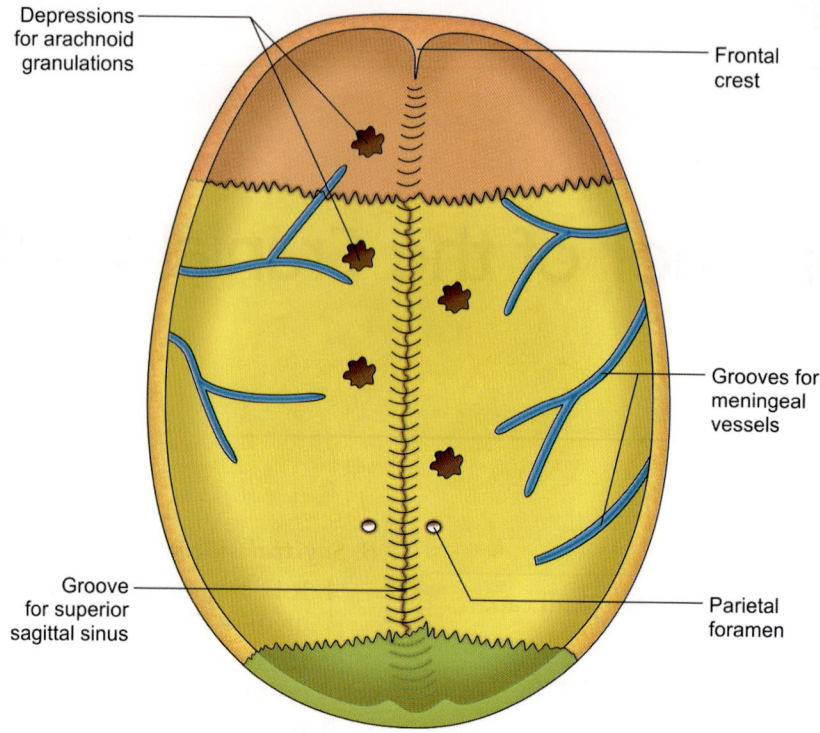

Fig. 42.1: Skull cap: Internal surface

2. Grooves for parietal twigs of middle meningeal vessels are more posteriorly placed. These run backwards and upwards.

G. Impressions for cerebral gyri
These are less marked in cranial vault in contrast to the interior of the base of skull where cerebral impressions are well defined.

Interior of the Base of the Skull

DEFINITION

It is the base of skull (neurocranium minus skull cap) observed from inside, i.e. the cavity side.

SUBDIVISIONS

Internal surface of the base of the skull is naturally demarcated into three fossae known as the anterior, middle and posterior cranial fossae.

I. ANTERIOR CRANIAL FOSSA

A. Boundaries

a. Anterior and lateral

Frontal bone.

b. Posterior

    i. *Posterior border of lesser wing of sphenoid.*
    ii. *Anterior clinoid process.*
    iii. *Anterior margin of sulcus chiasmatis.*

B. Floor

a. Median region

    i. Anteriorly: *Cribriform plate of ethmoid.*
    ii. Posteriorly: Anterior part of superior surface of body of sphenoid (*jugum sphenoidale*).

b. Lateral region

    i. Anteriorly: *Orbital plates of frontal bone.*
    ii. Posteriorly: *Lesser wings of sphenoid.*

C. Features and attachments (Figs 43.1 and 43.2)

a. Frontal crest

1. It is a median crest in the anterior wall of fossa.
2. It provides attachment to *falx cerebri.*

b. Crista galli of cribriform plate

1. It is an upward tooth like projection in the midline of cribriform plate just behind the frontal crest.
2. This projection receives attachment of *anterior end of falx cerebri.*

c. Foramen caecum

1. It is situated between crista galli and crest of frontal bone.
2. It is usually blind but sometimes may transmit an *emissary vein* from nasal cavity to superior sagittal sinus.

d. Cribriform plate of ethmoid on each side of crista galli

1. It is a sieve-like (perforated) bony plate.

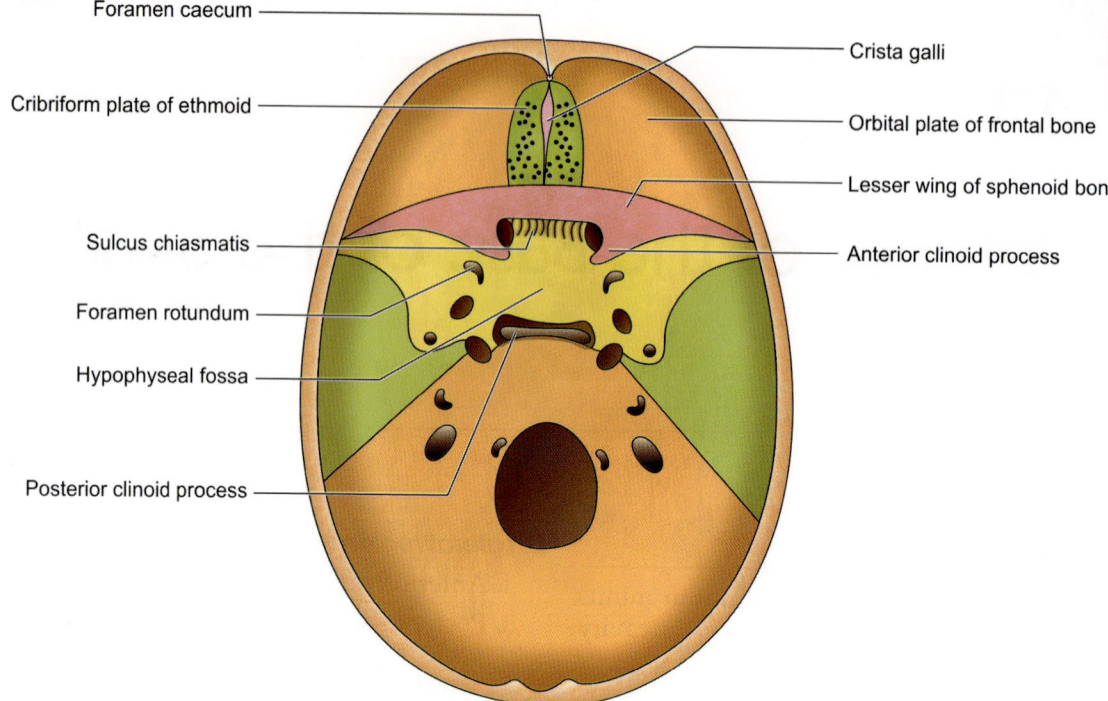

Foramen caecum

Cribriform plate of ethmoid

Sulcus chiasmatis

Foramen rotundum

Hypophyseal fossa

Posterior clinoid process

Crista galli

Orbital plate of frontal bone

Lesser wing of sphenoid bone

Anterior clinoid process

Fig. 43.1: Base of skull: Internal surface

2. 15–20 filaments of olfactory nerve pass through each perforate plate from olfactory mucosa of nose to olfactory bulb.
3. Groove just lateral to crista galli is related to:
    i. *Olfactory bulb.*
    ii. *Gyrus rectus.*
4. Anterior ethmoidal canal
    i. It opens in the *cribrofrontal suture* behind the crista galli.
    ii. *Anterior ethmoidal nerve and vessels* pass through it.
5. A *slit-like aperture* by the side of anterior part of crista galli is meant for a process of dura mater.
6. A foramen just lateral to anterior end of slit.
    Through this passage, *anterior ethmoidal nerve and vessels* enter the nose from anterior cranial fossa.

7. Posterior ethmoidal canal
    i. It is present in the posterolateral corner of cribriform plate.
    ii. It transmits *posterior ethmoidal vessels.*

e. Jugum sphenoidale
1. It is most anterior part of the superior surface of body of sphenoid.
2. Its anterior margin meets the posterior margin of cribriform plate.
3. Posteriorly it is limited by sulcus chiasmatis.
4. It separates anterior cranial fossa from two sphenoidal sinuses located in the body of sphenoid.

f. Orbital plates of frontal bone
1. Each of the two orbital plates separates anterior cranial fossa from corresponding orbit just lateral to cribriform plate.

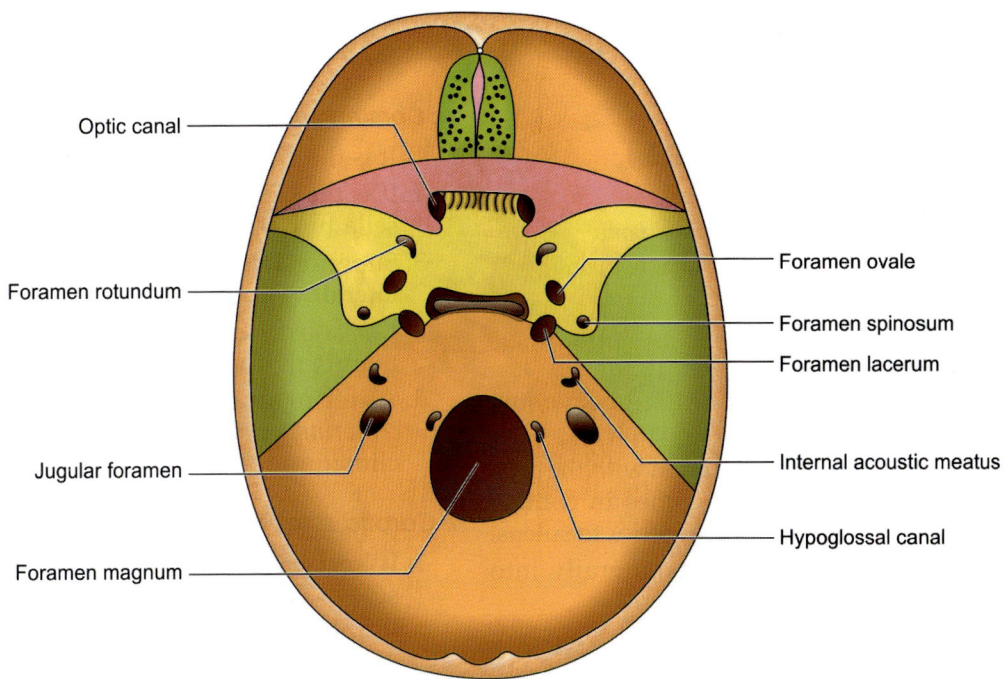

Fig. 43.2: Base of skull : Internal surface

2. It shows impressions for cerebral gyri.

3. It supports the orbital surface of frontal lobe of cerebrum.

4. Medially it covers the superior surface of ethmoidal labyrinth (anterior and posterior ethmoidal canals intervening between the two).

5. Posteriorly it meets the anterior margin of lesser wing of sphenoid.

g. Lesser wings of sphenoid

1. Jugum sphenoidale continues laterally with superior surface of lesser wing.

2. It is broad medially and tapers laterally.

3. Posterior margin of lesser wing is related to:

   i. *Sphenoparietal sinus.*

  ii. *Lateral sulcus* of cerebral hemisphere.

4. Posterior border of lesser wing ends medially into *anterior clinoid process*

which receives attachment of free margin of tentorium cerebelli.

II. MIDDLE CRANIAL FOSSA

A. Boundaries

a. Anterior

   i. Posterior border of *lesser wing of sphenoid*.

  ii. *Anterior clinoid process*.

 iii. Anterior border of *sulcus chiasmatis*.

b. Posterior

   i. Superior border of *petrous part of temporal bone*.

  ii. *Posterior clinoid process*.

 iii. *Dorsum sellae*.

c. Lateral (on each side)

   i. *Greater wing of sphenoid*.

  ii. Anteroinferior angle of *parietal bone*.

 iii. Squamous part of *temporal bone*.

B. Floor

a. Central portion

Body of sphenoid.

b. Lateral portion (on each side)

i. *Greater wing of sphenoid.*
ii. *Squamous part of temporal bone.*
iii. *Anterior surface of petrous temporal.*

C. Features and attachments

a. Sulcus chiasmatis

1. It is transversely running groove just behind the jugum sphenoidale.
2. It is named after its relation with the *optic chiasma* which never comes in contact with it but lies posterosuperior to sulcus.
3. Sulcus chiasmatis leads laterally into optic canals.

b. Optic canal

1. It connects the middle cranial fossa with the orbit.
2. It is bounded by anterior and posterior roots of lesser wing and body of sphenoid.
3. It transmits:
   i. *Optic nerve.*
   ii. *Ophthalmic artery.*
   iii. *Meninges.*

c. Tuberculum sellae

1. It forms an elevation just behind the sulcus chiasmatis.
2. *Middle clinoid processes* are the lateral prominent ends of tuberculum sellae.
3. It receives attachment of anterior margin of *diaphragma sellae*.

d. Sella turcica

1. It is the depressed area behind the tuberculum sellae.
2. It is shaped like a Turkish saddle and therefore named sella turcica.
3. *Hypophyseal fossa* is the deepest part in it. It lodges *pituitary gland*.

4. *Sphenoidal air sinus* is present below the floor of the hypophyseal fossa.

e. Dorsum sellae

1. It is the back of Turkish saddle.
2. It is the square plate of bone behind the sella turcica.
3. Superior angles of dorsum sellae project laterally into *posterior clinoid processes*.
4. *Diaphragma sellae* is attached to the upper margin of dorsum sellae.
5. Anterior end of attached margin of *tentorium cerebelli* is attached to posterior clinoid process.

f. Carotid sulcus

1. It is observed as a shallow groove on each side of the body of sphenoid.
2. It lodges *cavernous sinus* enclosing cavernous part of *internal carotid artery*.
3. It extends posteriorly up to foramen lacerum where it is deepened.
4. The lateral margin of carotid sulcus at its posterior end, projects backwards into tongue-shaped *lingula*.
5. Lingula lies over the *posterior opening of pterygoid canal*.

g. Superior orbital fissure

1. It is a triangular fissure connecting the lateral portion of middle cranial fossa with orbit.
2. It is bounded above by the *lesser wing*, below by the *greater wing* and medially by the *body of sphenoid*.
3. Common annular tendon (tendinous ring of Zinn) is attached to a small projection seen on the lower border of fissure.
4. Common annular tendon divides the fissure into lateral, middle and medial parts through which following structures traverse:

Through lateral part
   i. *Lacrimal nerve.*
   ii. *Frontal nerve.*

iii. *Trochlear nerve.*

iv. *Superior ophthalmic vein.*

 v. *Meningeal branch of lacrimal artery.*

vi. *Orbital branch of middle meningeal artery.*

Through common annular tendon, i.e. middle part

 i. Upper and lower divisions of *oculomotor nerve.*

 ii. *Nasociliary nerve.*

iii. *Abducent nerve.*

Through medial part

 i. *Inferior ophthalmic vein.*

 ii. *Sympathetic twigs* form internal carotid sympathetic plexus.

Note: *To remember structures passing through superior orbital fissure, remember 'I Slept One Night And Left For Tokyo' in which I—Inferior ophthalmic vein, S—Sympathetic twigs, Superior ophthalmic vein, O—Oculomotor nerve, N—Nasociliary nerve, A—Abducent nerve, L—Lacrimal nerve, F—Frontal nerve, T—Trochlear nerve.*

h. Foramen rotundum

1. It is present in the greater wing of sphenoid.
2. It is located just below and behind the medial end of superior orbital fissure.
3. It leads forwards into pterygopalatine fossa.
4. It transmits *maxillary nerve.*

Note: *Remember, it is not visible in norma basalis.*

i. Foramen ovale

1. It is located posterolateral to foramen rotundum.
2. It leads inferiorly into infratemporal fossa.
3. It transmits:
    i. *Mandibular nerve.*
    ii. *Accessory meningeal artery.*

iii. *Lesser petrosal nerve.*

iv. *Emissary vein.*

Note: *Remember Ovale—MALE, where M—Mandibular, A—Accessory, L—Lesser and E—Emissary.*

j. Foramen spinosum

1. It is situated posterolateral to foramen ovale.
2. It leads inferiorly into infratemporal fossa.
3. It transmits:
    i. *Middle meningeal artery.*
    ii. *Nervus spinosus.*
    iii. *Parietal trunk of middle meningeal vein.*

k. Foramen of Vesalius (sphenoidal emissary foramen)

1. It is inconstant.
2. It is located between foramen rotundum and foramen ovale.
3. It transmits emissary vein connecting the cavernous sinus and pterygoid venous plexus.

l. Foramen innominatum

1. This is also an inconstant foramen.
2. It is located between foramen ovale and foramen spinosum.
3. It transmits *lesser petrosal nerve.*

m. Foramen lacerum

1. It is a foramen with irregular margin between sphenoid and apex of petrous temporal.
2. *Carotid* and *pterygoid canals* open into it.
3. Only two structures pass through it, i.e. *meningeal branch of ascending pharyngeal artery* and *emissary vein.*
4. *Internal carotid artery* traverses its upper part *with its sympathetic and venous plexuses.*

5. *Nerve of pterygoid canal (Vidian nerve)* is formed in its upper part by the union of *greater superficial petrosal* and *deep petrosal nerves*.

n. Anterior surface of petrous temporal

1. *Trigeminal impression* is a depression for trigeminal ganglion adjacent to apex.
2. A ridge limits the trigeminal impression posteriorly.
3. *Roof of internal acoustic meatus* is a depressed area behind the ridge.
4. *Arcuate eminence* is a prominent elevation behind the second depression. It is produced by superior semicircular canal. Its posterior sloping lies over lateral and posterior semicircular canals.
5. Area anterolateral to trigeminal impression forms the *roof of anterior part of carotid canal*.
6. Area anterolateral to arcuate eminence forms *roof of vestibule and beginning of facial canal*.
7. Thin plate of bone between squamous temporal and features described above is called *tegmen tympani*. It forms roof of mastoid antrum, middle ear and canal for tensor tympani from posterior to anterior. Tegmen tympani projects downwards to form lateral walls of canal for tensor tympani and bony Eustachian tube and appears in norma basalis in the squamotympanic fissure.
8. A hiatus lateral to arcuate eminence leads into a *groove for greater superficial petrosal nerve* which runs towards foramen laerum on the tegmen tympani.
9. Lateral to aforementioned groove is present another *groove for lesser petrosal nerve* which runs towards foramen ovale.

o. Superior border of petrous temporal

1. It is gooved by the superior petrosal sinus.
2. Margins of groove provide attachment to tentorium cerebelli.

3. It is crossed by the trigeminal nerve near the apex of petrous temporal.

p. Lateral part of the fossa shows following additional features:

1. Markings for the middle meningeal vessels.
2. Depressions produced by the gyri of temporal lobe of cerebral hemisphere.

III. POSTERIOR CRANIAL FOSSA

It is the largest and the deepest of all cranial fossae. It lodges cerebellum, pons and medulla.

A. Boundaries

a. Anterior

　　i. *Dorsum sellae.*
　　ii. Posterior clinoid process.
　　iii. *Superior border of petrous temporal.*

b. Posterior

Squamous part of occipital bone.

c. Lateral

　　i. *Mastoid part of temporal bone.*
　　ii. Mastoid angle of parietal bone.

B. Floor

1. *Basisphenoid and basiocciput.*
2. Posterior surface of petrous temporal.
3. Mastoid part of temporal bone.
4. Posteroinferior angle of the parietal bone.
5. Squamous part of occipital bone.

C. Features and attachments

a. Clivus

1. It is sloping surface in front of foramen magnum.
2. It is formed by the superior surface of basilar part of occipital bone, posterior part of superior surface of body of sphenoid and dorsum sellae.
3. It supports *pons* and *medulla*.

4. It is related to *basilar plexus of veins* and *basilar artery*.
5. Its lower part receives attachments of following structures from above downwards:
   i. *Membrana tectoria*.
   ii. *Superior longitudinal band of cruciform ligament*.
   iii. *Apical ligament of dens*.

b. Petro-occipital fissure

1. It is the junction between clivus and petrous temporal.
2. It is grooved by the *inferior petrosal sinus*.

c. Foramen magnum

1. It is largest foramen.
2. It is located in the floor of posterior cranial fossa.
3. Its margins provide attachments to following structures:
   i. *Anterior margin: Anterior atlanto-occipital membrane*.
   ii. *Posterior margin: Posterior atlanto-occipital membrane*.
   iii. *Lateral margins: Alar ligaments*.
4. Structures passing through its anterior part are:
   i. *Apical ligament of dens*.
   ii. *Superior longitudinal band of cruciform ligament*.
   iii. *Membrana tectoria*.
5. Structures passing through its posterior part are:
   i. *Medulla oblongata*.
   ii. *Meninges*.
   iii. *Spinal roots of accessory nerves*.
   iv. *Meningeal branches of upper cervical nerves*.
   v. *Vertebral arteries*.
   vi. *Sympathetic plexuses around the vertebral arteries*.
   vii. *Anterior and posterior spinal arteries*.

d. Internal occipital protuberance

1. It is situated opposite the external occipital protuberance.
2. It is related to *confluence of dural venous sinuses*.
3. On each side it is grooved by *transverse sinus*.

e. Internal occipital crest

1. It is a midline crest between internal occipital protuberance and the foramen magnum.
2. *Falx cerebelli* is attached to it.
3. *Cerebellar hemisphere* occupies the deep fossa on each side of the internal occipital crest.

f. Vermian fossa

1. It is a midline fossa at the lower end of internal occipital crest adjacent to foramen magnum.
2. It is related to *inferior vermis of the cerebellum*.

g. Transverse sulcus

1. It runs laterally on each side from the internal occipital protuberance.
2. At the mastoid angle of the parietal bone it continues as sigmoid sulcus.
3. It lodges the *transverse sinus*.
4. *Attached margin of tentorium cerebelli* is attached to its lips.
5. Right transverse sulcus is wider than the left one and is continuous posteriorly with superior sagittal sulcus.

h. Sigmoid sulcus

1. It is downward continuation of transverse sulcus at the mastoid angle of parietal bone.
2. It ends at the lateral end of jugular foramen.
3. It lodges *sigmoid sinus* which enters the jugular foramen to continue with internal jugular vein.

i. Jugular foramen

1. It is located at the posterior end of *petro-occipital fissure*.
2. It is an interosseous foramen situated between the anterior margin of jugular process of occipital bone and posterior margin of petrous part of temporal bone.
3. It is divided into anterior, middle and posterior parts.
4. *9th, 10th and 11th cranial nerves* pass through its middle part.
5. *Inferior petrosal sinus* and *meningeal branch of ascending pharyngeal artery* traverse its anterior part.
6. Sigmoid sinus and meningeal branch of occipital artery pass through its posterior part.

j. Jugular tubercle

1. Medial to the lower margin of jugular foramen, there is a rounded elevation known as *jugular tubercle*.
2. It is located anterosuperior to the internal opening of hypoglossal canal.
3. It is grooved by the 9th, 10th and 11th cranial nerves.

k. Hypoglossal canal

1. Its internal opening is located just above the tubercle for alar ligament on the medial aspect of occipital condyle.
2. It transmits:
   i. *Hypoglossal nerve*.
   ii. *Meningeal branch of ascending pharyngeal artery*.
   iii. *Emissary vein from basilar venous plexus*.

l. Condylar canal

1. It is inconstant.
2. Its internal orifice is located postero-lateral to that of hypoglossal canal.
3. It transmits emissary vein from sigmoid sinus.

m. Internal acoustic meatus

1. Its *porus* (inlet or medial end) is present in the centre of the posterior surface of petrous temporal.
2. It is about 1 cm in length.
3. It transmits:
   i. *Facial nerve*.
   ii. *Vestibulocochlear nerve*.
   iii. *Labyrinthine vessels*.
4. *Fundus* of internal acoustic meatus is a plate of bone at its lateral end. The plate is divided into upper and lower areas by a transverse ridge (*crista falciformis*). The upper area is further divided into anterior and posterior areas by a vertical crest called *Bill's bar*. Anterior to bar is the *facial canal* for facial nerve. Area behind the bar is called *superior vestibular area* which presents number of small openings for the nerve fibres supplying utricle and superior and lateral semi-circular ducts.
   Below the transverse crest, anteriorly is the *cochlear area* (which possesses number of foramina called *tractus spiralis foraminosus*) and posteriorly is the *inferior vestibular area*. Fibres of cochlear nerve enter the cochlear area while nerve fibres supplying the saccule enter the inferior vestibular area. Below and behind the inferior vestibular area is *foramen singulare* for the passage of nerve to posterior semicircular duct (Fig. 43.3).

n. Aqueduct of vestibule

1. A slit behind the porus of internal acoustic meatus leads into aqueduct of vestibule.
2. Aqueduct of vestibule contains *saccus and ductus endolymphaticus* along with the small artery and vein.

o. Subarcuate fossa

1. It is an irregular depression located above and between the openings of internal acoustic meatus and aqueduct of vestibule.
2. It lodges a process of dura mater.

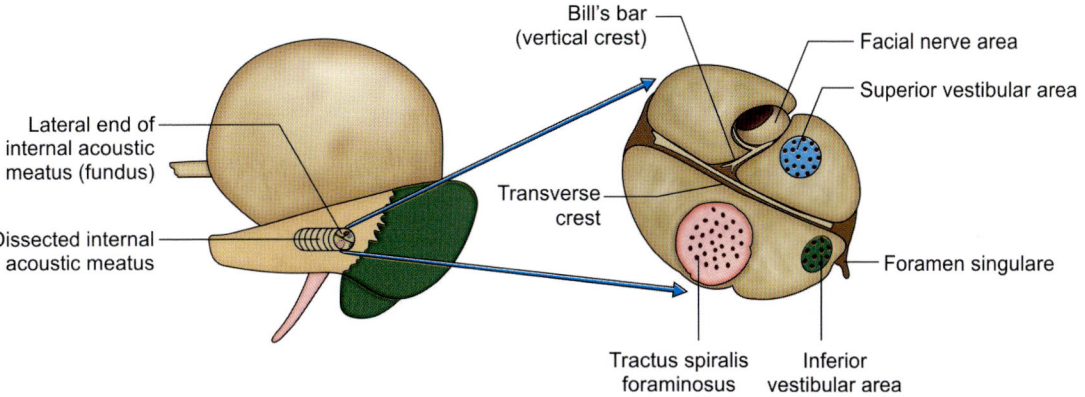

Fig. 43.3: Fundus of right internal acoustic meatus

Index